Singular Differential Equations and Special Functions

Mathematics and Physics for Science and Technology

Series Editor: L.M.B.C. Campos

Director of the Center for Aeronautical
and Space Science and Technology
Lisbon University

Volumes in the series:

Topic A – Theory of Functions and Potential Problems

Volume I (Book 1) – Complex Analysis with Applications to Flows and Fields
L.M.B.C. Campos

Volume II (Book 2) – Elementary Transcendentals with Applications to Solids and Fluids
L.M.B.C. Campos

Volume III (Book 3) – Generalized Calculus with Applications to Matter and Forces
L.M.B.C. Campos

Topic B – Boundary and Initial-Value Problems

Volume IV – Ordinary Differential Equations with Applications to Trajectories and Oscillations
L.M.B.C. Campos

Book 4 – Linear Differential Equations and Oscillators
L.M.B.C. Campos

Book 5 – Non-Linear Differential Equations and Dynamical Systems
L.M.B.C. Campos

Book 6 – Higher-Order Differential Equations and Elasticity
L.M.B.C. Campos

Book 7 – Simultaneous Differential Equations and Multi-Dimensional Vibrations
L.M.B.C. Campos

Book 8 – Singular Differential Equations and Special Functions
L.M.B.C. Campos

Book 9 – Classification and Examples of Differential Equations and their Applications
L.M.B.C. Campos

For more information about this series, please visit: https://www.crcpress.com/Mathematics-and-Physics-for-Science-and-Technology/book-series/CRCMATPHYSCI

Mathematics and Physics for Science and Technology

Volume IV

Ordinary Differential Equations with Applications to Trajectories and Oscillations

Book 8

Singular Differential Equations and Special Functions

By

L.M.B.C. Campos

Director of the Center for Aeronautical and Space Science and Technology

Lisbon University

CRC Press
Taylor & Francis Group
Boca Raton London New York

CRC Press is an imprint of the Taylor & Francis Group, an **informa** business

CRC Press
Taylor & Francis Group
6000 Broken Sound Parkway NW, Suite 300
Boca Raton, FL 33487-2742

Printed on acid-free paper

International Standard Book Number-13: 978-0-367-13723-6 (Hardback)

Library of Congress Cataloging-in-Publication Data

Names: Campos, Luis Manuel Braga da Costa, author.
Title: Singular differential equations and special functions / Luis Manuel Braga da Campos.
Description: Boca Raton : CRC Press, Taylor & Francis Group, 2018. | Includes bibliographical references and index.
Identifiers: LCCN 2018050996 | ISBN 9780367137236 (hardback : alk. paper)
Subjects: LCSH: Functions, Special. | Differential equations. | Mathematical analysis.
Classification: LCC QA351 .C2525 2018 | DDC 515/.5–dc23
LC record available at https://lccn.loc.gov/2018050996

Visit the Taylor & Francis Web site at
http://www.taylorandfrancis.com

and the CRC Press Web site at
http://www.crcpress.com

MIX
Paper from responsible sources
FSC™ C013985
www.fsc.org

Printed in the United Kingdom
by Henry Ling Limited

to Leonor Campos

Contents

Contents vii
Diagrams, List, Notes, and Tables xiii
Preface xvii
Acknowledgments xix
About the Author xxi
Notation for Functions xxiii

9. Existence Theorems and Special Functions 1
9.1 Existence, Unicity, Robustness, and Uniformity of Solutions 1
9.1.1 Existence of Solution and the Lipschitz Condition 2
9.1.2 Transformation of a Differential into an Integral Equation (Picard 1893) 3
9.1.3 Convergence of the Successive Approximations 4
9.1.4 Contraction Mapping and Fixed Point 5
9.1.5 Lipschitz (1864) or Contraction Condition, Continuity, and Differentiability 6
9.1.6 Continuity (Contraction) Condition on the Independent (Dependent) Variable 7
9.1.7 Uniform Convergence to a Continuous Solution 9
9.1.8 Theorem of Existence of Solution of a Differential Equation 10
9.1.9 Rectangle as the Domain of Successive Approximations 11
9.1.10 Theorem of Unicity of Solution of a Differential Equation 11
9.1.11 Robustness Relative to Perturbed Initial Conditions 12
9.1.12 Comparison of Successive Approximations to the Original and Perturbed Problems 14
9.1.13 Theorem of Robustness with Regard to the Initial Condition 15
9.1.14 Theorem on Uniformity with Regard to a Parameter in a Differential Equation 16
9.1.15 Simultaneous System of First-Order Differential Equations 16
9.1.16 Contraction or Lipschitz Condition for Several Variables 18
9.1.17 Combined Theorem of Existence, Unicity, Robustness, and Uniformity 19
9.1.18 Ordinary Differential Equation of Any Order 20

9.1.19 Linear Ordinary Differential Equation 21
9.1.20 Combined Theorem for an Ordinary Differential Equation 22
9.2 Autonomous Systems and Stability of Equilibria (Lyapunov 1954) 23
9.2.1 Local/Asymptotic Stability/Instability and Indifference 25
9.2.2 Positive/Negative Definite/Semi-Definite and Indefinite Function 28
9.2.3 Derivative along an Unsteady/Autonomous Differential System 29
9.2.4 Lyapunov (1966) Function and First Theorem 31
9.2.5 Proof of the Lyapunov Stability Theorem 34
9.2.6 Proof of the Theorem on Asymptotic Stability 35
9.2.7 Proof of the Theorem on Instability 36
9.2.8 Damped Oscillator with Parameters Dependent in Position 37
9.2.9 Damped Oscillator with Parameters Depending on Time 38
9.2.10 Stability of Undamped Oscillator with Parametric Resonance 40
9.2.11 Exponential Asymptotic Growth or Decay 40
9.2.12 Proof of the Second Lyapunov Theorem (1892) 41
9.2.13 Existence of at Least One Eigenvalue of an Autonomous System 43
9.2.14 Linear Differential Equation with Bounded Coefficients 44
9.2.15 Linear Autonomous System with Constant Coefficients 45
9.2.16 Linearized Differential System Near an Equilibrium Point 46
9.2.17 Fundamental Solution of an Autonomous Differential System 48
9.2.18 Properties of Positive-Definite Quadratic Forms 50
9.2.19 Stability Function and Its Derivative Following the Differential System 51
9.2.20 Third Lyapunov Theorem on Autonomous Systems 52
9.2.21 Stability of Solutions of an Autonomous Differential Equation 53
9.3 Linear Differential Equations with Periodic Coefficients (Floquet 1883; Lyapunov 1907) 54
9.3.1 Conditions for the Existence of Periodic Solutions (Floquet 1883) 54
9.3.2 Distinct and Coincident Eigenvalues and Exponents 55
9.3.3 Natural Integrals and Asymptotic Stability 56

9.3.4 Diagonal Matrices and Jordan Blocks 57
9.3.5 Invariant Second-Order Differential Equation 59
9.3.6 Growing/Decaying and Monotonic/Oscillatory Solutions 60
9.3.7 Fundamental Solution of a Linear Differential Equation 61
9.3.8 Eigenvalues of the Invariant Second Order Equation 62
9.3.9 Proof of the Fourth Lyapunov (1907) Theorem 63
9.4 Analytic Coefficients and Generalized Circular/Hyperbolic Functions 64
9.4.1 Singularities of Single-Valued Complex Functions 65
9.4.2 Regular Points, Poles, and Essential Singularities 68
9.4.3 Sheets of the Riemann Surface of a Multi-Valued Function 70
9.4.4 Principal Branch, Branch-Point, and Branch-Cut 72
9.4.5 Regular Points and Regular/Irregular Singularities 74
9.4.6 Analytic, Regular, and Irregular Integrals 75
9.4.7 Singularities and Integrals at the Point-at-Infinity 78
9.4.8 Linear Autonomous System with Analytic Coefficients 79
9.4.9 Linear Differential Equation with Analytic Coefficients 81
9.4.10 Calculation of the Coefficients of the Analytic Solution 82
9.4.11 Two Methods to Obtain the Recurrence Relation for the Coefficients 84
9.4.12 Generalized Hyperbolic Differential Equation 85
9.4.13 Generalized Hyperbolic Cosine and Sine 86
9.4.14 Airy (1838) Differential Equation and Functions 88
9.4.15 Generalized Circular Cosine and Sine 88
9.4.16 Generalized Circular Differential Equation 90
9.4.17 Complex Non-Integer Values of the Parameter 90
9.4.18 Differentiation of the Generalized Cosine and Sine Functions 92
9.4.19 Inequalities for Generalized Cosines and Sines 93
9.4.20 Generalized Secant, Cosecant, Tangent, and Cotangent 94
9.5 Regular Singularities and Integrals of Two Kinds (Fuchs 1860, Frobenius 1873) 96
9.5.1 Linear Autonomous System with a Regular Singularity 97
9.5.2 Indices and Coefficients of the Regular Natural Integrals 98
9.5.3 Two Related Sets of Regular Natural Integrals 99
9.5.4 Application of Compatibility and Initial Conditions 101

9.5.5 Linear Differential Equation with Regular Singularities (Fuchs 1868) ... 103
9.5.6 Indicial Equation and Recurrence Formula for the Coefficients ... 105
9.5.7 Regular Integrals of the First and Second Kinds ... 106
9.5.8 Second-Order Differential Equation with a Regular Singularity ... 107
9.5.9 Regular Integral of Second Kind First Type ... 109
9.5.10 Regular Integral of the Second Kind Second Type ... 111
9.5.11 Convergence of the Series in the Regular Integrals ... 113
9.5.12 Wronskian of a Linear Second-Order Differential Equation ... 115
9.5.13 Gamma Function (Weierstrass 1856) as a Generalization of the Factorial ... 117
9.5.14 Generalized Bessel Differential Equation (Campos et al. 2019) ... 118
9.5.15 Order and Degree of the Generalized Bessel Function ... 121
9.5.16 The Digamma Function as the Logarithmic Derivative of the Gamma Function ... 123
9.5.17 Generalized Neumann Function of Integer Order ... 125
9.5.18 Preliminary and Complementary Functions and Logarithmic Term ... 126
9.5.19 General Integral in the Case of Integer Order ... 129
9.5.20 Wronskians of Generalized Bessel and Neumann Functions ... 131
9.5.21 Generalized Neumann Function with Complex Order ... 133
9.5.22 Cylindrical Bessel Differential Equation (Euler 1764, Bessel 1824, Neumann 1867, Hankel 1869) ... 134
9.5.23 Spherical Bessel Differential Equation ... 135
9.5.24 Spherical Bessel and Neumann Functions ... 137
9.5.25 Classification of Six Cases of Regular Integrals ... 139
9.5.26 Relation between Spherical Bessel and Elementary Functions ... 140

9.6 Irregular Singularities and Asymptotic Normal Integrals (Thome 1883, Poincaré 1886, Campos 2001) ... 142
9.6.1 Regular/Irregular Integrals of a Linear Differential Equation ... 142
9.6.2 Regular Integral near an Irregular Singularity ... 144
9.6.3 Existence of a Normal Integral near an Irregular Singularity ... 145
9.6.4 Singularity of a Differential Equation at the Point at Infinity ... 147
9.6.5 Convergent Series versus Asymptotic Expansions ... 148

9.6.6 Spherical and Cylindrical Hankel (1869) Functions 150
9.6.7 Asymptotic Integrals of the Cylindrical Bessel Differential Equation (Campos 2001) 152
9.6.8 Asymptotic Expansions for Bessel, Neumann, and Hankel Functions 153
9.6.9 Generalized Hankel Function of the First Kind 155
9.6.10 Generalized Hankel Function of the Second Kind 158
9.6.11 Wronskians and Alternative General Integrals 160
9.6.12 Generalized versus Original Bessel Differential Equations 162
9.6.13 Parametric Discontinuity in the Asymptotic Integrals 165
9.6.14 Bifurcation for the Degree at the Point at Infinity 166
9.6.15 Numerical Computation for Small and Large Variable 168

9.7 Essential Singularities and Infinite Determinants 169
9.7.1 Existence of Eigenvalues and of Eigenintegrals 170
9.7.2 Irregular Integrals of the First Kind 172
9.7.3 Case of Indices Differing by an Integer 173
9.7.4 Irregular Integral of Second Kind 175
9.7.5 Regular Integrals of the Second Kind First/Second Type 178
9.7.6 Irregular, Regular, and Analytic Integrals 179
9.7.7 Infinite Linear System for the Coefficients 181
9.7.8 Indices as Roots of an Infinite Determinant 183
9.7.9 Five Types of Convergence of Infinite Determinants (Poincare 1886) 183
9.7.10 Convergence Theorem for Infinite Determinants (Von Koch 1892) 185
9.7.11 Parametric Resonance Forced by a Fundamental and Harmonics 186
9.7.12 Hill (1892) Differential Equation with Trigonometric Coefficients 187
9.7.13 Hill Differential Equation with Power Coefficients 188
9.7.14 Infinite Linear System for the Coefficients 189
9.7.15 Exact Analytic Evaluation of the Hill Determinant 192
9.7.16 Indices as Roots of a Transcendental Equation 194

9.8 Kernel and Path of Integral Transforms (Laplace 1812; Bateman 1909) 195
9.8.1 Eulerian Integral of the Second Kind (Euler 1772) 196
9.8.2 Permutations and Properties of the Beta Function 198
9.8.3 Relation between the Gamma and Beta Functions 199
9.8.4 Evaluation of Integrals via Gamma and Beta Functions 202
9.8.5 Kernel and Path of a General Integral Transform 203
9.8.6 Generalized Laplace Transform in the Complex Plane 205
9.8.7 Depression of the Degree of the Coefficients of a Differential Equation 207

9.8.8 Application to the Generalized Bessel Differential Equation 208
9.8.9 Integral Representation for the Generalized Bessel Function........ 210
9.8.10 Application to the Original Bessel Differential Equation 212
9.8.11 Integral Representation for the Bessel Function 214
9.8.12 Partial Differential Equation for the Bateman (1909) Kernel........ 216
9.8.13 Adjoint Operator and Bilinear Concomitant 218
9.8.14 Integral Representations for the Two Hankel Functions........ 219
9.8.15 Integral Representation for the Neumann Function 221
9.8.16 Second Integral Representation for the Bessel Function........ 223
9.9 Continued Fractions as Solutions of Differential Equations 225
9.9.1 Continued Fraction Associated with a Differential Equation 225
9.9.2 Logarithmic Derivative of the Solution of a Differential Equation 226
9.9.3 Solution as a Terminating Continued Fraction 227
9.9.4 Confluent Hypergeometric Differential Equation (Kummer 1830) 228
9.9.5 Convergence of Simple Infinite Continued Fractions........ 229
9.9.6 Continued Fraction for the Confluent Hypergeometric Function 230
9.9.7 Generalized Bessel and Confluent Hypergeometric Differential Equations........ 231
9.9.8 Confluent Hypergeometric Series 231
9.9.9 Continued Fraction for the Generalized Bessel Function........ 233
9.9.10 Recurrence and Differentiation Relations for Cylinder Functions 234
9.9.11 Cylinder Functions with Integer Order Difference 235
9.9.12 A Continued Fraction for Cylinder Functions........ 236
9.9.13 Special Limit Periodic Continued Fractions 237
9.9.14 Convergence of Complex Continued Fractions........ 238
9.9.15 Convergence of Special Continued Fractions 240
Conclusion 9 315

Bibliography........ **319**

Index **323**

Diagrams, List, Notes, and Tables

Diagrams

D 9.1 Methods of Solution of Differential Equations 244
D 9.2 Relations Among Special Functions 281
D 9.3 Classes of Functions 313

List

L 9.1 Notation for Some Special Functions 315

Notes

N 9.1 Classes of Differential Equations with Exact Analytical Solutions 241
N 9.2 Existence, Unicity, and Regularity Theorems 242
N 9.3 Qualitative Theory of Differential Equations 243
N 9.4 Approximate Numerical and Analytic Solutions of Differential Equations 244
N 9.5 Ordinary and Partial Differential Equations 245
N 9.6 Non-Cartesian, Inhomogenous, and Unsteady Problems 245
N 9.7 Special or Higher Transcendental Functions 246
N 9.8 Methods of One or Two Characteristic Polynomials 248
N 9.9 Method of Two Polynomials of Homogenous Derivatives 249
N 9.10 Generalized Hypergeometric Functions of Type ${}_2F_2$ 252
N 9.11 Asymptotic Regular Series Solutions 253
N 9.12 Generalized Hypergeometric Asymptotic Series 255
N 9.13 Analytic Continuation between the Interior and Exterior of the Unit Disk 255
N 9.14 The Gaussian Hypergeometric Series (Gauss 1812) and Differential Equation 260

N 9.15 Gaussian Hypergeometric Function of the First Kind 261
N 9.16 Gaussian Hypergeometric Function of the Second Kind 262
N 9.17 Preliminary and Complementary Gaussian Hypergeometric Functions 264
N 9.18 General Integral of the Gaussian Hypergeometric Differential Equation.. 266
N 9.19 Analytic and Logarithmic Cases, Poles, and Polynomials 268
N 9.20 Legendre (1785) Differential Equation... 270
N 9.21 Ultraspherical Legendre Differential Equation.............................. 272
N 9.22 Associated Legendre Differential Equation.................................... 274
N 9.23 Hyperspherical Associated Legendre Differential Equation........ 276
N 9.24 A Hierarchy of Legendre Functions and Differential Equations... 278
N 9.25 Hyperspherical Legendre Differential Equation (Campos & Cunha 2012)... 282
N 9.26 Jacobi (1859) Functions and Differential Equation......................... 283
N 9.27 Chebychev (1859) Differential Equation of the First Type 284
N 9.28 Chebychev (1947) Differential Equation of the Second Type 286
N 9.29 Confluent Hypergeometric Differential Equation (Kummer 1839) 289
N 9.30 Laguerre (1879) Functions and Differential Equation 291
N 9.31 Associated Laguerre Differential Equation 292
N 9.32 Hermite (1864) Functions and Differential Equation 293
N 9.33 Subhypergeometric and Bessel Differential Equations 294
N 9.34 Superhypergeometric and Generalized Hill Differential Equations... 295
N 9.35 Extended Gaussian Hypergeometric Differential Equation (Campos 2000) 297
N 9.36 Extended Gaussian Hypergeometric Functions (Campos 2001a)... 298
N 9.37 Extended Confluent Hypergeometric Differential Equation (Campos 2001b) 300
N 9.38 Doubly Extended Bessel Differential Equation.............................. 301
N 9.39 Self-Adjoint and Invariant Differential Equations......................... 303
N 9.40 Whittaker (1904) Functions and Differential Equation 304
N 9.41 Self-Adjoint and Invariant Generalized Bessel Differential Equations... 305
N 9.42 Gaussian Hypergeometric, Jacobi, and Legendre Forms.............. 307
N 9.43 Chebychev, Laguerre, and Hermite Forms 308
N 9.44 Transformations of the Generalized Bessel Differential Equation (Malmsten 1850, Lommel 1868)....................................... 309
N 9.45 Two Classes of Combined Changes of Variable (Lommel 1879, Pearson 1880) 311
N 9.46 Algebraic and Elementary/Higher Transcendental Functions..... 312
N 9.47 Special Functions and Differential Equations 314

Tables

T 9.1 Stability of an Equilibrium Position 27
T 9.2 Stability of Conservative System 28
T 9.3 First-Order Linear Differential Equation: Classification of Points and Integrals 74
T 9.4 Second-Order Linear Differential Equation: Linearly Independent Particular Integrals 143
T 9.5 Alternative General Integrals of the Generalized Bessel Differential Equation 163
T 9.6 Bessel Differential Equation: Original and Generalized 163
T 9.7 Linear Second-Order Differential Equation: Integrals of the First and Second Kind 177
T 9.8 Second Linear Differential Equation: Classification of Points and Integrals 180
T 9.9 Method of Characteristic Polynomials 248

Preface

Volume IV (*"Ordinary Differential Equations with Applications to Trajectories and Oscillations"*) is organized like the preceding three volumes of the series *Mathematics and Physics for Science and Technology*: volume III, *Generalized Calculus with Applications to Matter and Forces*; volume II, *Transcendental Representations with Applications to Solids and Fluids*; and volume I, *Complex Analysis with Applications to Flows and Fields*. The books of volume IV correspond to books 4 to 7 of the series and consist of the chapters 1 to 8 of volume IV. The first book of volume IV is *Linear Differential Equations and Oscillators*; the second, *Non-Linear Differential Equations and Dynamical Systems*; the third, *Higher-Order Differential Equations and Elasticity*; and the fourth *Simultaneous Differential Equations and Multi-Dimensional Vibrations*. The present book, *Singular Differential Equations and Special Functions* is the fifth of volume IV and eighth of the series and consists of chapter 9 of volume IV.

Chapters 1 to 8 of volume IV considered mostly ordinary differential equations and simultaneous systems for which exact analytical solutions can be obtained in finite terms using only elementary functions. Chapter 9 starts with general classes of differential equations and simultaneous systems for which the properties of the solutions can be established *a priori*, such as existence and unity of solution, robustness and uniformity with regard to changes in boundary conditions, and parameters, and stability and asymptotic behavior. Chapter 9 proceeds to consider the most important class of linear differential equations with variable coefficients, that be analytic functions or have regular or irregular singularities. The solution of singular differential equations by means of (i) power series, (ii) parametric integral transforms, and (iii) continued fractions lead to more than 20 special functions; among these is given greater attention to generalized circular, hyperbolic, Airy, Bessel, and hypergeometric differential equations and the special functions that specify their solutions.

Organization of the Book

Volume IV consists of ten chapters: (i) the odd-numbered chapters present mathematical developments; (ii) the even numbered chapters contain physical applications; and (iii) the last chapter is a set of 20 detailed examples of (i) and (ii). The chapters are divided into sections and subsections, for example chapter 9, section 9.1, and subsection 9.1.1. The formulas are numbered by chapters in curved brackets; for example, (9.2) is equation 2 of chapter 9. When referring to volume I, the symbol I is inserted at the beginning, for example: (i) chapter I.36, section I.36.1, subsection I.36.1.2; (ii) equation (I.36.33a). The final part of each chapter includes: (i) a conclusion referring to the figures as a kind of visual summary; (ii) the note(s), list(s), table(s), diagram(s) and classification(s) as additional support. The latter (ii) apply at the end of each chapter, and are numbered within the chapter (for example diagram D9.2, list L9.1, note N9.27, table T9.8); if there is more than one they are numbered sequentially (for example, notes 9.1 to 9.47). The chapter starts with an introductory preview, and related topics may be mentioned in the notes at the end. The lists of mathematical symbols and physical quantities appear before the main text, and the index of subjects and bibliography at the end of the book. The "Series Preface," information "About the Author," and "Mathematical Symbols" from the first book of volume IV are not repeated, and the "Notation for Functions," "Bibliography," "References," and "Index" are focused on the present fifth book of volume IV.

Acknowledgments

The fourth volume of the series justifies renewing some of the acknowledgments also made in the first three volumes, to those who contributed more directly to the final form of the volume: Ms. Ana Moura, L. Sousa, and S. Pernadas for help with the manuscripts; Mr. J. Coelho for all the drawings; and at last, but not least, to my wife as my companion in preparing this work.

About the Author

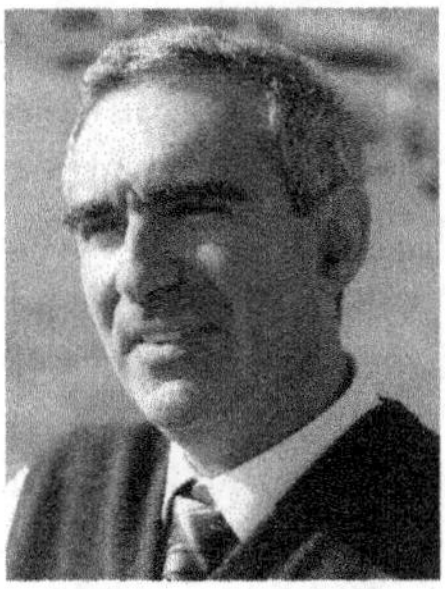

L.M.B.C. Campos was born on March 28, 1950, in Lisbon, Portugal. He graduated in 1972 as a mechanical engineer from the Instituto Superior Tecnico (IST) of Lisbon Technical University. The tutorials as a student (1970) were followed by a career at the same institution (IST) through all levels: assistant (1972), assistant with tenure (1974), assistant professor (1978), associate professor (1982), chair of Applied Mathematics and Mechanics (1985). He has served as the coordinator of undergraduate and postgraduate degrees in Aerospace Engineering since the creation of the programs in 1991. He is the coordinator of the Scientific Area of Applied and Aerospace Mechanics in the Department of Mechanical Engineering. He is also the director and founder of the Center for Aeronautical and Space Science and Technology.

In 1977, Campos received his doctorate on "waves in fluids" from the Engineering Department of Cambridge University, England. Afterwards, he received a Senior Rouse Ball Scholarship to study at Trinity College, while on leave from IST. In 1984, his first sabbatical was as a Senior Visitor at the Department of Applied Mathematics and Theoretical Physics of Cambridge University, England. In 1991, he spent a second sabbatical as an Alexander von Humboldt scholar at the Max-Planck Institut fur Aeronomic in Katlenburg-Lindau, Germany. Further sabbaticals abroad were excluded by major commitments at the home institution. The latter were always compatible with extensive professional travel related to participation in scientific meetings, individual or national representation in international institutions, and collaborative research projects.

Campos received the von Karman medal from the Advisory Group for Aerospace Research and Development (AGARD) and Research and Technology Organization (RTO). Participation in AGARD/RTO included serving as a vice-chairman of the System Concepts and Integration Panel, and chairman of the Flight Mechanics Panel and of the Flight Vehicle Integration Panel. He was also a member of the Flight Test Techniques Working Group. Here he was involved in the creation of an independent flight test capability, active in Portugal during the last 30 years, which has been used in national and international projects, including Eurocontrol and the European Space Agency. The participation in the European Space Agency (ESA) has afforded Campos the opportunity to serve on various program boards at the levels of national representative and Council of Ministers.

His participation in activities sponsored by the European Union (EU) has included: (i) 27 research projects with industry, research, and academic institutions; (ii) membership of various Committees, including Vice-Chairman of the Aeronautical Science and Technology Advisory Committee; (iii) participation on the Space Advisory Panel on the future role of EU in space. Campos has been a member of the Space Science Committee of the European Science Foundation, which works with the Space Science Board of the National Science Foundation of the United States. He has been a member of the Committee for Peaceful Uses of Outer Space (COPUOS) of the United Nations. He has served as a consultant and advisor on behalf of these organizations and other institutions. His participation in professional societies includes member and vice-chairman of the Portuguese Academy of Engineering, fellow of the Royal Aeronautical Society, Astronomical Society and Cambridge Philosophical Society, associate fellow of the American Institute of Aeronautics and Astronautics, and founding and life member of the European Astronomical Society.

Campos has published and worked on numerous books and articles. His publications include 10 books as a single author, one as an editor, and one as a co-editor. He has published 152 papers (82 as the single author, including 12 reviews) in 60 journals, and 254 communications to symposia. He has served as reviewer for 40 different journals, in addition to 23 reviews published in *Mathematics Reviews*. He is or has been member of the editorial boards of several journals, including *Progress in Aerospace Sciences, International Journal of Aeroacoustics, International Journal of Sound and Vibration*, and *Air & Space Europe*.

Campos's areas of research focus on four topics: acoustics, magnetohydrodynamics, special functions, and flight dynamics. His work on acoustics has concerned the generation, propagation, and refraction of sound in flows with mostly aeronautical applications. His work on magnetohydrodynamics has concerned magneto-acoustic-gravity-inertial waves in solar-terrestrial and stellar physics. His developments on special functions have used differintegration operators, generalizing the ordinary derivative and primitive to complex order; they have led to the introduction of new special functions. His work on flight dynamics has concerned aircraft and rockets, including trajectory optimization, performance, stability, control, and atmospheric disturbances.

The range of topics from mathematics to physics and engineering fits with the aims and contents of the present series. Campos's experience in university teaching and scientific and industrial research has enhanced his ability to make the series valuable to students from undergraduate level to research level.

Campos's professional activities on the technical side are balanced by other cultural and humanistic interests. Complementary non-technical interests include classical music (mostly orchestral and choral), plastic arts (painting, sculpture, architecture), social sciences (psychology and biography), history (classical, renaissance and overseas expansion) and technology (automotive, photo, audio). Campos is listed in various biographical publications, including *Who's Who in the World* since 1986, *Who's Who in Science and Technology* since 1994, and *Who's Who in America* since 2011.

Notation for Functions

The list of notations separates ordinary, generalized, auxiliary, and special functions

1 Ordinary Functions

- cos($x;m$) – generalized circular cosine with parameter m: IV.9.4.15, II.5.1.1
- cosh($x;m$) – generalized hyperbolic cosine with parameter m: IV.9.4.13, II.5.1.1
- cot($x;m$) – generalized circular cotangent with parameter m: 9.4.20, II.5.2.1
- coth($x;m$) – generalized circular hyperbolic cotangent with parameter m: IV.9.4.20, II.5.2.1
- csc($x;m$) – generalized circular cosecant with parameter m: 9.4.20, II.5.2.1
- csch($x;m$) – generalized hyperbolic cosecant with parameter m: IV.9.4.20, II.5.2.1
- exp(x) – exponential: II.3.1
- log(x) – logarithm of base e: II.3.5
- $\log_a(x)$ – logarithm of base a: II.3.7
- sec($x;m$) – generalized circular secant with parameter m: IV.9.4.20, II.5.2.1
- sech($x;m$) – generalized hyperbolic secant with parameter m: IV.9.4.20, II.5.2.1
- sin($x;m$) – generalized general circular sine with parameter m: IV.9.4.20, II.5.2.1
- sinh($x;m$) – generalized hyperbolic sine with parameter m: IV.9.4.13, II.5.1.1
- tan($x;m$) – generalized circular tangent with parameter m: IV.9.4.20, II.5.2
- tanh($x;m$) – generalized hyperbolic tangent with parameter m: IV.9.4.20, II.5.2

2 Generalized Functions

$H(x)$ – Heaviside unit jump: III.1.2
$G(x;\xi)$ – Green's function: N1.5
$\delta(x)$ – Dirac unit impulse: III.1.3
$\text{sgn}(x)$ – sign function: I.36.4.1, III.1.7.1

3 Auxiliary Functions

$\text{erf}(x)$ – error function: III.1.2.2
$\sin(x;k)$ – elliptic sine of modulus k: IV.4.4.9, I.39.9.2
$\tilde{y}(k)$ – Fourier transform of $y(x)$; N.IV.1.11
$\bar{y}(s)$ – Laplace transform of $y(x)$: N.IV.1.15
$A(q)$ – Anharmonic factor: IV.4.4.10
$A(\mu,\nu)$ – Extended matching coefficient: IV.9.5.21
$W(y_1,\ldots,y_N)$ – Wronskian of a set of functions: IV.1.2.3
$\psi(x)$ – Digamma function: IV.9.5.16, I.29.5.2
$\Gamma(x)$ – Gamma function: IV.9.5.13, N.III.1.8

4 Special and Extended Functions: See List 9.1

9

Existence Theorems and Special Functions

The preceding chapters have focused mostly on (i) obtaining explicit analytically exact solutions (ii) in terms of elementary functions for certain classes of differential equations and systems that do admit such solutions (chapters 1, 3, 5, and 7), including a fairly wide range of applications (chapters 2, 4, 6, and 8). Some problems, like sound in Gaussian and power law horns (notes 7.39–7.45), or the separation of variables in the Laplace operator in hypercylindrical and hyperspherical coordinates (notes 8.11–8.17), do not have solutions in terms of elementary functions (ii), and require special functions specified by series (sections 9.5–9.7), parametric integrals (section 9.8), or continued fractions (section 9.9); the special functions appear as solutions of linear differential equations with variable coefficients that may not have (or may have) singularities [section(s) 9.4 (9.5–9.9)]. The singular and non-linear differential equations can be solved by analytical (numerical) approximate methods [notes 5.15–5.20 (4.8–4.13)]. When applying approximate methods to differential equations it is necessary to know that a solution exists, under which conditions it is unique, and possibly other properties to validate the method; it is not safe to assume *a priori* that a solution exists, is unique, and that the chosen method converges to it. The existence, unicity, uniformity, and robustness theorems (section 9.1) apply to much wider classes of differential equations than those that can be solved analytically, but in many cases do not help to find a solution. Even if an explicit solution is not available, the qualitative theory of differential equations can indicate some properties, such as stability of a system (section 9.2). The forms of a differential equation may indicate what type of solutions are possible for example periodic solutions (section 9.3), and guide the construction of methods of solution such as power series (sections 9.4–9.7) or parametric integrals (section 9.8) or continued fractions (section 9.9).

9.1 Existence, Unicity, Robustness, and Uniformity of Solutions

Most of the present volume IV has concentrated on methods to obtain analytical solutions of ordinary (chapters 1 to 6) and simultaneous (chapters 7 and 8) differential equations, including general methods (chapters 1, 3, 5, 7) and typical applications (chapters 2, 4, 6, 8); the class of equations for which the existence of a solution can be proved is much wider than the set of equations that can be solved analytically, and the knowledge that a solution does exist is a starting point for numerical or analytical methods of approximation. Even if an analytical solution of a differential equation has been obtained, the possibility remains that other solutions could exist, such as the special integrals (sections 5.1–5.4); the latter possibility is excluded by a unicity theorem that involves imposing some initial conditions. The solution is robust if the result of small changes in the initial conditions is bounded; non-robustness can lead to solutions that differ substantially for close initial conditions; for example, if there are bifurcations, discontinuities, or chaotic cases. Another useful property is uniformity or differentiability with regard to a parameter; for example, it was used to obtain linearly independent particular integrals [chapter 1 (7)] of linear differential equations (simultaneous systems) with constant [sections 1.3–1.4 (7.4–7.5)] and power [sections 1.6–1.7 (7.6–7.7)] coefficients, when the characteristic polynomial has multiple roots or there is resonance [subsections 1.4.1, 1.7.1 (7.5.2, 7.7.2)]. The proof of the theorems of existence, unicity, robustness, and uniformity is based on replacing the differential equation by an equivalent integral equation which is solved by successive approximations. The requirement that the successive approximations converge to a limit function that satisfies the differential equation is met by imposing a contraction condition; the latter ensures that in the limit as the number of approximations tends to infinity; the iterations converge to a fixed point which specifies the solution. A sufficient condition for the convergence to a fixed point is that the form of the differential equation is specified by a Lipschitz function. It is sufficient to prove the existence, unicity, robustness, and uniformity for a system of simultaneous first-order differential equations because a differential equation of any order or a simultaneous system can always be reduced to a set of first-order simultaneous equations.

9.1.1 Existence of Solution and the Lipschitz Condition

The theorems of existence (subsections 9.1.1–9.1.8), unicity, robustness and uniformity subsections (9.1.9–9.1.14) of solutions will be proved first for a first-order differential equation; similar methods apply (subsections 9.1.15–9.1.20) to higher order equations and systems. The Picard method replaces the differential equation by an integral equation (subsection 9.1.2), leading to a Markov chain that can be solved iteratively. The successive iterations converge (subsection 9.1.3) to a fixed point (subsection 9.1.4), that specifies the solution (subsection 9.1.5) in the case when they correspond to a contraction mapping (subsection 9.1.7); the Lipschitz condition (subsection 9.1.5) on the form of the differential equation (subsection 9.1.6) acts as the contraction condition.

The method of successive approximations (subsections 9.1.1–9.1.8) applies in a rectangle (subsection 9.1.9) and can be used to prove: (i) the existence of solution (subsections 9.1.1–9.1.8) of the differential equation; (ii) its unicity (subsection 9.1.10) with the boundary condition; (iii) the robustness of the solution (subsection 9.1.11), that is, its differentiability with regard to the initial conditions (subsection 9.1.13); and (iv) the uniformity of the solution (subsection 9.1.14), that is, its differentiability with regard to parameters in the differential equation. The proofs of (iii) [(iv)] use again the Lipschitz or contraction condition (subsection 9.1.4), in the original form (subsection 9.1.5) [for the parameter in the differential equation (subsection 9.1.14)]. Both proofs are based on the comparison (subsection 9.1.12) of the original and modified successive approximations to the solution of the differential equation.

The theorems of existence (subsections 9.1.1–9.1.8) and also unicity, robustness, and uniformity (subsections 9.1.9–9.1.14) of solution can be extended from a single differential equation of first order to any system of simultaneous differential equations of any order that can always be reduced to a system of first order equations (subsections 9.1.15–9.1.17); in particular a single differential equation of order N can be reduced (subsections 9.1.18–9.1.20) to a system N of first-order equations. Thus, by generalizing the Lipschitz or contraction condition to a set of functions of several variables (subsection 9.1.16), the theorems of existence, unicity, robustness, and uniformity of solution can be extended to a system of first-order equations (subsections 9.1.15–9.1.17) and hence also to a single differential equation of any order (subsections 9.1.18–9.1.20).

9.1.2 Transformation of a Differential into an Integral Equation (Picard 1893)

Consider a differential equation of first order and first degree that can be solved for the derivative (9.1a):

$$\frac{dy}{dx} = f(x,y), \qquad y(x_0) = y_0, \tag{9.1a, b}$$

and whose unicity usually requires (subsection 1.1.5) the specification of the initial value of the solution at one point (9.1b). The designations boundary (initial) value(s) or condition(s) may be applied indeferently to an ordinary differential equation or simultaneous system since there is only one independent variable; in physical and engineering problems the word boundary (initial) is usually associated with the independent variable being a position (time). Examples have been given of singular differential equations of first-order first-degree (sections 3.1–3.4) for which $f(x, y)$ is not a continuous function of x or y; for example, through the point of discontinuity passes no solution (pass an infinite number of solutions) such as [subsection 4.1.8 (4.1.7)] a center (focal or nodal point). Thus, in order that existence and unicity be possible, it is required that the function $f(x, y)$ in the ordinary differential equation of first-order first-degree (9.1a) is integrable (9.2a) in x, y so that the differential equation together with the initial condition (9.1b), is equivalent to the **integral equation** (9.2b):

$$f(x,y) \in \mathcal{E}\left((x_0,x),(y_0,y)\right): \qquad y(x) = y_0 + \int_{x_0}^{x} f\left(t, y(t)\right) dt. \tag{9.2a, b}$$

The integral equation (9.2b) lends itself to solution by the **method of successive approximations**: (i) the first approximation is obtained by replacing the initial condition (9.1b) in the integral (9.2b) leading to (9.3a):

$$y_1(x) = y_0 + \int_{x_0}^{x} f(t, y_0) dt, \quad y_{j+1}(x) = y_0 + \int_{x_0}^{x} f\left(t, y_j(t)\right) dt; \quad \lim_{j\to\infty} y_j(x) = y(x), \tag{9.3a–c}$$

(ii) each successive approximation follows from the preceding in the same way (9.3b). The system (9.3a, b) can be interpreted as a Markov chain where each element depends only on the preceding. Its solution exists if the method of successive approximations succeeds, that is if: (i) the sequence (9.3a, b) tends to a limit function (9.3c); and (ii) that limit function satisfies the original integral equation (9.2b). Thus the **Picard (1893) method** *applies (standard CCII) to a first-order differential equation solvable for the slope (9.1a) with an initial condition (9.1b) and: (i) replaces it with an integral equation (9.2b) involving an integrable function (9.2a); (ii) leads to a system of finite difference-integral equations (9.3a, b) that can be solved by recurrence; and (iii) depends on the existence of a limit function (9.3c) that satisfies the integral (9.2b) or differential (9.1a) equation.* Before considering conditions for which (iii) hold (subsections 9.1.4–9.1.8), an example is given (subsection 9.1.3) of the application of the Picard method of successive approximations.

9.1.3 Convergence of the Successive Approximations

As an example, consider the differential equation (9.4a) with initial condition (9.4b):

$$\frac{dy}{dx} = y, \qquad y(0) = 1: \qquad y(x) = 1 + \int_0^x y(t) dt, \tag{9.4a–c}$$

it is equivalent to integral equation (9.4c) with (9.5a) for which (9.3a, b) the successive approximations are (9.5b, c):

$$f(x,y) = y: \quad y_1(x) = 1 + \int_0^x dt = 1 + x, \quad y_2(x) = 1 + \int_0^x (1+t) dt = 1 + x + \frac{x^2}{2}; \tag{9.5a, b}$$

proceeding by induction (9.6a):

$$y_j(x) = \sum_{q=0}^{j} \frac{x^q}{q!}, \qquad y_{j+1}(x) = 1 + \sum_{q=0}^{j} \int_0^x \left(\frac{t^q}{q!} \right) dt = \sum_{q=0}^{j+1} \frac{x^q}{q!}, \tag{9.6a, b}$$

it follows that the n-th approximation is given by (9.6b). Thus the limit function exists (9.7a) and coincides with the exponential (9.7b):

$$y(x) \equiv \lim_{j \to \infty} y_j(x) = \sum_{q=0}^{\infty} \frac{x^q}{q!} = e^x. \tag{9.7a, b}$$

The exponential function (chapter II.5) can be defined by the properties (9.4a, b) ≡ (II.1.25a, b) and the Picard method shows that it has the power series representation (9.7a). However, the Picard method does not prove the convergence of the series (9.7a) for the exponential; that can be established by other methods such as: (a) the D'Alembert convergence test (subsection I.29.3.2); (b) noting that (9.4a) implies that the exponential is an analytic function (section I.1.2) and (9.7a) is its MacLaurin series (I.23.34b). In addition, it is necessary to prove that the series satisfies: (i) the boundary condition (9.4b); and (ii) the differential equation (9.4a). The latter proof relies on the series (9.7a) being uniformly convergent (section I.21.6) and hence differentiable term-by-term (9.8b):

$$m = q-1: \quad \frac{d}{dx}\left(e^x\right) = \frac{d}{dx}\left\{ \sum_{q=0}^{\infty} \frac{x^q}{q!} \right\} = \sum_{q=0}^{\infty} \frac{1}{q!} \frac{d}{dx}\left(x^q\right) = \sum_{q=1}^{\infty} \frac{x^{q-1}}{(q-1)!} = \sum_{m=0}^{\infty} \frac{x^m}{m!} = e^x, \tag{9.8a, b}$$

where was used the change of variable of summation (9.8a). These additional proofs of convergence of the sequence of functions to the solution of the differential equation with boundary condition are equivalent to the existence of a **fixed point** (9.3c) that satisfies the differential (9.4a, b) and integral (9.4c) equations. This simple example indicates the way towards the proof in the general case (9.3a, b); that is, to prove that a fixed point exists (subsection 9.1.4).

9.1.4 Contraction Mapping and Fixed Point

The preceding example suggests that the method of successive approximations leads to a unique solution if the difference between successive iterations (9.9a) reduces (Figure 9.1a) as the number of approximations increases:

$$y_j(x) - y_{j-1}(x) = \frac{x^j}{j!}, \qquad y_j(x) = y_0 + \sum_{q=1}^{j} \left\{ y_q(x) - y_{q-1}(x) \right\}, \tag{9.9a, b}$$

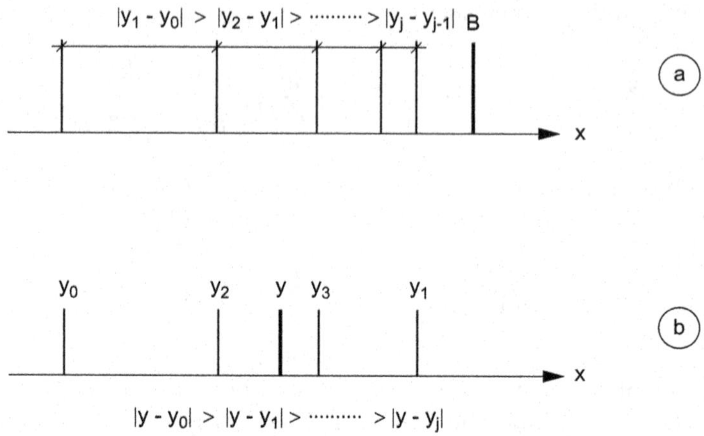

FIGURE 9.1
The method of successive approximations proves the existence, unicity and other properties of the solution of a differential equation by using a contraction mapping that converges to a fixed point that is the unique solution. The convergence can be (a) monotonic from one side or (b) alternating from both sides.

sufficiently fast for the series (9.9b) to have a bound B independent of x as $j \to \infty$. In that case, the series is uniformly convergent (section I.21.4) and specifies a continuous limit function (9.3c); also, the series can be integrated (differentiated) term-by-term, proving that the limit function satisfies the original integral (differential) equation. One way to form a uniformly convergent sequence is to impose (Figure 9.1b) a **contraction mapping** (9.10a):

$$k < 1: \quad \left| y_j(x) - y_{j-1}(x) \right| < k \left| y_{j-1}(x) - y_{j-2}(x) \right| < k^{j-1} \left| y_1(x) - y_0(x) \right|, \qquad \text{(9.10a, b)}$$

that specifies a **fixed point** (9.3c) in the limit (9.10b). The condition (9.10a) for the existence of a fixed point is generalized by the Lipschitz condition (subsection 9.1.5).

9.1.5 Lipschitz (1864) or Contraction Condition, Continuity, and Differentiability

An example of contraction property applied to a function is (9.11c) the **Lipschitz (1864) condition** with **coefficient** (9.11a) and **exponent** (9.11b):

$$k > 0, \alpha \in |R: \qquad \mathcal{K}_k^\alpha(x_0, x) \equiv \left\{ f(x): \quad \left| f(x) - f(x_0) \right| < k \left| x - x_0 \right|^\alpha \right\}. \qquad \text{(9.11a–c)}$$

The condition (9.11c) specifies (standard CCIII) the set of Lipschitz or contraction functions (9.11a, b). From (9.11c) it follows that:

$$k > 0: \qquad \lim_{x \to x_0} \left| f(x) - f(x_0) \right| \begin{cases} = 0 & \text{if} \quad \alpha > 0, & (9.12a) \\ \le k & \text{if} \quad \alpha = 0, & (9.12b) \\ = \infty & \text{if} \quad \alpha < 0, & (9.12c) \end{cases}$$

a Lipschitz or contraction function (9.11a–c): (i) is continuous for (9.12a); (ii) is bounded but may be discontinuous for (9.12b); and (iii) may be unbounded or singular for (9.12c). Also:

$$k > 0: \qquad \lim_{x \to x_0} \left| \frac{f(x) - f(x_0)}{x - x_0} \right| \begin{cases} = 0 & \text{if} \quad \alpha > 1, & (9.13a) \\ \le k & \text{if} \quad \alpha = 1, & (9.13b) \\ = \infty & \text{if} \quad \alpha < 1, & (9.13c) \end{cases}$$

a Lipschitz or contraction function (9.11a–c): (i) has vanishing derivative for (9.12a); (ii) has bounded incremental ratio for (9.13b); and (iii) may have unbounded incremental ratio for (9.13c). Thus the Lipschitz functions with (9.14a) include the differentiable functions and are contained in the continuous functions (9.14b):

$$0 < \alpha \le 1: \qquad C \supset \mathcal{K}^{\alpha} \supset \mathcal{D}; \qquad \left| f(x) - f(x_0) \right| \le k \left| x - x_0 \right|^{\frac{1}{2}}; \qquad (9.14a\text{–}c)$$

for example, the function (9.14c) is continuous, non-differentiable, and belongs (does not belong) to Lipschitz space $\mathcal{K}^{\alpha}$ with $\alpha \ge \frac{1}{2} - \varepsilon \left(\alpha \le \frac{1}{2} + \varepsilon \right)$ with $\varepsilon > 0$. The Lipschitz condition (9.11a–c) can be applied either to the dependent y or to the independent x variable (subsection 9.1.6), to prove the uniform convergence of the Picard sequence of successive approximations to a continuous solution (subsection 9.1.7), hence establishing the existence and unicity of solution of the differential equation (subsection 9.1.8).

9.1.6 Continuity (Contraction) Condition on the Independent (Dependent) Variable

In order to prove the existence and unicity of solution of the differential (9.1a, b) or integral (9.2a, b) equation, it is assumed that the function $f(x, y)$ is continuous in x (9.15a, b) [Lipschitz in y with (9.15c, d) exponent $\alpha = 1$] in the neighborhood of $x = x_0 \left(y = y_0 \right)$:

$$\left| x - x_0 \right| \le a: \qquad f(x, y) \in C, \qquad \left| y - y_0 \right| \le b: \qquad f(x, y) \in \mathcal{K}^1. \qquad (9.15a\text{–}d)$$

The Lipschitz condition (9.15d) implies that the function $f(x,y)$ is also continuous in y, and hence: (i) integrable (9.2a) along the x-axis (9.2b) as required in the Picard method of successive approximations (9.3a–c); (ii) bounded (9.16c) in the rectangle (9.16a, b):

$$x_0 - a \le x \le x_0 + a, \qquad y_0 - b \le y \le y_0 + b: \qquad |f(x,y)| \le B. \tag{9.16a–c}$$

If $B > b/a \left(B \le b/a\right)$ the Lipschitz condition (9.17b) is applied in the smaller (Figure 9.2a) [same (Figure 9.2b)] rectangle (9.17a):

$$|x - x_0| \le h \equiv \min\left(a, \frac{b}{B}\right): \qquad |f(x,Y) - f(x,y)| \le k|Y - y|. \tag{9.17a, b}$$

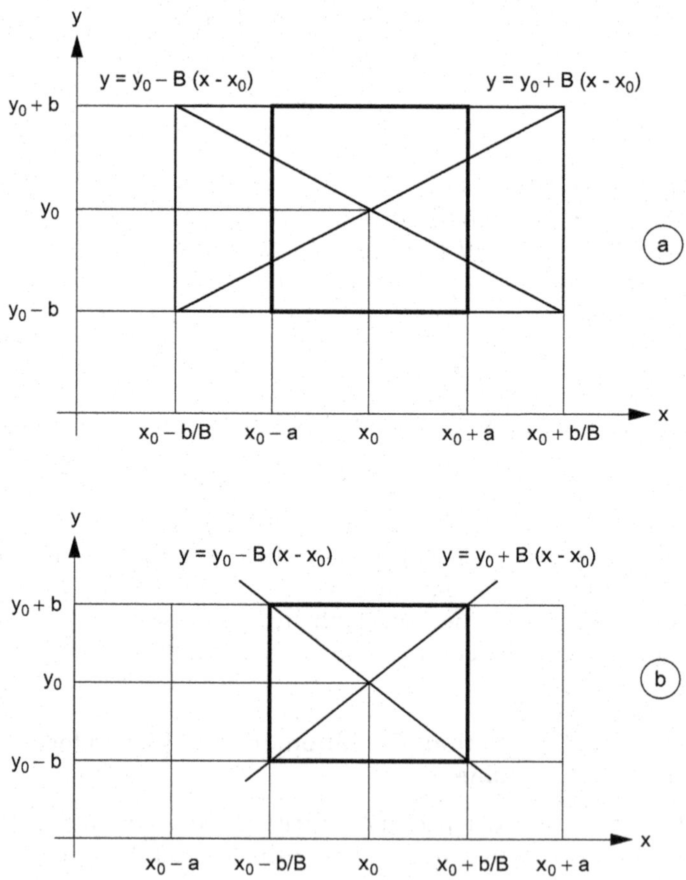

FIGURE 9.2
The region of convergence of the successive approximations to the unique solution of a differential equation is an interval (Figure 9.1) both for the dependent y and independent x variables, leading to a rectangle (Figure 9.2) in the (x, y) plane. The size of the rectangle may be driven (a) either by the independent or (b) by the dependent variable.

These conditions are applied to the successive approximations: (i) the first (9.3a):

$$|y_1(x)-y_0| \le \int_{x_0}^{x} |f(t,y_0)|\,dt \le B\int_{x_0}^{x} dt = B|x-x_0|, \tag{9.18a}$$

uses only continuity; (ii) all of the following:

$$\begin{aligned} |y_2(x)-y_1(x)| &\le \int_{x_0}^{x} |f(t,y_1(t))-f(t,y_0)|\,dt < k\int_{x_0}^{x} |y_1(t)-y_0|\,dt \\ &< kB\int_{x_0}^{x} |t-x_0|\,dt = \frac{kB}{2}|x-x_0|^2, \end{aligned} \tag{9.18b}$$

use the Lipschitz property.

9.1.7 Uniform Convergence to a Continuous Solution

It follows from (9.18b) by induction that the difference between the *j*-th successive approximations has an upper bound:

$$|y_j(x)-y_{j-1}(x)| \le \frac{k^{j-1}}{j!} B|x-x_0|^j, \tag{9.19}$$

since: (i) for $j=1$ $(j=2)$ the formula (9.19) reduces to (9.18a) [(9.18b)]; (ii) if (9.19) holds for *j*, then in also holds (9.20) for $j+1$:

$$\begin{aligned} |y_{j+1}(x)-y_j(x)| &\le \int_{x_0}^{x} |f(t,y_j(t))-f(t,y_{j-1}(t))|\,dt \le k\int_{x_0}^{x} |y_j(t)-y_{j-1}(t)|\,dt \\ &< B\frac{k^j}{j!}\int_{x_0}^{x} |t-x_0|^j\,dt = B\frac{k^j}{(j+1)!}|x-x_0|^{j+1}. \end{aligned} \tag{9.20}$$

Using the identity (9.9b) it follows that *j*-th approximation has an upper bound (9.21a):

$$|y_j(x)| \le |y_0| + \sum_{q=1}^{j} |y_q(x)-y_{q-1}(x)| \le |y_0| + B\sum_{q=1}^{j} \frac{k^{q-1}h^q}{q!}, \tag{9.21a, b}$$

where (9.17a; 9.19) were used in (9.21b). Taking the limit $j \to \infty$ in (9.21b) leads to (9.22a):

$$\lim_{j\to\infty} \left| y_j(x) \right| \le \left| y_0 \right| + \frac{B}{k} \sum_{q=1}^{\infty} \frac{(kh)^q}{q!} = \left| y_0 \right| + \frac{B}{k} \left[\exp(kh) - 1 \right], \qquad (9.22\text{a, b})$$

where the exponential (9.7b) was used in (9.22b). This proves that $y_j(x)$ tends to a limit function $y(x)$ as $j \to \infty$, and the convergence is uniform (section I.21.5) because it is independent of x. Thus the limit may be taken under the integral sign in (9.3b), to prove:

$$y(x) = \lim_{j\to\infty} y_j(x) = y_0 + \int_{x_0}^{x} \lim_{j\to\infty} f\left(t, y_{j-1}(t)\right) dt = y_0 + \int_{x_0}^{x} f\left(t, y(t)\right) dt, \qquad (9.23\text{a–c})$$

that the limit function (9.23a) satisfies (9.23b, c) the integral equation (9.2a, b). It follows that the limit functions satisfies the differential equation (9.1a) and initial condition (9.1b); also it is continuous (9.24b) in the rectangle of Figure 9.2a because it is (section I.21.5) the limit of a uniform convergent series (9.24a):

$$y(x) = \lim_{j\to\infty} y_j(x) = \lim_{j\to\infty} \left\{ y_0 + \sum_{q=1}^{j} \left\{ y_q(x) - y_{q-1}(x) \right\} \right\} \in C\left(\left| x - x_0 \right| < h \right), \qquad (9.24\text{a, b})$$

of continuous functions. This completes the proof of the existence theorem that is stated next (subsection 9.1.8).

9.1.8 Theorem of Existence of Solution of a Differential Equation

Thus has been proved the **theorem of existence and unicity:**

$$f(x,y) \in C\left(x_0 - a \le x \le x_0 + a \right): \qquad \left| f(x,y) \right| \le B; \qquad (9.25\text{a, b})$$

if (standard CCIV) the function $f(x,y)$ is: (i) continuous in an interval (9.15a, b) ≡ (9.25a) with upper bound (9.16c) ≡ (9.25b); (ii) Lipschitz (9.17b) ≡ (9.26c) with exponent unity in y in a rectangle (9.16b) ≡ (9.26a) and (9.17a) ≡ (9.26b):

$$\left| y - y_0 \right| \le b, \quad \left| x - x_0 \right| \le h \equiv \min\left\{ a, \frac{b}{B} \right\}: \qquad \left| f(x,Y) - f(x,y) \right| < k \left| Y - y \right|, \qquad (9.26\text{a–c})$$

then the differential equation (9.1a) with initial condition (9.1b), and the equivalent integral equation (9.2a, b), have a unique solution in the rectangle (Figure 9.2a, b) that is a continuous function (9.24b) in the closed interval (9.26b). Since only existence of a solution was proved before (subsections 9.1.2–9.1.8) next (subsections 9.1.9–9.1.14) are addressed the questions of unicity together with robustness (uniformity) with regard to the initial condition (parameters in the differential equation).

9.1.9 Rectangle as the Domain of Successive Approximations

The preceding results imply the following theorem: *the successive approximations (9.3a, b) to the solution of the differential (9.1a, b) [integral (9.2a, b)] equation with bounded function (9.27a) satisfy (standard CCV) the inequality (9.27b):*

$$\left|f\left(x,y_j(x)\right)\right|\leq B: \qquad \left|y_j(x)-y_0\right|\leq b, \tag{9.27a, b}$$

and thus lie (Figure 9.2a, b) in the rectangle (9.26a, b). The first condition (9.27a) is an assumption; the latter condition (9.27b) follows from the former (9.27a), and can be proved by induction, by noting that: (i) it holds for $j = 1$:

$$\left|y_1(x)-y_0\right|\leq\int_{x_0}^{x}\left|f\left(t,y_0\right)\right|dt\leq B\int_{x_0}^{x}dt=B\left|x-x_0\right|\leq Bh\leq b; \tag{9.28}$$

(ii) if it holds for j in (9.27b), then using (9.29) it follows that:

$$\left|y_{j+1}(x)-y_0\right|\leq\int_{x_0}^{x}\left|f\left(t,y_j(t)\right)\right|dt\leq B\int_{x_0}^{x}dt\leq B\left|x-x_0\right|\leq Bh\leq b, \tag{9.29}$$

it also holds for $j + 1$.

9.1.10 Theorem of Unicity of Solution of a Differential Equation

Concerning unicity, must be excluded the possibility that a function $Y(x)$ exists, distinct from the limit function $y(x)$, and satisfying the same differential equation (9.30a) and initial condition (9.30b):

$$dY/dx=f(Y,x), \qquad Y(x_0)=y_0, \tag{9.30a, b}$$

as well as the continuity and Lipschitz conditions. Such a function $Y(x)$ would satisfy the integral equation:

$$Y(x)=y_0+\int_{x_0}^{x}f\left(t,Y(t)\right)dt, \tag{9.31}$$

but need not be obtained by the method of successive approximations; some other method could conceivably lead to a different solution. To see that this is not the case, compare the new solution $Y(x)$ with the successive approximations of $y(x)$, namely: (i) the first (9.31) using (9.16c) leading to (9.32):

$$\left|Y(x)-y_0\right| \le \int_{x_0}^{x} \left|f(t,Y(t))\right| dt \le B \int_{x_0}^{x} dt = B\left|x-x_0\right|; \tag{9.32}$$

(ii) the second using (9.3a; 9.17b; 9.32) leading to (9.33):

$$\begin{aligned} \left|Y(x)-y_1\right| &\le \int_{x_0}^{x} \left|f(t,y(t))-f(t,y_0)\right| dt \le k \int_{x_0}^{x} \left|Y(t)-y_0\right| dt \\ &\le kB \int_{x_0}^{x} \left|t-x_0\right| dt = \frac{Bk}{2}\left|x-x_0\right|^2; \end{aligned} \tag{9.33}$$

(iii) the j-th approximation (9.34) using (9.17a):

$$\left|Y(x)-y_j(x)\right| \le \frac{Bk^j}{(j+1)!}\left|x-x_0\right|^{j+1} \le \frac{Bk^j h^{j+1}}{(j+1)!} \le b\frac{(kh)^j}{(j+1)!}. \tag{9.34}$$

The upper bound (9.34) vanishes uniformly in x as $j \to \infty$ in (9.35a):

$$0 = \lim_{j\to\infty} b\frac{(kh)^j}{(j+1)!} = \lim_{j\to\infty}\left|Y(x)-y_j(x)\right|, \quad Y(x) = \lim_{j\to\infty} y_j(x) = y(x), \tag{9.35a, b}$$

showing that the function $Y(x)$ coincides (9.35b) with the limit function $y(x)$ of the sequence of successive approximations; thus the latter is the unique solution. It has been proved that *the differential equation (9.1a) where the function is continuous (9.25a) with upper bound (9.25b) [Lipschitz (9.26c) in the rectangle (9.26a, b)] in the independent (dependent) variable has (standard CCVI) a unique solution satisfying the condition (9.1b).* A similar method proves robustness (subsections 9.1.11–9.1.13) with regard to initial conditions; that is, that a small perturbation in the initial condition leads to a small perturbation in the solution. The reverse can be true in the case of chaotic systems (sections 4.8–4.9).

9.1.11 Robustness Relative to Perturbed Initial Conditions

Consider the same differential equation (9.36a) ≡ (9.1a):

$$\frac{dY}{dx} = f(x,Y), \qquad Y(x_0) = y_0 + \varepsilon \equiv Y_0, \tag{9.36a, b}$$

with an initial condition (9.1b) perturbed by a small ε to (9.36b). The solution is **robust** relative to small perturbations in the initial condition (9.37a) if these entail a small perturbation (9.37b) in the solution (Figure 9.3a):

$$\left|Y(x_0)-y(x_0)\right| \le \varepsilon \Rightarrow \left|Y(x)-y(x)\right| \le \delta. \qquad (9.37a, b)$$

The solution (9.38a) of the differential equation (9.1a) depends on the initial condition (9.1b), and if it is differentiable (9.38b) it leads to (9.38d):

$$y = y(x;y_0) \in \mathcal{D}(|R): \quad |\zeta - y_0| < |Y_0 - y_0|: \quad |Y(x)-y(x)| = \left|\frac{\partial y}{\partial \zeta}\right| |Y_0 - y_0| = \varepsilon \left|\frac{\partial y}{\partial \zeta}\right| < \delta, \qquad (9.38a–f)$$

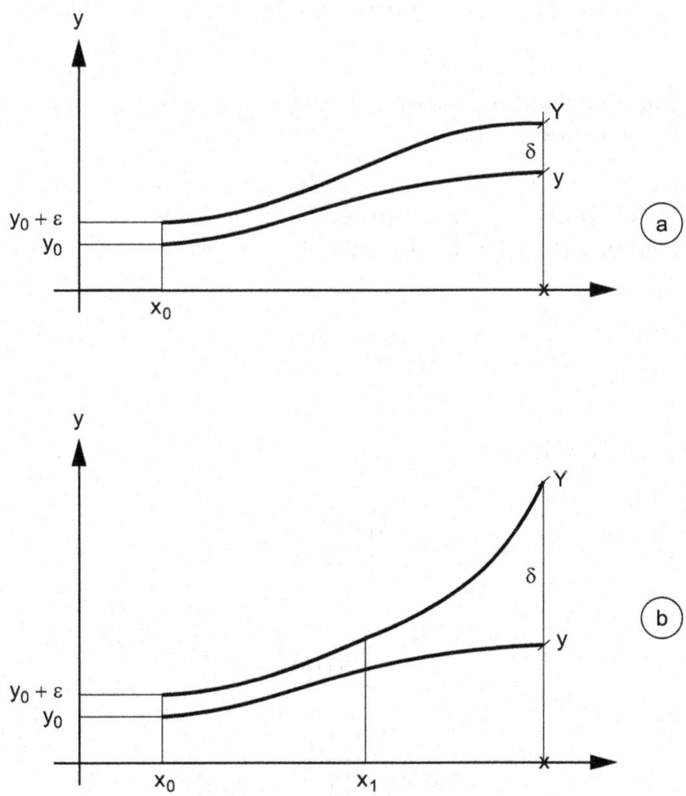

FIGURE 9.3
The solution of a differential equation is (a) robust [(b) has a bifurcation] with regard to the initial conditions if a small initial deviation ε remains small δ (grows larger) as the independent variable increases.

where: (i) the mean value theorem (I.23.40) ≡ (9.38d) with (9.38c) was used (section I.23.8); (ii) then follows (9.38e) the upper bound (9.37b) ≡ (9.38f) that is consistent with (9.37b). Thus, *a sufficient condition for robustness (9.37a, b) is (standard CCVII) that the solution (9.38a) of the differential equation (9.1a) be differentiable (9.38b, c) with regard to the initial coordinate.* In the case (Figure 9.3b) of non-robustness, a small perturbation in the initial condition (9.36b) would lead to solutions differing significantly after some $x > x_1$, for example $x = x_1$ could be a bifurcation (chapter 4). The condition of robustness of the solution of a differential (9.1a, b) or integral (9.2a, b) equation can be compared with the perturbed problem (9.39a):

$$Y_1(x) = y_0 + \varepsilon + \int_{x_0}^{x} f(t, y_0 + \varepsilon)\,dt, \qquad Y_{j+1}(x) = y_0 + \varepsilon + \int_{x_0}^{x} f(t, Y_j(t))\,dt, \tag{9.39a, b}$$

for example via their respective successive approximations (9.39b).

9.1.12 Comparison of Successive Approximations to the Original and Perturbed Problems

In order to implement the preceding ideas, the approximations of the same order in the two problems unperturbed (9.3a, b) and perturbed (9.39a, b) are compared, leading to: (i) for the first order:

$$|Y_1(x) - y_1(x)| \le |\varepsilon| + \int_{x_0}^{x} |f(t, Y_0) - f(t, y_0)|\,dt \le |\varepsilon| + k|\varepsilon| \int_{x_0}^{x} dt = |Y_0 - y_0| \left\{1 + k|x - x_0|\right\}; \tag{9.40}$$

(ii) for the second order:

$$\begin{aligned} |Y_2(x) - y_2(x)| &\le |\varepsilon| + \int_{x_0}^{x} |f(t, Y_1(t)) - f(t, y_1(t)|\,dt \\ &\le |\varepsilon| + k \int_{x_0}^{x} |Y_1(t) - y_1(t)|\,dt \\ &\le |\varepsilon| + |\varepsilon|\,k \int_{x_0}^{x} \{1 + k|t - t_0|\}\,dt \\ &\le |\varepsilon| \left\{1 + k|x - x_0| + \frac{k^2}{2}|x - x_0|^2\right\}; \end{aligned} \tag{9.41}$$

(iii) for the j-th approximation:

$$\left|Y_j(x) - y_j(x)\right| \le |\varepsilon| \sum_{q=0}^{j} \frac{k^q}{q!} \left| x - x_0 \right|^q. \tag{9.42}$$

From (9.42) it follows that the j-th approximation:

$$\left|\frac{\partial y_j}{\partial y_0}\right| = \lim_{\epsilon \to 0} \left|\frac{Y_j(x) - y_j(x)}{\varepsilon}\right| \le \sum_{q=0}^{j} \frac{k^q}{q!} |x - x_0|^q \le \sum_{q=0}^{j} \frac{(kh)^q}{q!} \le e^{kh}, \tag{9.43}$$

is uniformly differentiable with regard to the initial condition. Thus (9.9b) the series:

$$\lim_{j \to \infty} \frac{\partial y_j}{\partial y_0} = 1 + \sum_{q=1}^{\infty} \frac{\partial}{\partial y_0} \left[y_q(x) - y_{q-1}(x) \right] = \frac{\partial y}{\partial y_0}, \tag{9.44}$$

is uniformly convergent to its sum $\partial y / \partial y_0$, showing that the differentiability with regard to y_0 is uniform in x as stated next (subsection 9.1.13).

9.1.13 Theorem of Robustness with Regard to the Initial Condition

Thus has been proved a **theorem of robustness** *(standard CCVIII): if the function $f(x,y)$ is: (i) continuous in the independent variable for (9.25a) with upper bound (9.25b); and (ii) Lipschitz in the dependent variable (9.26a) in the rectangle (9.26a, b) ≡ (9.45a, b), then the solution of the differential (9.1a) or integral (9.2b) equation is uniformly differentiable with regard to the initial condition (9.45):*

$$\frac{\partial y(x; y_0)}{\partial y_0} = g(x; y_0) \in C\left(|x - x_0| < h, |y - y_0| < y\right), \tag{9.45}$$

and a small perturbation in the initial condition (9.36a, b) leads to a robust solution (9.37a, b) with upper bound (9.38a–f) on the perturbation of the solution. A similar situation arises if, instead of perturbing the initial condition (9.36b) and leaving the differential equation unchanged (9.36a), a parameter λ introduced in the latter (9.46a):

$$\frac{dy}{dx} = f(x, y; \lambda), \qquad y(x_0) = y_0, \tag{9.46a, b}$$

and the boundary conditions is left unchanged (9.46b) ≡ (9.1b). This case is considered next, leading to a theorem of uniformity of solution with regard to a parameter in the differential equation (subsection 9.1.14).

9.1.14 Theorem on Uniformity with Regard to a Parameter in a Differential Equation

In the case (9.46a, b), the equivalent integral equation is (9.47):

$$y(x;\lambda) = y_0 + \int_{x_0}^{x} f(t, y(t); \lambda)\, dt, \tag{9.47}$$

and the proof of differentiability of the solution with regard to the parameter $\partial y(x;\lambda)/\partial\lambda$ follows as in the subsection 9.1.12, on the assumption that the function $f(x,y;\lambda)$ is Lipschitz in λ:

$$|x - x_0| < h, |y - y_0| < b, \quad |\lambda - \lambda_0| \le d: \quad |f(x,y;\lambda) - f(x;y;\lambda_0)| \le k_0 |\lambda - \lambda_0|. \tag{9.48a–d}$$

This establishes a **theorem of parametric uniformity** *(standard CCIX): if the function $f(x,y;\lambda)$ is continuous in x for (9.25a) with upper bound B in (9.25b); (ii) Lipschitz (9.26c) in y in the rectangle (9.26a, b); and (iii) Lipschitz (9.48c) in the parameter λ in (9.48a, b); then the differential equation with parameter λ (9.46a) and initial condition (9.46b) has a solution $y(x;\lambda)$ that is uniformly differentiable (9.49) with regard to λ:*

$$\frac{\partial y(x;\lambda)}{\partial \lambda} = G(x;\lambda) \in C|x - x_0| < h, |\lambda - \lambda_0| \le d, \tag{9.49}$$

in the domain of validity of (ii, iii). The theorems of existence (subsections 9.1.1–9.1.8), unicity (subsections 9.1.9–9.1.10), and robustness (uniformity) with regard [subsections 9.1.11–9.1.13 (9.1.14)] to the initial condition (parameters in the differential equation) can be extended from a first-order differential equation (subsections 9.1.1–9.1.14) to [subsections 9.1.15–9.1.17 (9.1.18–9.1.20)] a simultaneous system (differential equation of any order).

9.1.15 Simultaneous System of First-Order Differential Equations

Next is considered the extension of the ordinary differential equation of first order first degree (9.1a) to a **generalized autonomous system** (9.50a):

$$m, n = 1, \ldots, M: \qquad \frac{dy_m}{dx} = f_m(x; y_n), \qquad y_m(x_0) = y_{m,0}, \tag{9.50a–c}$$

that involves only first-order derivatives (9.50b) of each dependent variable, explicitly as functions of the independent variable x and all dependent variables together with M boundary conditions (9.50c) specifying the initial value of each dependent variable for a given value of the independent variable. The system (9.50a–c) can be written explicitly:

$$\frac{dy_1}{dx} = f_1(x; y_1, y_2, \ldots, y_M), \qquad y_1(x_0) = y_{1,0}, \tag{9.51a}$$

$$\frac{dy_2}{dx} = f_2(x; y_1, y_2, \ldots, y_M), \qquad y_2(x_0) = y_{2,0}, \tag{9.51b}$$

$$\frac{dy_M}{dx} = f_M(x; y_1, y_2, \ldots, y_M), \qquad y_M(x_0) = y_{M,0}. \tag{9.51c}$$

If all the functions (9.50a, b) are integrable (9.52) in a rectangle:

$$f_n(x; y_m) \in \mathcal{E}\left(|x - x_0| < a, \quad |y - y_{m,0}| < b_m\right), \tag{9.52}$$

the system of differential equations (9.50a, b) with initial conditions (9.50c) is equivalent to the system of finite difference integral equations (9.53):

$$y_m(x) = y_{m,o} + \int_{x_0}^{x} f\left(t; y_1(t), \ldots, y_M(t)\right) dt. \tag{9.53}$$

The latter system can be solved by the method of successive approximations:

$$y_{m,1}(x) = y_{m,o} + \int_{x_0}^{x} f\left(t; y_{1,o}, \ldots, y_{M,o}\right) dt, \tag{9.54a}$$

$$y_{m,j+1}(x) = y_{m,o} + \int_{x_0}^{x} f\left(t; y_{1,j}(t), \ldots, y_{M,j}(t)\right) dt. \tag{9.54b}$$

It is clear that (9.1a, b; 9.2a, b; 9.3a, b) are the particular case $M = 1$ in (9.50a) of (9.50b, c; 9.52, 9.53; 9.54a, b). Thus the Picard method of successive approximations (subsection 9.1.2) can be extended to an generalized autonomous system (9.50a) of first-order differential equations (9.50b) with initial conditions (9.50c) by: (i) transforming to an equivalent system of integral equations (9.53) involving integrable functions in a rectangle (9.52); (ii) the latter can be solved iteratively as a Markov chain or iterative sequence of equations (9.54a, b). The proof of the convergence of (9.54a, b) as j tends to infinity.

$$\lim_{j \to \infty} y_{m,j}(x) = y_m(x), \tag{9.54c}$$

to the solution of the differential (9.50a–c) and integral (9.53) of the solution of the finite difference-integral equations (9.54a, b) uses the extension of the Lipschitz condition (subsection 9.1.5) to several variables (subsection 9.1.16).

9.1.16 Contraction or Lipschitz Condition for Several Variables

In order to prove the theorems of existence and unicity of solution and robustness (uniformity) with regard to a perturbation of the initial conditions (parameters in the differential equations) for generalized autonomous systems of ordinary differential equations, is needed (9.17a, b) the **generalized of the Lipschitz condition** (9.55a, b):

$$|Y_\ell - y_\ell| \le b_\ell, \; |x - x_0| \le h: \; \left| f_m(x;Y_\ell) - f_m(x;y_\ell) \right| < \sum_{\ell=1}^{L} k_{m,\ell} |Y_\ell - y_\ell|; \tag{9.55a–c}$$

stating that the set of M functions (9.56a) in L variables (9.56b) has the Lipschitz or contraction property (9.55c) in (L + 1)-dimensional hyper parallelepiped (9.55a, b) where hold (9.56c, d):

$$m = 1, \ldots, M: \qquad \ell = 1, \ldots, L: \;\; k_{m,\ell} > 0, \;\; h \equiv \min\left(a, \frac{b_\ell}{B}\right): \;\; \left| f_m(x,y) \right| < B. \tag{9.56a–e}$$

The Lipschitz condition (9.55a–c) implies that the functions (9.50b) are continuous (9.12a) with regard to y, and if they are also continuous with regard to x they are bounded (9.56e). The generalized contraction or Lipschitz condition (9.55a–c; 9.56a–d) is used next with number of functions $M = L$ equal to the number of variables. From the Lipschitz condition (9.55c), applied together with (9.56e) in (9.55a, b), it follows by induction that the difference of successive approximations (9.54b) has the upper bound (9.57a, b):

$$k_m \equiv \sum_{n=1}^{M} k_{m,n}: \qquad \left| y_{m,j}(x) - y_{m,j-1}(x) \right| \le \frac{B(k_m)^{j-1}}{j!} |x - x_0|^j; \tag{9.57a, b}$$

thus the proofs of the theorems of existence (unicity) of solution [subsections 9.1.4–9.1.8 (9.1.9–9.1.10)] is extended to the present case. The same can be said of (9.58a–c) the extension of the proof of robustness of the solution with regard to perturbation in initial conditions:

$$m, n = 1, \ldots, N: \qquad \frac{dY_m}{dx} = f_m(x;Y_n), \qquad Y_m(x_0) = y_{m,o} + \varepsilon_m. \tag{9.58a–d}$$

The uniformity of the solution of the autonomous system with regard to parameter:

$$m, n = 1, \ldots, M: \qquad \frac{dY_m}{dx} = f_m(x;Y_n;\lambda), \qquad y_m(x_0) = y_{m,0}, \tag{9.59a–c}$$

also follows (subsection 9.1.14) from:

$$|\lambda - \lambda_0| \le c: \qquad \left| f_m(x;y_n;\lambda) \right| - f_m(x;y_n;\lambda_0) < k_{m,0} |\lambda - \lambda_0|, \tag{9.60a, b}$$

which is the Lipschitz condition for the parameter analogous to (9.48a, b). The preceding results may be combined in a theorem covering the (i) existence, (ii) unicity, (iii) robustness, and (iv) uniformity of a generalized autonomous system of ordinary differential equations (subsection 9.1.17).

9.1.17 Combined Theorem of Existence, Unicity, Robustness, and Uniformity

The preceding results may be condensed into a **combined theorem of existence, unicity, robustness, and uniformity**: *if the functions (9.50a, b) are: (i) continuous (9.61a) in x in a hyper parallelepiped with upper bound (9.61b):*

$$f(x;y_m)\in C\left(\left|x-x_0\right|\le a;\quad \left|y_m-y_{m,0}\right|\le b_m\right):\qquad \left|f(x;y_m)\right|<B; \tag{9.61a, b}$$

(ii) Lipschitz in a sub-hyper parallelepiped (9.55a–c; 9.56a–d) ≡ (9.62a–f):

$$m,n=1,\dots,M;\qquad \left|x-x_0\right|\le h,\qquad \left|y_n-y_{n,0}\right|\le b_n:$$
$$\left|f_m(x;Y_n)-f_n(x;y_n)\right|<\sum_{n=1}^{M}k_{m,n}\left|Y_n-y_n\right|,\ k_{m,n}>0,\ h=\min\left\{a,\frac{b_m}{B}\right\}. \tag{9.62a–f}$$

Then the generalized autonomous system of differential equations (9.50a, b) with initial conditions (9.50c), or the equivalent system of integral equations (9.53) has (standard CCXI) a unique solution (9.63a) that is continuous in the dependent variable (9.63b):

$$m=1,\dots,M;\qquad y_m(x;y_{m,o})\in C\left(\left|x-x_0\right|\le h\right),\qquad \frac{\partial Y_m}{\partial y_{s,0}}=g_{m,s}(x;y_{s,o}), \tag{9.63a–c}$$

and (standard CCXII) uniformly differentiable (9.63c) with regard to the initial conditions. A perturbation ε_m in the m-th initial condition (9.58d) causes (9.64a) a perturbation in the robust solution not exceeding (9.64b):

$$\left|\zeta_m-x_0\right|<h:\qquad \left|Y_m(x)-y_m(x)\right|=\left|\sum_{n=1}^{M}\varepsilon_n\frac{\partial Y_m}{\partial \zeta_n}\right|\equiv\delta_m<\sum_{s=0}^{M-1}\varepsilon_n\,k_{m,n}. \tag{9.64a, b}$$

If the generalized autonomous system of differential equations involves a parameter λ and the functions f_m are (9.60a, b) Lipschitz in λ, then the solution is (standard CCXIII) uniformly differentiable with regard to the parameter (9.65a):

$$\frac{\partial Y_m(x;\lambda)}{\partial\lambda}=G_m(x;\lambda)\in C\left(\left|x-x_0\right|\le h,\ \left|y_s-y_{s,0}\right|\le b_s,\ \left|\lambda-\lambda_0\right|\le c\right), \tag{9.65a, b}$$

in the region of validity of the results is (9.65b). An ordinary differential equation of order N can be transformed to a generalized autonomous system of N ordinary differential equations, so that the combined theorem of existence, unicity, robustness, and uniformity of solution (subsections 9.1.15–9.1.17) for the latter also applies to the former (subsections 9.1.18–9.1.20).

9.1.18 Ordinary Differential Equation of Any Order

An ordinary differential of order N, explicit in the derivative of highest order (9.66a, b):

$$y^{(N)}(x) \equiv \frac{d^N y}{dx^N} = F\left(x; y(x),\, y'(x),\dots, y^{(N-1)}(x)\right), \qquad (9.66a, b)$$

is equivalent to an autonomous system of N first-order differential equations (9.67a–d):

$$\frac{dy}{dx} = y_1(x), \quad \frac{d^2y}{dx^2} = y_2(x) = y_1'(x),\dots, \frac{d^{N-1}y}{dx^{N-1}} = y_{N-1}(x) = y_{N-2}'(x), \qquad (9.67a–c)$$

$$y^{(N)}(x) = \frac{dy_{N-1}}{dx} = F\left(x; y(x), y_1(x),\dots, y_{N-1}(x)\right). \qquad (9.67d)$$

The same statement (9.66a, b) ≡ (9.67a–d) can be made more compactly as (9.68a–d):

$$s = 0,\dots, N-1: \qquad y^{(N)}(x) = F\left(x; y^{(s)}(x)\right) \Leftrightarrow y_{N-1}' = F\left(x; y_s(x)\right),$$
$$y_s(x) \equiv y^{(s)}(x) = y_{s-1}'(x), \qquad (9.68a–d)$$

and more extensively as (9.69a–d):

$$\frac{dy}{dx} = y_1, \quad \frac{dy_1}{dx} = y_2, \quad \frac{dy_2}{dx} = y_3, \quad \frac{dy_{N-2}}{dx} = y_{N-1}, \quad \frac{dy_{N-1}}{dx} = F\left(x; y, y_1, y_3, \dots y_{N-1}\right). \qquad (9.69a–d)$$

Thus the theorems of existence, unicity, robustness, and uniformity of solution for an autonomous system of differential equations extend to the ordinary differential equation (9.66a, b) of order N provided that the corresponding conditions be met: (i) the initial conditions (9.50c), for (9.67a–c) specify the value of the dependent variable and its first $N-1$ derivatives at a point x_0:

$$y^{(s)}(x_0) = y_{s,o} \equiv \left\{ y(x_0) = y_0, \quad y'(x_0) = y_0', \dots, y^{(N-1)}(x_0) = y_0^{(N-1)} \right\}; \qquad (9.70a, b)$$

(ii) the function in (9.66b) is continuous (9.71a, b) in x in a hyper parallelepiped with center at $\left(x_0, y_0, \ldots, y_0^{(N-1)}\right)$, with upper bound (9.71c):

$$s = 0, \ldots, N-1: \quad F\left(x; y^{(s)}\right) \in C\left(\left|x - x_0\right| < a, \quad \left|y^{(s)}(x) - y_0^{(s)}\right| < b_s\right), \left|F\left(x, y^{(s)}\right)\right| < B; \tag{9.71a–c}$$

(iii) since the functions in (9.67a–c) ≡ (9.68a, c, d) ≡ (9.69a–c) are all Lipschitz, the generalized Lipschitz condition (9.62a–f) applies only to (9.66b) ≡ (9.69d) leading to (9.72e):

$$\left|x - x_0\right| \le h \equiv \min\left\{a, \frac{b_s}{B}\right\}, \qquad \left|y - y_s\right| \le b_s, \quad k_s > 0:$$
$$\left|F\left(x; Y^{(s)}(x)\right) - F\left(x; y^{(s)}(x)\right)\right| < \sum_{s=0}^{N-1} k_s \left|Y^{(s)}(x) - y^{(s)}(x)\right|, \tag{9.72a–e}$$

whose region of validity is (9.72a–c) for the contraction parameter (9.72d). A particularly important sub-case is that of linear ordinary differential equations (subsection 9.1.19).

9.1.19 Linear Ordinary Differential Equation

In the case of a linear differential equation of order N:

$$\sum_{n=1}^{N} A_n(x) \frac{d^n y}{dx^n} = 0, \tag{9.73a}$$

the function F in (9.66b) is (9.73b, c):

$$s = 0, \ldots, N-1: \qquad \frac{d^N y}{dx^N} = F\left(x; y_s\right) = -\sum_{s=1}^{N-1} \frac{A_s(x)}{A_N(x)} y_s(x). \tag{9.73b, c}$$

Since the functions $y_s(x)$ are continuous, otherwise $d^N y/dx^N$ would not exist, the conditions of continuity (9.71a–c) and Lipschitz (9.72a–e) are met if all coefficients in (9.73a) are continuous functions (9.73d):

$$A_0(x), \ldots, A_N(x) \in C\left(x_0 - h \le x \le x_0 + h\right); \qquad \left|x - x_0\right| \le h: \quad A_N(x) \ne 0, \tag{9.73d–f}$$

and the highest order coefficient (9.73f) has no zeros in the same range (9.73e). The condition (9.73f) is not met at a singularity of the differential equation (section 9.5) when (9.73c) fails to determine the highest order derivative.

The same conditions ensure robustness with regard to perturbations in initial conditions:

$$s = 0,\dots,N-1: \qquad \frac{d^n Y}{dx^n} = F\left(x; Y^{(s)}(x)\right), \qquad Y^{(s)}(x_0) = y_o^{(s)} + \varepsilon_s. \tag{9.74a–c}$$

Also the differentiability with regard to a parameter λ in the differential equation:

$$s = 0,\dots,N-1: \qquad \frac{d^n Y}{dx^n} = F\left(x; Y^{(s)}(x); \lambda\right), \qquad Y^{(s)}(x_0) = y_o^{(s)}, \tag{9.74d–f}$$

follows from the Lipschitz condition in λ:

$$|\lambda - \lambda_0| \le c: \qquad \left| F\left(x; Y^{(s)}(x);\ \lambda\right) - F\left(x; Y^{(s)}(x); \lambda_0\right) \right| < k_s |\lambda - \lambda_0|. \tag{9.74g, h}$$

In the case of the parametric linear differential equation (9.75b) of order N in (9.75a):

$$n = 1,\dots,N: \qquad \sum_{n=0}^{N} A_n(x;\lambda) \frac{d^n Y}{dx^n} = 0, \tag{9.75a, b}$$

the Lipschitz condition (9.75d) may be applied with regard to the parameter:

$$s = 0,\dots,N-1: \qquad \left| A_s(x;\lambda) - A_s(x;\lambda_0) \right| < k_s |\lambda - \lambda_0|, \tag{9.75c, d}$$

to all the coefficients in (9.75b) except the last (9.75c). These results may be summarized in a combined existence, unicity, robustness, and uniformity theorem (subsection 9.1.20) for ordinary differential equations of any order, both in the general non-linear (particular linear) cases [subsection 9.1.18 (9.1.19)].

9.1.20 Combined Theorem for an Ordinary Differential Equation

The preceding conclusions are summarized in **the theorem of existence, unicity, stability, and uniformity of solution for an ordinary non-linear (linear) differential equation** *(9.66a, b) [(9.73a)]: if the function is (coefficients are) continuous (9.71a–c) [(9.73d)] in an hyper parallelepiped (9.71a–c) [interval (9.73e)]; and (ii) Lipschitz in a sub-hyper parallelepiped (9.72a–e) [the coefficient of highest order is non-zero (9.73f)], then the ordinary differential equation of order N, non-linear with explicit highest order derivative (9.66a, b) [linear (9.73a)] with initial conditions (9.70a, b) specifying the dependent variable and its derivatives of order up to N – 1 at x_0, has: (i–ii) a unique solution* *[standard CCXIV (CCXVII)] that has continuous N-th derivative in a neighborhood of x_0 in (9.76a):*

$$y\left(x;y_0,\dots,y_0^{(N-1)}\right)\in C^N\left(|x-x_0|\le h\right);\quad \frac{\partial y}{\partial y_{0,m}}=g_m\left(x;y,\dots,y^{(N-1)}\right),$$
$$\frac{\partial y}{\partial\lambda}=h\left(x;y,\dots,y^{(N-1)}\right), \tag{9.76a–c}$$

(iii) the solution is [standard CCXV (CCXVIII)] robust (9.76b) with regard to a perturbation of the initial conditions (9.74a–c); and (iv) the solution is uniform, that is differentiable [standard CCXVI (CCXIX)] with regard to a parameter (9.76c) assuming that the Lipschitz condition (9.74g, h) [(9.75c, d)] is met. In the case of the linear ordinary differential equation (9.73a) at a point x_* where the coefficient of the highest-order derivative would vanish $A_N(x_*)=0$, the derivative of order N would be (9.73b, c) infinite if all of the other coefficients did not vanish or possibly indeterminate if some did vanish; in either case the highest order derivative could not be determined and the point would be a singularity of the differential equation (sections 9.4–9.7). Before addressing singular ordinary differential equations (sections 9.5–9.9) some additional general properties are considered (sections 9.1–9.3), with the stability of autonomous systems next (section 9.2).

9.2 Autonomous Systems and Stability of Equilibria (Lyapunov 1954)

Another important property of differential equations is stability of an equilibrium point, that is a point where all derivatives vanish and the system is at rest. The equilibrium will be (subsection 9.2.1) stable if for any small perturbation the system returns to the equilibrium position; it is indifferent it neither returns to the equilibrium nor moves more away from it; it is unstable if for some perturbations it may move away from the equilibrium. The stability/indifference/instability is asymptotic if it is established after an infinite time. The stability of equilibria can be determined from the solution of the differential equation, if it is available; if not, a first integral like the energy may be sufficient to establish stability (subsection 9.2.2). An extension of the concept of energy is that of a Lyapunov or stability function that, if it exists, can specify the stability of an equilibrium position without solving the differential equation (subsection 9.2.3). A suitable choice of Lyapunov function can be used to prove the stability or otherwise of certain classes of differential equations such as: (i/ii) linear equations with bounded (subsections 9.2.11–9.2.14) or periodic (section 9.3) coefficients; (iii–iv) autonomous systems (subsections 9.2.4–9.2.10 and 9.2.15–9.2.21). The stability results relate to some approximate solutions of differential equations (note 5.10); for example, near a turning point (note 5.11) where the solution changes between oscillatory and monotonic (note 5.12).

The first Lyapunov theorem (subsections 9.2.6–9.2.7) applies to an autonomous system with an equilibrium point where all the derivatives in the differential equation vanish and the stability is determined by the solution in its neighborhood. The stability (instability) implies (subsection 9.2.1) that all paths remain (some paths do not remain) close to the equilibrium point. The stability of an equilibrium point follows from the potential, if it exists (subsection 9.2.2). A more general approach is to use a Lyapunov function (subsection 9.2.4) whose derivative along the differential system (subsection 9.2.3) can specify stability or instability (subsection 9.2.5); an example is a damped oscillator for which the resilience and friction coefficients are not constant and depend [subsection 9.2.8 (9.2.9)] on position (time). An important special case of oscillator with coefficients dependent on time is parametric resonance (subsection 9.2.10).

The asymptotic stability of an autonomous system (subsections 9.2.1–9.2.10) corresponds to solutions which decay to zero at infinity. This is one case of asymptotic behavior of the solution of a differential equation. For an equation or simultaneous system that is linear and has constant coefficients the solutions cannot grow or decay faster than an exponential at infinity (subsection 9.2.11). There is a broadly similar extension to linear equations (simultaneous systems) with bounded non-constant coefficients [subsection 9.2.14 (9.2.13)]. This second theorem of Lyapunov is proved (subsection 9.2.12) using a quadratic stability function and its derivative following the differential system.

The first Lyapunov theorem establishes the stability of an autonomous (and some non-autonomous) differential system provided (subsections 9.2.1–9.2.10) that a suitable stability function can be found. The second Lyapunov theorem (subsections 9.2.11–9.2.14) involves a specific choice of Lyapunov function for a linear differential system with bounded coefficients. The third Lyapunov theorem builds up on the preceding two; using a specific stability function (subsection 9.2.16), which is a positive-definite quadratic form (subsection 9.2.17); inequalities are obtained (subsection 9.2.18) for its time derivative with regard to a non-linear autonomous system (subsection 9.2.19). The latter prove [subsection 9.2.20 (9.2.21)] the asymptotic stability of autonomous differential systems (equations) by showing that it is specified by the linearization (subsection 9.2.15) in the neighborhood of an equilibrium point. The theorem basically states that the stability of a non-linear system near an equilibrium point (chapter 4) is the same as that of the system linearized (chapter 2) in its neighborhood (subsection 9.2.20).

9.2.1 Local/Asymptotic Stability/Instability and Indifference

From a physical point of view there are seven possible cases of an **physical equilibrium** position (Figure 9.4a), depending (standard CCXX) on the evolution with time (Figure 9.4b) illustrated by a one-dimensional system for which: (i) the position is a continuously differentiable function of time (9.77a) with initial position (9.77b) at time $t = 0$; (ii) the velocity is continuous (9.77c) and vanishes (9.77d) at the equilibrium point $x = 0$:

$$x(t)\in C^1(|R), \quad x(0) = x_0: \qquad v(t) \equiv \dot{x}(t) \equiv \frac{dx}{dt} \in C(|R), \quad \dot{x}(0) = 0. \qquad (9.77a\text{–}d)$$

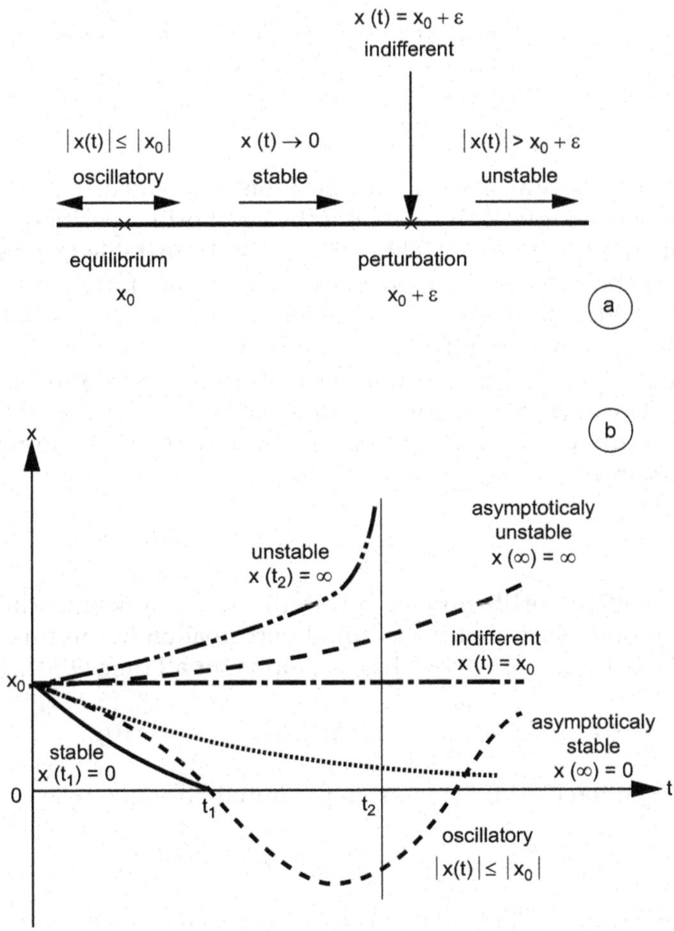

FIGURE 9.4
The (a) stability of an equilibrium position is determined by (b) the temporal evolution after an initial disturbance (Table 9.1).

There are seven cases of **physical equilibrium and stability**:

$$\text{physical stability} \begin{cases} x(t) = x_0: & \textit{indifferent}, & (9.78a) \\ 0 < t_1 < \infty: & x(t_1) = 0 \;\; \textit{stable}, & (9.78b) \\ \lim_{t\to\infty} x(t) = 0: & \textit{asymptotically stable}, & (9.78c) \\ |x(t)| \le x_0,\; x(t) >< 0 & \textit{oscillatory}, & (9.78d) \\ 0 < t_2 < \infty: & |x(t_2)| = \infty: \;\; \textit{unstable}, & (9.78e) \\ \lim_{t\to\infty} |x(t)| = \infty & \textit{asymptotically unstable}, & (9.78f) \\ \lim_{t\to\infty} x(t) = \pm\infty: & \textit{overstable}, & (9.78g) \end{cases}$$

namely: (I) **indifferent** if the initial position is retained over time (9.78a); (II–III) **stable (asymptotically stable)** if the equilibrium position is regained after a finite (infinite) time (9.78b) [(9.78c)]; (V/VI) **unstable (asymptotically unstable)** if the displacement diverges after a finite (infinite) time (9.78e) [(9.78f)]; (IV/VII) **oscillatory (overstable)** if there is an oscillation with bounded (9.78d) [unbounded (9.78g)] amplitude.

There are five cases of **mathematical equilibrium and stability** that apply (standard CCXXI) (Lyapunov) to a simultaneous differential system of first-order first-degree ordinary differential equations (9.79b) with an equilibrium point (9.79c), in vector notation (9.79a):

$$\vec{x} \equiv (x_1, \ldots, x_N): \qquad \dot{\vec{x}} = \vec{F}(\vec{x}, t), \qquad \vec{F}(0,t) = 0. \qquad (9.79a\text{–}c)$$

There is **stable equilibrium** (case I) if: (i) there is a neighborhood of the equilibrium point such that if the initial perturbation lies in this neighborhood (9.80a, b) the system (9.79b) has a solution for all time (9.80c):

$$\exists_{\varepsilon>0}: \qquad |\vec{x}_0| < \varepsilon \Rightarrow 0 \le t < \infty: \qquad \vec{x} = \vec{x}(t; \vec{x}_0), \qquad \vec{x}_0 \equiv \vec{x}(0), \qquad (9.80a\text{–}e)$$

where the solution (9.80d) depends on the initial position (9.80e);

$$I - \textit{stable}: \qquad \forall_{\delta>0}\, \exists_{\varepsilon>0}: \qquad |\vec{x}_0| < \varepsilon \Rightarrow |\vec{x}(t)| < \delta. \qquad (9.80f\text{–}i)$$

(ii) given any ε however small (9.80f) a δ can be found (9.80g) such that if the initial perturbation is a neighborhood of order ε of equilibrium $\vec{x}_0 \in V_\varepsilon(\vec{a})$ in (9.80h) then the solution is in a neighborhood of order δ of equilibrium $\vec{x} \in V_\delta(\vec{a})$ on (9.80i). The remaining four cases of mathematical stability are: (II) **instability** if the displacement increases with time, that is, for every δ

however large (9.81a) there is a ε such that for an initial position within a distance ε of equilibrium (9.81b) the position can be farther than δ after a finite time (9.81a):

$$II-unstable: \qquad \forall_{\delta>0}\ \exists_{\varepsilon>0}: \qquad |\bar{x}_0|<\varepsilon \Rightarrow |\bar{x}(t)|>\delta; \tag{9.81a–c}$$

(III/IV) **asymptotic stability (instability)** if after an infinite time the equilibrium position is regained (9.81d) [the deviation from the equilibrium position is infinite (9.81e)]:

$$III-asymptotically\ stable: \qquad \lim_{t\to\infty}\bar{x}(t)=0; \tag{9.81d}$$

$$IV-asymptotically\ unstable: \ \lim_{t\to\infty}\bar{x}(t)=\infty; \quad V-indifferent: \ \bar{x}(t)=x_0. \tag{9.81e, f}$$

(v) **indifferent** if there is no deviation from the disturbed position (9.81f).

The mathematical definition of stability does not quite coincide with the physical definition of stability in every case (Table 9.1). For example, consider an undamped oscillator (9.82a) ≡ (2.54c) for which the solution (9.82d) ≡ (2.56a) with initial conditions (9.82b, c) satisfies (9.82e):

$$\ddot{x}+\omega^2x=0, \qquad x_0\equiv x(0)\neq 0=\dot{x}_0(0)\equiv\dot{x}_0, \quad x(t)=x_0\cos(\omega t), \quad |x(t)|\le x_0, \ x(t)><0; \tag{9.82a–f}$$

physically this is an oscillatory case (9.82f) because the system never stays again at the equilibrium position $x=0$, even though it crosses it every half-period $\tau/2=\pi/\omega$; mathematically both (9.80a–i) are met with $\varepsilon > x_0 \ge |x(t)| < \delta$, that is, $\delta=\varepsilon$ so the equilibrium position is stable.

TABLE 9.1

Stability of an Equilibrium Position

		Stability	
Case	**Condition**	**Physical**	**Mathematical**
I	$x(t)=x_0$	indifferent	indifferent
II	$x(t_1)=a$	stable	stable
III	$\lim_{t\to\infty}x(t)=a$	asymptotically stable	asymptotically stable
IV	$\lvert x(t)-a\rvert \le \lvert x_0-a\rvert$	oscillatory	stable
V	$x(t_2)=\infty$	unstable	unstable
VI	$\lim_{t\to\infty}x(t)=\infty$	asymptotically unstable	asymptotically unstable
VII	$\lim_{t\to\infty}x(t)=\pm\infty$	overstable	asymptotically unstable

Position; $x(t)$; velocity $\dot{x}(t)$;
initial position: $x(0)=x_0$: equilibrium position $\dot{x}(a)=0$

TABLE 9.2

Stability of Conservative System

Case	Figure	Condition	Potential	Stability
I	9.5a	$\Phi(x) > 0$	positive definite	stable
II	9.5b	$\Phi(x) \geq 0$	positive semi-definite	indifferent
III	9.5c	$\Phi(x) < 0$	negative definite	unstable
IV	9.5d	$\Phi(x) \leq 0$	negative semi-definite	unstable
V	9.5e	$\Phi(x) = 0$	zero	indifferent
VI	9.5f	$\Phi(x) <=> 0$	indefinite	unstable

9.2.2 Positive/Negative Definite/Semi-Definite and Indefinite Function

The following classification (Table 9.2) will be shown shortly to be relevant to the assessment of equilibria:

$$\forall_{\vec{x} \in D}: \qquad \Phi(\vec{x}) \begin{cases} > 0 & \textit{positive definite}, & (9.83a) \\ \geq 0 & \textit{positive semi-definite}, & (9.83b) \\ <> 0 & \textit{indefinite} & (9.83c) \\ \leq 0 & \textit{negative indefinite}, & (9.83d) \\ < 0 & \textit{negative definite}, & (9.83e) \end{cases}$$

namely the classification of a function defined in a domain (standard CCXXII) as: (i/ii) positive (negative) definite if it positive (negative) at all points (9.83a) [(9.83e)]; (iii/iv) positive (negative) semi-definite if it is non-negative (non-positive), that is zero at least one point and positive (negative) at all other points (9.83b) [(9.83d)]; and (v) indefinite if it has no fixed sign, that is, there is at least one point where it is positive and another where it is negative, and it may or may not take zero values. This classification is exhaustive. The definitions of **extended positive (negative) definite** function (standard CCXXIII) apply to a function depending also on other parameters, for example time:

$$0 \leq t < \infty: \quad \Psi(\vec{x},t) \text{ is extended} \begin{cases} \text{positive definite:} & \Psi(\vec{x},t) \geq \Phi(\vec{x}) > 0, & (9.84a) \\ \text{negative definite:} & \Psi(\vec{x},t) \leq \Phi(\vec{x}) < 0, & (9.84b) \end{cases}$$

if it has a lower (upper) bound that is positive (negative) definite (9.84a) [(9.84b)].

Consider a mechanical system (9.85a) under **conservative forces** that are minus the gradient of a potential function (9.85b):

$$m\ddot{\vec{x}} = \vec{F} = -\nabla\Phi \equiv -\frac{\partial\Phi}{\partial\vec{x}}; \qquad 0 = \vec{F}(0) = \nabla\Phi|_{\vec{x}=0}. \qquad (9.85\text{a–d})$$

an equilibrium position (9.85c) corresponds to a zero force, that is a stationary point of the potential and (standard CCXXIV) six cases arise (Figure 9.5a–f): (i) if the equilibrium position is a minimum of the potential (Figure 9.5a) the potential is positive definite in its neighborhood, it is stable mathematically, and stable or oscillatory physically; (ii) if the equilibrium position is a maximum (Figure 9.5c) it is **unconditionally unstable**, that is, unstable for every perturbation, because the potential is negative definite in its neighborhood; (iii/iv) if the potential is positive (negative) semi-definite [Figure 9.5b(d)] the equilibrium is indifferent (unstable); (v) there is also instability, though not unconditional instability, if the potential is indefinite (Figure 9.5f); and (vi) the trivial case of zero potential (Figure 9.5e) corresponds to indifferent equilibrium. In conclusion, *the sign of the potential in the neighborhood of (standard CCXXV) the equilibrium point determines the stability:*

$$\Phi(\vec{x})\begin{cases} >0 & \text{stable:} \quad \text{positive-definite} & (9.86\text{a}) \\ \geq & \text{indifferent:} \quad \text{positive semi-definite} & (9.86\text{b}) \\ \leq, >< & \text{unstable:} \quad \text{negative semi-definite or indefinite.} & (9.86\text{c}) \end{cases}$$

as follows: (i) there is stability for a positive potential (9.86a); (ii) indifference if the potential can be zero but is never negative (9.86b); and (iii) instability if the potential can be negative (9.86c). In the case of a non-conservative system, such as an unsteady or an autonomous differential system (subsection 9.2.3), the potential can be replaced by a stability function (subsection 9.2.4) in order to assess the stability of an equilibrium position.

9.2.3 Derivative along an Unsteady/Autonomous Differential System

The derivative with regard to time of the potential (9.87a, b) equals minus the work per unit time or activity or power (9.87c, d) of the conservative force (9.85b):

$$\frac{d\Phi}{dt} = \frac{\partial\Phi}{\partial\vec{x}}.\frac{d\vec{x}}{dt} = -\vec{F}.\vec{v} = -\frac{F.d\vec{x}}{dt} = -\frac{dW}{dt}. \qquad (9.87\text{a–d})$$

Near a stable equilibrium position the force points toward the equilibrium and it is necessary to overcome the negative work in a displacement.

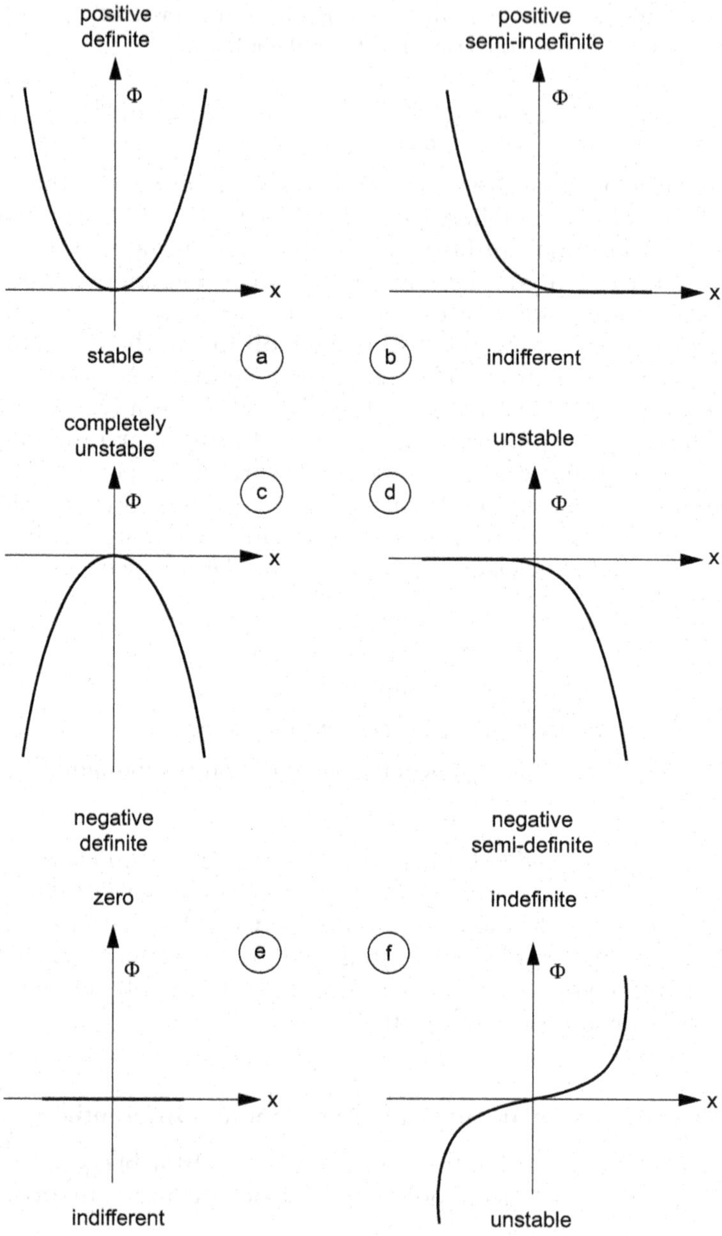

FIGURE 9.5
In the case of a conservative dynamical system, the stability of an equilibrium position (Figure 9.4) is determined (Table 9.2) by the shape of the potential function in the neighborhood of the equilibrium position.

A similar idea is (9.88b) the (standard CCXXVI) **derivative** (9.88b, c) **following an autonomous or steady differential system** (9.88a):

$$\dot{\vec{x}} = \vec{G}(\vec{x}): \qquad \frac{dH}{dt} = \frac{\partial H}{\partial \vec{x}} \cdot \frac{d\vec{x}}{dt} = \vec{G}.\nabla H, \tag{9.88a–c}$$

where the function H could be the potential $H = \Phi$ if it exists; if the potential does not exist, some other **Lyapunov or stability function** could be used instead. A further extension is (standard CCXXVII) a **generalized or unsteady autonomous system** that does depend explicitly on time (9.89a):

$$\dot{\vec{x}} = \vec{F}(\vec{x},t): \qquad \frac{dH}{dt} = \frac{\partial H}{\partial t} + \frac{\partial H}{\partial \vec{x}} \cdot \frac{d\vec{x}}{dt} = \frac{\partial H}{\partial t} + \vec{F}.\nabla H\,; \tag{9.89a–c}$$

the derivative becomes (9.89b, c), adding to (9.88b, c) the partial derivative with regard to time. An intermediate case between a general unsteady (9.89a–c) and an autonomous or steady (9.88a–c) differential system is (standard CCXXVIII) an **asymptotically autonomous system** (9.90a):

$$\dot{\vec{x}} = \vec{F}(\vec{x},t): \qquad \lim_{t\to\infty} \vec{F}(\vec{x},t) = \vec{G}(\vec{x}), \tag{9.90a, b}$$

for which the force tends uniformly to a function independent of time (9.90b).

9.2.4 Lyapunov (1966) Function and First Theorem

The derivative with regard to time of a Lyapunov or stability function H following a differential system has the following geometrical interpretation (Figures 9.6a–c): (i) the stability function is zero (9.91a) at the equilibrium position (9.89b) and positive definite (9.91c) in its neighborhood (9.91a):

$$|\vec{x}| < \varepsilon: \qquad H(0) = 0, \qquad H(\vec{x} \neq 0) > 0; \qquad H(\vec{x}) = c > 0, \tag{9.91a–d}$$

(ii) the equation (9.91d) specifies a surface with at least one element surrounding the equilibrium point; (iii) there may be other elements of the surface that can be excluded by choosing a sufficiently small neighborhood of the equilibrium point; (iv) the normal to the surface has the direction of ∇H and the tangent to the integral curves has the direction of $\dot{\vec{x}}$ leading to three cases:

$$\dot{\vec{x}}.\nabla H \begin{cases} < 0 & \text{for all } \vec{x}\text{:} \quad \textit{stable}, & (9.92a) \\ = 0 & \text{for all } \vec{x}\text{:} \quad \textit{indifferent}, & (9.92b) \\ > 0 & \text{for some } \vec{x}\text{:} \quad \textit{unstable}; & (9.92c) \end{cases}$$

(v) if (9.92a) holds at all points, the paths point inward and the equilibrium is stable (Figure 9.6a); (vi) if (9.92b) holds at all points the paths are tangential (Figure 9.6b) and the equilibrium is indifferent; and (vii) if (9.92c) holds at some points, some paths point outward (Figure 9.6c) and the equilibrium is unstable.

These remarks suggest a stability criterion which generalizes the potential (subsection 9.4.2) and may be stated as the **Lyapunov first theorem**: *consider the autonomous differential system (9.88a) ≡ (9.93b) where $\vec{F}$ has continuous first derivative (9.93c) with an equilibrium position (9.93a), and choose H to be a stability or Lyapunov function that is zero at the equilibrium position (9.93d) and positive definite in its neighborhood (9.93e):*

$$F(\vec{a})=0: \qquad \dot{\vec{x}}=F(\vec{x})\in C^1\left(|R^N\right); \qquad H(\vec{a})=0, \qquad H\left(|\vec{x}-\vec{a}|>0\right)>0; \tag{9.93a–e}$$

then (standard CCXXIX): (i/ii) if at all points in the neighborhood (9.94a, b) the derivative of the Lyapunov or stability function is negative semi-definite (9.94c) [definite (9.94d)] the equilibrium is stable (asymptotically stable):

$$\exists_{\varepsilon>0}: \quad \forall_{|\vec{x}-\vec{a}|<\varepsilon}: \quad \dot{H}\equiv\frac{dH}{dt}=\vec{F}.\nabla H\begin{cases}\le 0: & \textit{stable},\\ <0: & \text{asymptotically stable};\end{cases} \tag{9.94a–d}$$

(iii) if the stability function is positive (negative) at all points (9.95a) and its derivative is positive (negative) at some points (9.95b) there is instability:

$$\forall_{\vec{x}\in D}: \qquad H(\vec{x})>(<)0; \qquad \exists_{\vec{b}\in D}: \qquad \dot{H}\left(\vec{b}\right)>(<)0\Rightarrow \textit{unstable}. \tag{9.95a, b}$$

The stability (i/ii) [instability (iii)] applies (iv) to a generalized or unsteady system (9.89a, b) using the extension of positive (9.84a) [negative (9.84b)] definiteness applicable for all time. The asymptotic stability (ii) applies (v) for a stability function with an infinitesimal upper bound:

$$\forall_{\delta>0} \qquad \exists_{\varepsilon>0}: \qquad \forall_{t>0}: \qquad |\vec{x}|<\varepsilon\Rightarrow\left|H(\vec{x},t)\right|<\delta, \tag{9.96a–e}$$

that is, if given an δ however small there is a ε such that the stability function is (9.96e) less than δ in a neighborhood (9.96d) of order ε of $\vec{a}$ for all time (9.96c).

If the stability function $H\equiv E$ is identified with the energy of a physical system, the interpretation of the first Lyapunov theorem is: (i) if the energy decays with time the system returns to the equilibrium position and is asymptotically stable; (ii) if the energy cannot increase with time, a perturbation the system cannot move further away from the equilibrium position, that is thus stable; and (iii) if for some initial condition the energy increases steadily with time the system moves further away from equilibrium and is

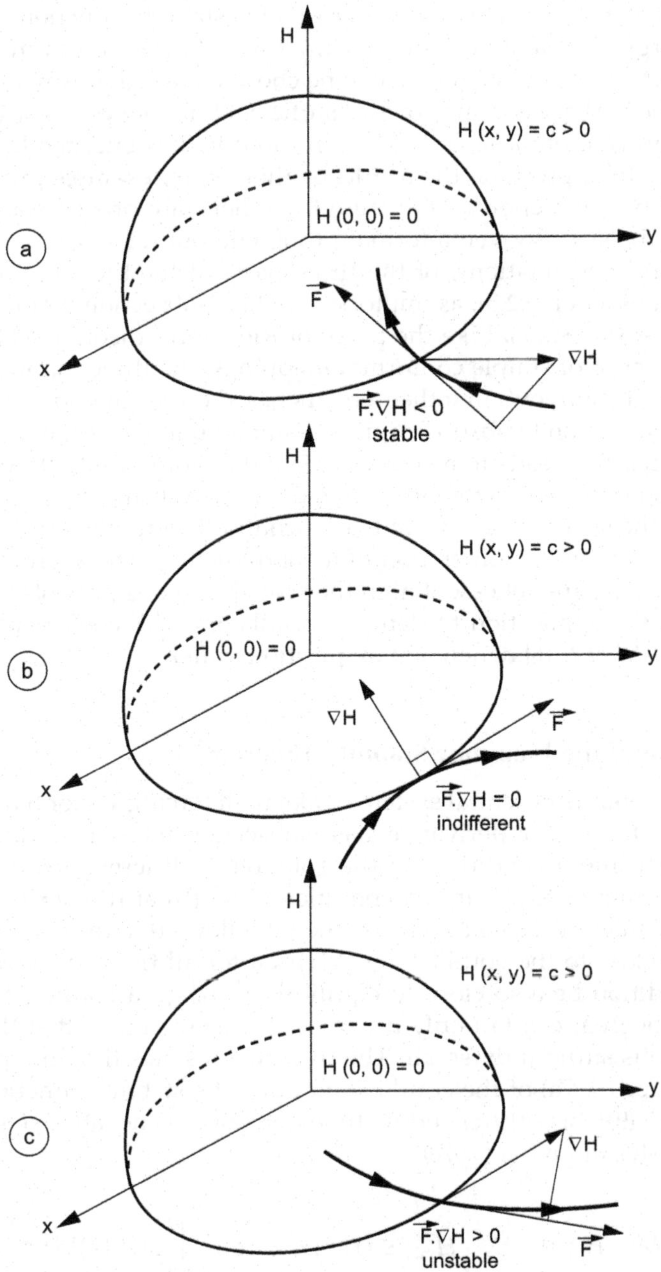

FIGURE 9.6
The stability of an equilibrium position (Figure 9.4) may be considered not only for conservative dynamical systems that have a potential function (Figure 9.5) but also for non-conservative dynamical systems with a Lyapunov stability function with suitable properties similar to those of a potential.

unstable. The theorem applies to any suitable stability function: (i) it could be the energy or potential if it exists; (ii) it might be another function if the energy exists; or (iii) it would have to be chosen in another way if an energy is not defined. The theorem provides sufficient but not necessary conditions for stability, asymptotic stability, and instability; thus one stability function may be able to improve on the results of another, for example prove asymptotic stability (subsection 9.2.6) where the other only proved stability (subsection 9.2.5). Next is given a formal proof, without reference to physical or geometrical interpretations, of the three parts of the theorem; namely, on stability (subsection 9.2.5), asymptotic stability (subsection 9.2.6), and instability (subsection 9.2.7). Like the proof of Riemann's theorem (chapter I.37) on the existence of simple conformal mappings, the three following proofs constituting Lyapunov's first theorem are based on the method of *reductio ad absurdum* (reduction to absurd): (i) it is assumed that the result is false; (ii) it is shown that this leads to a contradiction; therefore (iii) it follows that the result must be true. Thus the proof by reduction to absurd is based on showing that if the stated result is not true, a contradiction follows; thus the key to the proof is the demonstration of a contradiction. These proofs (subsections 9.2.5–9.2.7) are not essential in the sequel, and it is possible to progress directly to the application to damped oscillators with coefficients [subsection 9.2.8 (9.2.9–9.2.10)] dependent on position (time).

9.2.5 Proof of the Lyapunov Stability Theorem

The autonomous differential system (9.93b) with forcing vector having (9.93c) continuous first-order derivative has (subsection 9.1.8) a unique solution $\vec{x}(t;x_0)$ with initial condition $\vec{x}_0$; the solution is differentiable (subsection 9.1.12) with regard to the initial condition $\vec{x}_0 = \vec{x}(0)$ at time $t = 0$ and holds over a time interval $0 \le t \le t_1$. If $t_1 = \infty$ then it follows that the solution will be arbitrarily close to the equilibrium $\left|\vec{x}(t)\right| < \delta$ for all time provided that the initial condition be also close to equilibrium $|\vec{x}_0| < \varepsilon$ according to (9.80f–i). Thus the theorem can fail only if $t_1 < +\infty$. It is shown next that this cannot occur if $|\vec{x}_0|$ is sufficiently small. The hypothesis states that in a punctured neighborhood (9.97a) of the equilibrium point the stability function is positive definite (9.97b) ≡ (9.91c) and its time derivative is negative semi-definite (9.97c) ≡ (9.94c), implying (9.97e):

$$0 < \varepsilon < |\vec{x}| \le M: \quad H > 0 \ge \dot{H}, \quad H_{\min} \le H(\vec{x}) = H(\vec{x}_0) - \int_0^t \dot{H}(\vec{x}(s))ds \le H(\vec{x}_0). \tag{9.97a–e}$$

Since the stability function $H(\vec{x})$ is continuous in the annulus (9.97a) it must have a minimum in (9.97d). Also, since the stability function vanishes at the origin (9.91b) and is positive elsewhere (9.93e) there exists (9.98a) a positive ε such that if $\vec{x}_0$ is in a neighborhood of order ε of $\vec{a}$ then $H(\vec{x}_0)$ does not exceed H_{min}:

$$\exists_{\varepsilon>0}: \qquad |\vec{x}_0 - \vec{a}| < \delta \Rightarrow |H(\vec{x}_0)| < H_{min}, \quad H_{min} > |H(\vec{x}_0)| \geq H_{min}. \qquad (9.98a\text{–}d)$$

If $t_1 < \infty$ then both of (9.97e) and (9.98c) must hold, leading to a contradiction (9.98d). The only way to avoid the contradiction is to set $t_1 = \infty$, in which case the theorem is proved. QED.

9.2.6 Proof of the Theorem on Asymptotic Stability

The hypotheses of the theorem on asymptotic stability are the same (9.93a–e) as for stability, except that $\dot{H} \leq 0$ in (9.94c) is tightened to $\dot{H} < 0$ in (9.94d). Thus the preceding proof holds and the autonomous system (9.93b) has a solution (9.99b) valid for all time (9.99b) implying that the limit (9.99c) exists:

$$0 < t < \infty: \qquad \vec{x} = \vec{x}(t;\vec{x}_0) \Rightarrow \lim_{t\to\infty} H(\vec{x}(t;\vec{x}_0)) = b = 0. \qquad (9.99a\text{–}d)$$

It remains to prove that the limit is zero (9.99d); for example, by showing that if it is not zero, then a contraction follows. Assume then that the limit (9.99c) is not zero (9.100a), implying (9.100b–d):

$$b \neq 0: \qquad \exists_{\eta>0}: \qquad 0 < t < \infty \Rightarrow H(\vec{x}(t;\vec{x}_0)) > \eta. \qquad (9.100a\text{–}d)$$

However, as before (9.98a–c), given η there is a $\varepsilon > 0$ such that if $\vec{x}$ is (9.101b) in a neighborhood (9.101a) of order ε of $\vec{a}$ then H cannot (9.101c) exceed η:

$$\exists_{\delta>0}: \qquad |\vec{x}| < \varepsilon \Rightarrow |H(\vec{x})| < \eta; \qquad t > 0 \Rightarrow |\vec{x} - \vec{a}| > \varepsilon, \qquad (9.101a\text{–}e)$$

comparing (9.101c) with (9.100b) it follows that the latter can hold only for solutions such that (9.101d, e) hold. Since the solution $\vec{x}(t;\vec{x}_0)$ exists in the annulus (9.97a), and the hypothesis on $\vec{F}$ and H imply that $\dot{H}$ in (9.94d) is continuous negative definite, so $-\dot{H}$ has positive minimum (9.102a):

$$0 < -\dot{H}_{min} = \min_{\varepsilon<|\vec{x}|\leq r} \dot{H}(\vec{x}); \qquad H(\vec{x}) = \dot{H}(\vec{x}_0) - \int_0^t \dot{H}(\vec{x}(s))ds \leq H(\vec{x}_0) - \dot{H}_{min}\, t, \qquad (9.102a\text{–}c)$$

this implies (9.102b) so that $H < 0$ for a (9.102c) sufficiently long time. This contradicts the assumption (9.93e), so (9.100a) cannot be true, implying (9.99d) that is asymptotic stability. QED.

9.2.7 Proof of the Theorem on Instability

To complete the proof of Lyapunov first theorem there remains only the case (iii) of instability. Consider the case when stability function is positive definite (9.95a) for all $\vec{x}$, and for some $\vec{b}$ has positive derivative (9.95b); a similar proof can be made in the opposite case $H(\vec{x})<0$ and $\dot{H}(\vec{b})<0$ replacing H by $-H$. The condition (9.103b) implies (9.103c):

$$0<\left|\vec{x}-\vec{b}\right|<\varepsilon: \qquad \dot{H}>0 \Rightarrow H(\vec{x}_0)\equiv H(\vec{x}(0)) = H(\vec{x}(t)) - \int_0^t \dot{H}(\vec{x}(s))ds < H(\vec{x}(t)) \le M < \infty, \tag{9.103a–d}$$

where H has (9.103d) an upper bound M, valid for all $\vec{x}$ in a neighborhood (9.103a) of $\vec{b}$. By hypothesis (9.95a) holds (9.104a):

$$H(\vec{b})>0: \qquad \exists_{\varepsilon>0}: \qquad |\vec{x}-\vec{a}|<\varepsilon \Rightarrow H(\vec{x})<H(\vec{b}), \tag{9.104a–d}$$

implying (9.104d), that is there is a neighborhood of order ε of the equilibrium point for which H does not exceed the value $H(\vec{b})$. The conditions of the theorem of existence and unicity (subsection 9.1.8) apply to $\vec{x}(t;\vec{b})$ and the solution (9.105b) with initial value (9.105c) holds for some time interval (9.105a):

$$0\le t<t_1: \qquad x=\vec{x}(t;\vec{b}), \qquad \vec{x}(0)=\vec{b}; \qquad H(\vec{x}(t;\vec{b}))>H(\vec{b})>0, \tag{9.105a–d}$$

also, (9.103d) implies (9.105d). Since (9.105d) contradicts (9.104d) it can hold only if (9.106b) is valid in the time span (9.105a) ≡ (9.106a):

$$0\le t<t_1: \qquad \left|\vec{x}(t;\vec{b})-\vec{a}\right|>\varepsilon; \qquad 0<\dot{H}_{\min}\equiv \min_{\left|\vec{x}-\vec{b}\right|<\varepsilon} \dot{H}(\vec{x}), \tag{9.106a–c}$$

since $\dot{H}$ is positive definite in (9.95b) the neighborhood of $\vec{b}$ it has a minimum (9.106c). The latter (9.103c) implies (9.107a):

$$H(\vec{x}(t;\vec{c}))>H(\vec{a})+\dot{H}_{\min}\,t>M \quad \text{if} \quad t>t_2 \Rightarrow x(t_2,\vec{c})>\varepsilon, \tag{9.107a–c}$$

that violates (9.103d) after a sufficiently long time; this means that the solution (9.105b, c) must reach the boundary (9.107c) in a finite time (9.107b) and will stay outside for all subsequent time. Thus the system is unstable. QED.

Having completed the proof (subsections 9.2.5–9.2.7) of the Lyapunov first theorem (subsection 9.2.4) it is applied next to a damped oscillator (sections 2.2–2.5) whose resilience and friction coefficients [subsection (9.2.9) 9.2.8] depend on (time) position including the case of parametric resonance (subsection 9.2.10). Although an explicit solution is not available, the conditions for stability can be established using the Lyapunov first theorem with a suitable stability function; in this case the stability function is chosen to be the total energy, that is the sum of the kinetic and potential energies.

9.2.8 Damped Oscillator with Parameters Dependent in Position

The unforced damped harmonic oscillator (2.15) ≡ (9.108a) has been considered (sections 2.1–2.4) with constant mass m, friction coefficient μ, and spring resilience k:

$$m\ddot{x}+\mu\dot{x}+kx=0: \qquad \mu\begin{cases} >0: & \textit{decay}, \\ <0: & \textit{amplification}; \end{cases} \qquad k\begin{cases} >0: & \text{oscillatory}, \\ <0: & \text{monotonic}. \end{cases} \tag{9.108a–c}$$

showing that: (i) positive (negative) friction (9.108b) leads to decay (amplification) because the linear friction force (2.8c) opposes (favors) the motion; and (ii) a positive (negative) resilience (9.108c) leads to an oscillatory (monotonic) motion because the restoring force (2.5c) acts as an attractor toward (repeller away from) the origin. Next are considered the extensions [subsections 9.2.7 (9.2.8)] of the unforced damped harmonic oscillator (9.108a) still with constant mass, but with friction coefficient and spring resilience a function of position (9.109a) [time (9.109b)]:

$$m\ddot{x}+\mu(x)\dot{x}+k(x)x=0, \qquad m\ddot{x}+\mu(t)\dot{x}+k(t)x=0. \tag{9.109a, b}$$

Although the general integral is not known for either of the differential equations (9.109a, b) the stability can be established by using the total energy as the Lyapunov stability function.

The friction coefficient (spring resilience) being a function of position imply that the friction (2.8c) ≡ (9.110a) [restoring (2.5c) ≡ (9.110b)] force remains a linear (becomes a non-linear) function of velocity (position):

$$h(x,\dot{x})=-\mu(x)\dot{x}, \quad j(x)=-k(x)\,x; \quad \Phi(x)=-\int^x j(\xi)d\xi=\int^x k(\xi)\xi d\xi, \tag{9.110a–d}$$

the potential of the restoring force (9.110c) is thus given by (9.110d). The unforced damped harmonic oscillator with friction coefficient and spring resilience a function of position (9.109a) is equivalent to the autonomous system:

$$\dot{x}=v, \qquad m\dot{v}=-\mu(x)\,v-k(x)\,x; \qquad E_t-\Phi(x)=\frac{1}{2}m\dot{x}^2=E_v, \tag{9.111a–d}$$

the total energy (9.111c) is the sum of the potential (9.110d) and kinetic (9.111d) energies. Thus the total energy (9.111c, d; 9.110d) is given by (9.112a):

$$E_t = \frac{1}{2} m \dot{x}^2 + \int^x k(\xi)\, \xi \, d\xi = \frac{1}{2} m v^2 + \int^x k(\xi) \xi d\xi \equiv H(x, v), \qquad \text{(9.112a–c)}$$

and is chosen (9.112b) as the stability function (9.112c); the stability function (9.112c) depends on the position and on the velocity but not on time, because the differential system (9.111a, b) is steady or autonomous, since the coefficients do not depend on time.

The derivative of the stability function (9.112c) along the autonomous differential system (9.111a, b) is given by (9.113a–c):

$$\dot{H} \equiv \frac{dH}{dt} = \frac{\partial H}{\partial x}\frac{dx}{dt} + \frac{\partial H}{\partial v}\frac{dv}{dt} = k\, x\, v + m v \left(\frac{-\mu\, v - k\, x}{m} \right) = -\mu\, v^2 = -h(\dot{x})\, \dot{x} = -\Psi, \qquad \text{(9.113a–f)}$$

and equals minus the dissipation function (9.113f) ≡ (2.8b) that coincides with the activity (9.113d) or work or power per unit time (9.113e) of the friction force (9.110a). Applying the first Lyapunov stability theorem (9.93a–e; 9.94a–d) it follows that *the unforced damped harmonic oscillator (9.109a) with constant mass and friction coefficient (9.110a) [spring resilience (9.110b)] a function of position is stable (standard CCXXX) if: (i) the friction coefficient is positive (9.114b) so that the stability function (9.112c) has negative (9.114a) derivative (9.113d); and (ii) the spring resilience is positive (9.114d) so that the stability function (9.112c) is positive definite (9.114c):*

$$\dot{H} < 0 \quad \Rightarrow \quad \mu(x) > 0; \qquad H > 0 \quad \Rightarrow \quad k(x) > 0. \qquad \text{(9.114a–d)}$$

Failure of at least one of the conditions (9.114d) [(9.114b)] leads to instability due to the repulsive force (9.108c) [amplification (9.108b)]. It is expected that the oscillator (9.109a) is asymptotically stable for positive friction $\mu > 0$ and any initial position or velocity; using the energy (9.113a–c) as Lyapunov function proves asymptotic stability for $v \neq 0$ but fails to prove more than stability for $v = 0$. In order to prove asymptotic stability also for $v = 0$, a stability function "improving" on the energy must be used (see Example 10.19). The unforced undamped harmonic oscillator with friction coefficient and spring resilience a function of position (9.109a) [time (9.109b)] leads to a steady or autonomous (unsteady or general) differential system [subsection 9.2.8 (9.2.9)] so the stability conditions may not coincide.

9.2.9 Damped Oscillator with Parameters Depending on Time

The unforced damped oscillator (9.109b) with friction coefficient and linear spring with resilience dependent in time leads to friction (9.115a) [restoring (9.115b)] force that is a linear function of velocity (position):

$$h(\dot{x}, t) = -\mu(t)\, \dot{x}, \qquad j(x, t) = -k(t)\, x; \quad \dot{x} = v, \quad m\dot{v} = -\mu(t)\, v - k(t) x, \qquad \text{(9.115a–d)}$$

since the coefficients depend on time the equivalent differential system (9.115c, d) is unsteady. The restoring force, a linear function of position (9.115b) ≡ (2.5c) leads to a potential (2.5b) that is a quadratic function of position; it adds to the kinetic energy (9.111d) that is a quadratic function of velocity, in the total energy (9.116a):

$$E_t = \frac{1}{2}k(t)x^2 + \frac{1}{2}m\dot{x}^2 = \frac{1}{2}k(t)x^2 + \frac{1}{2}mv^2 = H(x,v,t). \qquad (9.116a, b)$$

The total energy is chosen as the stability function (9.116b) that depends on the position, velocity, and time.

The time derivative of the stability function (9.116b) along the unsteady differential system (9.115c, d) is given by (9.117a–c):

$$\dot{H} \equiv \frac{dH}{dt} = \frac{\partial H}{\partial t} + \frac{\partial H}{\partial x}\frac{dx}{dt} + \frac{\partial H}{\partial v}\frac{dv}{dt} = \frac{x^2}{2}\frac{dk}{dt} + kxv + mv\left(\frac{-\mu v - kx}{m}\right)$$
$$= -\mu v^2 + \frac{x^2}{2}\frac{dk}{dt} = -\Psi + \frac{x^2}{2}\frac{dk}{dt}, \qquad (9.117a–d)$$

adds to minus the dissipation function (9.113e, f) a term that is also negative if the spring resilience decays with time $dk/dt < 0$. Applying the first Lyapunov theorem (9.93a–e; 9.94a–d) it follows hat *the unforced undamped harmonic oscillator (9.109b) with constant mass and friction coefficient (spring resilience) a function of time (9.115a) [(9.115b)] is stable (standard CCXXXI) if: (i) the friction coefficient is positive (9.118b) so that there is dissipation (9.118a); (ii) the spring resilience is positive (9.118d) so that the stability function (9.116b) is positive definite (9.118c); and (iii) the spring resilience must decay with time (9.118f) so that the time derivative (9.117c) of the stability function (9.116b) is negative (9.118e):*

$$\Psi > 0 \Rightarrow \mu(t) > 0, \qquad H > 0 \Rightarrow k(t) > 0, \qquad \dot{H} < 0 \Rightarrow \frac{dk}{dt} < 0. \qquad (9.118a–f)$$

Violation of any of the three conditions (9.118b, d, f) can lead to instability. The comparison of the unforced damped harmonic oscillators with friction coefficient and spring resilience a function of position (9.114a–d) [time (9.118a–f)] shows that two conditions coincide (9.114b, d) ≡ (9.118b, d), but the latter unsteady case introduces a third condition (9.118f), that can be illustrated (subsection 9.4.10) by the case of parametric resonance (section 4.3).

9.2.10 Stability of Undamped Oscillator with Parametric Resonance

As an example of the condition (9.118f) (subsection 9.2.9) consider the parametric resonance (section 4.3) of an undamped harmonic oscillator, for which the equation of motion (4.88) ≡ (9.119a) involves a time dependent resilience (9.119b):

$$m\ddot{x} + k(t)x = 0, \qquad k(t) = \omega_0^2 m\left[1 + 2h\cos(\omega_e t)\right], \tag{9.119a, b}$$

specified by the natural frequency ω_0, and the excitation frequency ω_e and amplitude h. The excitation amplitude is small (9.120a), so the resilience is positive (9.120b) and the potential energy (2.5b) is positive definite as well as (9.111d) the total energy (9.120):

$$2h < 1 \quad \Rightarrow \quad k(t) > 0, \qquad \Phi = \frac{k(t)}{2}x^2 > 0, \qquad E_t \equiv H > 0, \tag{9.120a–d}$$

so the stability condition (9.118c, d) is met. However (9.119b) implies (9.121):

$$\frac{dk}{dt} = -2m\omega_0^2 h\omega_e \sin(\omega_e t) >< 0, \tag{9.121}$$

that the time derivative of the resilience of the spring does not have fixed sign. This confirms that *standard (CCXXXII) parametric resonance is unstable (section 4.3) since the oscillating support can feed energy into the mass spring system* (Figure 4.4). Thus the qualitative stability theory based on the Lyapunov first theorem confirms (subsections 9.2.1–9.2.10) the instability of parametric resonance demonstrated before (section 4.3) by two other methods: (i) exact solution of the Mathieu equation (subsections 4.3.1–4.3.19); (ii) approximate solutions in terms of elementary functions (subsections 4.3.11–4.3.20). The time derivative of the resilience has no fixed sign (9.121) and the same applies to the differential equation for the harmonic oscillator with parametric resonance (9.119a) has coefficients that are periodic functions of time (9.119b) so that the Floquet and fourth Lyapunov theorem apply (section 9.3). The coefficients are also bounded functions of time and thus the second (third) Lyapunov theorems [subsections 9.2.11–9.2.14 (9.2.15–9.2.20)] also apply.

9.2.11 Exponential Asymptotic Growth or Decay

Considering a single (simultaneous system of) ordinary differential equation(s) linear with constant coefficients (1.54) ≡ (9.122a) [(7.50) ≡ (9.123a)] for which the degree of the characteristic polynomial (1.52b) ≡ (9.122b) [(7.58c) ≡ (9.123b)] specifies the order N of the system:

$$\sum_{n=0}^{N} A_n \frac{dy^n}{dx^n} = 0: \qquad 0 = P_N(a) = \sum_{n=0}^{N} A_n a^n; \tag{9.122a, b}$$

$$\sum_{n=0}^{N} P_{nm}\left(\frac{d}{dx}\right) y_m(x) = 0: \qquad P_N(a) = Det\{P_{nm}(a)\}. \tag{9.123a, b}$$

The characteristic polynomial (7.71a, b) in both cases has roots (9.124a), whose multiplicities (9.124b) must add (9.124c) to N:

$$I \le s \le S: \qquad P_N(a) = A\prod_{s=1}^{S}(a-a_s)^{\alpha_s}, \qquad \sum_{s=1}^{S}\alpha_s = N. \tag{9.124a–c}$$

To each root or eigenvalue a_s corresponds (7.71c, d) a number of linearly independent normal integrals (9.125b) equal to the multiplicity (9.125a):

$$\beta_s = 0,\dots,\quad \alpha_s - 1: \qquad q_{s,\beta_s}(x) = x^{\beta_s - 1}\exp(a_s x). \tag{9.125a, b}$$

In the case of single roots, $\alpha_s = 1$ in (9.124b) and $\beta_s = 0$ in (9.125a) and the solution (9.125b) is an exponential (7.64a–d). In the case of multiple roots $\alpha_s \ge 2$ in (9.124b), two real numbers $(\underline{b}, \bar{b})$ can be chosen so that the real part of the eigenvalue lies between them (9.126a) and all normal integrals (9.125b) lie asymptotically in modulus between the corresponding exponentials (9.126b, c):

$$\bar{b} > \mathrm{Re}(a_s) > \underline{b}: \qquad \lim_{x\to\infty} e^{-\bar{b}x}\left|q_{s,\beta_s}(x)\right| = \lim_{x\to\infty} x^{\beta_s}\exp\left\{\left[\mathrm{Re}(a_s) - \bar{b}\right]x\right\} = 0, \tag{9.126a, b}$$

$$\lim_{x\to\infty} e^{-\underline{b}x}\left|q_{s,\bar{b}_s}(x)\right| = \lim_{x\to\infty} x^{\beta_s}\exp\left\{\left[\mathrm{Re}(a_s) - \underline{b}\right]x\right\} = \infty. \tag{9.126c}$$

Thus is proved the theorem: *consider (standard CCXXXIII) a single (simultaneous system of) ordinary differential equation(s) linear with constant coefficients (9.122a) [(9.123a)] with characteristic polynomial (9.122b) [(9.123b)] whose roots are the eigenvalues a_s in (9.124a–c); for any two real numbers such that the real parts of all eigenvalues (9.127a) lie between them (9.127b) the asymptotic solution in modulus lies (Figure 9.7) between the corresponding exponentials (9.127c, d):*

$$s = 1,\dots,S: \qquad \bar{b} > \mathrm{Re}(a_s) > \underline{b} \Rightarrow \lim_{x\to\infty} e^{-\bar{b}x} y(x) = 0, \quad \lim_{x\to\infty} e^{-\underline{b}x} y(x) = \infty. \tag{9.127a–d}$$

A broadly similar theorem is proved next for non-uniform bounded coefficients.

9.2.12 Proof of the Second Lyapunov Theorem (1892)

Any system of simultaneous ordinary differential equations can be reduced (subsection 7.1.2) to a system of first-order equations (9.128a, b):

$$m, n = 1,\dots,M: \quad \sum_{m=1}^{M} A_{nm}(x) y_m(x) = \frac{dy_n}{dx} \equiv y_n'(x), \quad A_{nm}(x) \in \mathcal{B}(|R), \tag{9.128a–d}$$

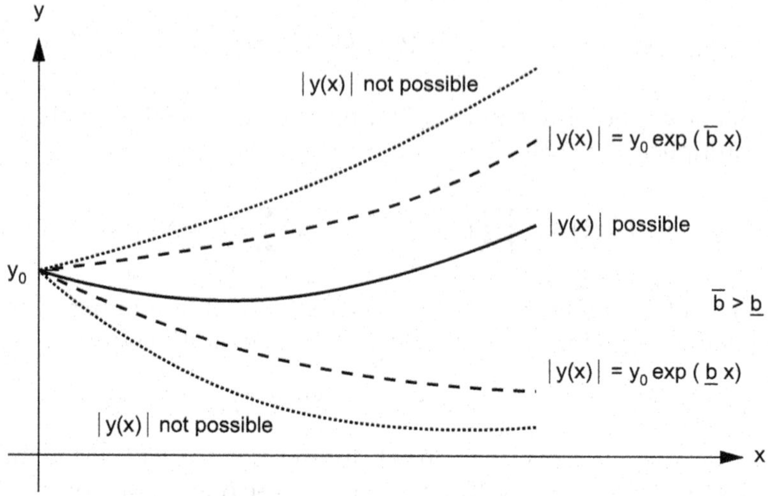

FIGURE 9.7
The asymptotic solutions for large independent variable of a linear differential equation with bounded variable coefficients must lie between two exponentials.

for example linear (9.128c) with non-uniform bounded coefficients (9.128d). The stability function (9.123b) that is a sum of squares multiplied by a real exponential (9.129a, c) is positive definite:

$$a \in \mathbb{R}: \qquad H(y_n;x) = \frac{e^{-2ax}}{2}\sum_{n=1}^{N}\left[y_n(x)\right]^2 = \frac{1}{2}\sum_{n=1}^{N}\left[e^{-ax}\,y_n(x)\right]^2 > 0; \qquad (9.129\text{a, b})$$

the derivative of the stability function (9.129b) following the differential system (9.128a, b), is specified by:

$$H' = \frac{dH}{dx} = \frac{\partial H}{\partial x} + \sum_{n=1}^{N}\frac{\partial H}{\partial y_n}\frac{dy_n}{dx} = e^{-2ax}\left[-a\sum_{n=1}^{N} y_n^2 + \sum_{n=1}^{N} y_n'\,y_n\right]$$
$$= e^{-2ax}\sum_{m,nn=1}^{N}\left(A_{nm} - a\delta_{nm}\right)y_n y_m, \qquad (9.130\text{a–d})$$

where δ_{nm} is the identity matrix. If a is chosen to be a large enough positive number (9.131a, b) then (9.130d) is negative (9.131c), and the positive definite stability function (9.129b) must decay asymptotically to zero (9.131d):

$$\exists_{\bar{b}>0}: \qquad 0 < a > \bar{b} \Rightarrow H' < 0, \quad \lim_{x\to\infty} H(x) = 0; \qquad \forall_{1\le m\le M}: \ \lim_{x\to\infty} y_m(x)\,e^{-ax} = 0, \qquad (9.131\text{a–e})$$

it follows that every function y_n in the sum (9.129b) is dominated by the exponential (9.131e). If a is chosen to be a negative number large enough in modulus (9.132a, b), then (9.130d) is positive (9.132c) and the stability function (9.129b) diverges at infinity (9.132d):

$$\exists_{\underline{b}<0}: \quad 0 > a < \underline{b} \Rightarrow H' > 0; \quad \lim_{x\to\infty} H(x) = \infty; \quad \exists_{1\le m\le M}: \quad \lim_{x\to\infty} e^{-ax}\, y_m(x) = \infty, \tag{9.132a–e}$$

it follows from (9.132d) and (9.129b) that at least one y_m dominates asymptotically the exponential (9.132e). The results (9.131e; 9.132e) contain the second Lyapunov theorem that: (i) generalizes the preceding theorem (subsection 9.2.11) from constant to bounded coefficients in the linear autonomous system of differential equations (9.128a–d); and (ii) is re-stated next (subsection 9.2.13) together with some consequences.

9.2.13 Existence of at Least One Eigenvalue of an Autonomous System

From the preceding proof (subsection 9.2.12) follows the direct form of the **second Lyapunov theorem**: *consider (standard CCXXXIV) a linear autonomous system of differential equations (9.128a–c) with bounded coefficients (9.128d) in Figure 9.7: (i) there is a positive number (9.133a) such that the corresponding exponential dominates all functions asymptotically (9.133b, c):*

$$\exists_{\bar{b}>0}: \qquad \exists_{1\le m\le M}: \qquad \lim_{x\to\infty} e^{-\bar{b}x}\, y_m(x) = 0; \tag{9.133a–c}$$

$$\exists_{\underline{b}<0}: \qquad \exists_{1\le m\le M}: \qquad \lim_{x\to\infty} e^{-\underline{b}x}\, y_m(x) = \infty, \tag{9.134a–e}$$

and (ii) there exists also a negative number (9.134a) such that the corresponding exponential is dominated (9.134b, c) by at least one of the functions.

The system of simultaneous differential equations of first order (9.135a, b) has an **eigenvalue** a if the corresponding exponential for $a+\varepsilon$ $(a-\varepsilon)$ for any ε however small (9.135c) has at least one solution dominated by (9.135d) [which dominates (9.135e)] the exponential:

$$n, m = 1, \dots, M; \quad f_n(y_m) = y_n': \quad \exists_{1\le m\le n}\ \forall_{\varepsilon>0}: \quad \lim_{x\to\infty} y_m(x) \exp\left[-(a+\varepsilon)x\right] = 0,$$

$$\lim_{x\to\infty} y_m(x) \exp\left[-(a-\varepsilon)x\right] = \infty. \tag{9.135a–e}$$

This definition (9.135a–e) together with the second Lyapunov theorem (9.133a–c; 9.134a–c) shows that: *an autonomous system of linear first-order equations with bounded coefficients (9.128a–d) has (standard CCXXXV) at least one*

eigenvalue *or characteristic number (9.135a–e)*. The results (subsections 9.2.11–9.2.13) for linear autonomous systems of differential equations also apply to: (i) general simultaneous systems of differential equations (7.6a–c) because it can be transformed (subsection 7.1.2) to an autonomous system; and (ii) to a linear ordinary differential equation of any order (subsection 9.2.14), because it is a particular case of (i), and is also reducible to an autonomous system.

9.2.14 Linear Differential Equation with Bounded Coefficients

A linear ordinary differential equation (9.129a) of order N with non-uniform coefficients (9.136b, c):

$$\sum_{n=0}^{N} A_n(x)\frac{d^n y}{dx^n} = 0; \qquad n = 0,\dots,N: \qquad A_n(x) \in \mathcal{B}(R), \tag{9.136a, b}$$

is equivalent to a system of N simultaneous linear differential equations (9.131a–d):

$$y_0(x) = y(x), \quad y_1(x) = y'(x) = y_0'(x), \quad y_2(x) = y_1'(x) = y''(x), \dots, \ y_{N-1}(x) = y^{(N-1)}(x), \tag{9.137a–c}$$

$$A_N(x)y_{N-1}'(x) = A_N(x)y^{(N)}(x) = -A_0(x)y(x) - A_1(x)y_1(x) - \dots - A_{N-1}(x)y_{N-1}(x), \tag{9.137d}$$

that can be put in the autonomous form (9.138a–d):

$$y'(x) = y_1(x), \quad y_1'(x) = y_2(x), \dots, y_{N-2}'(x) = y_{N-1}(x), \quad y_{N-1}'(x) = -\sum_{s=0}^{N-1} C_s(x)y_s(x), \tag{9.138a–d}$$

with coefficients (9.139b, d) that are bounded (9.133e):

$$A_N(x) \neq 0: \quad s = 0,\dots,N-1: \quad |C_s(x)| < B, \quad |C_s(x)| = \left|\frac{A_s(x)}{A_N(x)}\right| < \frac{B}{|A_N(x)|}, \tag{9.139a–e}$$

because the (9.139c) are bounded (9.136b, c) excluding (9.139a) singularities of the differential equation.

The conditions (9.133a–e) [(9.134a–c)] for the second Lyapunov theorem apply to show that:

$$\exists_{\bar{b}\in|R}\ \forall_{0\le s\le N-1}: \qquad \lim_{x\to\infty} e^{-\bar{b}x}\, y_s(x) = \lim_{x\to\infty} e^{-\bar{b}x}\, y^{(s)}(x) = 0, \tag{9.140a–c}$$

$$\exists_{\underline{b}\in R}\ \exists_{0\le s\le N-1}: \qquad \lim_{x\to\infty} e^{\bar{b}x}\, y_s(x) = \lim_{x\to\infty} y^{(s)}(x) = \infty, \tag{9.141a–c}$$

thus, *given a linear ordinary differential equation (9.136a) of order N with bounded coefficients (9.136b, c), there exists (standard CCXXXVI) a real number (9.140a) [(9.141a)] such that the solution (9.140b) [(9.141b)] and all derivatives (9.140c) [(9.141c)] up to order N − 1 at a non-singular point (9.139a) are dominated asymptotically by (dominate asymptotically an) the exponential.* This implies, for example:

$$y(x) = e^{ax}, x^a, \exp\left(a\sqrt{x}\right); \quad y(x) = \exp\left(-x^2\right), \exp\left(x^2\right), x^x, \tag{9.142a–f}$$

that (9.142a–c) are [(9.142d–f) are not] possible solutions of a linear ordinary differential equation with bounded coefficients because the possible solutions must lie in modulus between two exponentials (Figure 9.7). The first Lyapunov theorem concerns the stability of non-linear autonomous systems (subsections 9.2.1–9.2.10) and the second the exponential dominance of linear autonomous systems (subsections 9.2.11–9.2.14). Combining the two leads to the third Lyapunov theorem (subsections 9.2.15–9.2.20) stating that the stability of a non-linear autonomous system is dominated by the linear terms.

9.2.15 Linear Autonomous System with Constant Coefficients

A linear autonomous system of differential equations with constant coefficients (9.143a, b) can be eliminated (subsection 7.3.1) for any of the dependent variables leading to a linear differential equation with constant coefficients that has (section 1.3) exponential solutions (9.143c):

$$m, n = 1, \dots, M: \qquad \dot{x}_n = \sum_{m=1}^{M} A_{nm}\, x_m, \qquad x_n(t) = B_n\, e^{at}. \tag{9.143a–c}$$

Substitution of (9.143c) in (9.143b) leads to (9.144a):

$$0 = e^{at} \sum_{m=1}^{M} \left(A_{nm}\, B_m - a\, B_n\right) = x_n(t) \sum_{m=1}^{M} \left(A_{nm}\, B_m - a\, \delta_{mn}\right), \tag{9.144a, b}$$

using the identity matrix (6.305a–d) in (9.144b). A non-trivial solution (9.145a) requires that the determinant of the coefficients vanishes (9.145b):

$$\left\{x_1(t), x_2(t), \ldots, x_M(t)\right\} \neq \left\{0, 0, \ldots, 0\right\}: \qquad 0 = Det\left(A_{mn} - a\,\delta_{mn}\right) = P_M(a), \tag{9.145a–c}$$

thus the exponents a are the eigenvalues (9.145b) of the matrix of coefficients in (9.143b), and are specified by the roots of the characteristic polynomial (9.145c). If all roots are distinct (9.146a) the general integral for any of the dependent variables is a linear combination of exponentials (9.146b):

$$P_M(a) = (-)^N \prod_{m=1}^{M}(a - a_m): \qquad x_n(t) = \sum_{m=1}^{M} C_{nm}\, e^{a_m t}. \tag{9.146a, b}$$

The roots a_s of multiplicity α_s of the characteristic polynomial (9.147a, b) introduce (1.91a–c) power coefficients (9.147c) with exponents up to $\alpha_m - 1$:

$$\sum_{s=1}^{S}\alpha_s = M; \quad P_M(a) = (-)^N \prod_{s=1}^{S}(a - a_s)^{\alpha_s}: \quad x_n(t) = \sum_{s=1}^{S} e^{a_s t} \sum_{\beta=0}^{\alpha_s - 1} t^{\beta}\, C_{n,s,\beta}. \tag{9.147a–c}$$

Thus *the linear autonomous system of differential equations with constant coefficients (9.143a, b) has (standard CCXXXVII) eigenvalues (9.145b) that are the roots of the characteristic polynomial (9.145c). The general integral for each dependent variable is: (i) a linear combination of exponentials (9.146b) if all eigenvalues are distinct (9.146a); and (ii) multiple (9.147a) eigenvalues (9.147b) introduce power factor in the general integral (9.147c). The* N^2 *constant coefficients* $C_{n,m}\left(C_{n,s,\beta}\right)$ *in (9.146b) [(9.147c)] are specified by compatibility and initial conditions.* Bearing in mind that the modulus of an exponential equals the exponential of its real part:

$$\begin{aligned} \left|\exp(at)\right| &= \left|\exp\left\{t\left[\operatorname{Re}(a) + i\operatorname{Im}(a)\right]\right\}\right| \\ &= \left|\exp\left[t\operatorname{Re}(a)\right]\right|\left|\exp\left[it\operatorname{Im}(a)\right]\right| = \exp\left[t\operatorname{Re}(a)\right], \end{aligned} \tag{9.148a–c}$$

the real part of the eigenvalues specifies the stability of the equilibrium point; this extends to non-linear autonomous systems linearized in a neighborhood of an equilibrium point, leading to the third Lyapunov theorem (subsection 9.2.16).

9.2.16 Linearized Differential System Near an Equilibrium Point

Consider a non-linear autonomous differential system (9.149a, b) with forcing vector with continuous second-order derivatives (9.149c) near an equilibrium point (9.149d), chosen to be the origin (this can be ensured by a translation, so there is no loss of generality):

$$m,n,p,q = 1,\ldots,M: \qquad \dot{x}_n = F_n(x_m) \in C^2\left(\left|\vec{x}\right| < \varepsilon\right), \qquad F_n(0) = 0. \tag{9.149a–d}$$

The mean value theorem (section I.23.9) applies to (I.23.44b) the forcing vector to second-order (9.149a–c):

$$\dot{x}_n = \sum_{m=1}^{M} A_{n,m}\, x_m + R_n(x_m): \qquad A_{n,m} = \lim_{x_p \to 0} \frac{\partial F_n}{\partial x_m}, \tag{9.150a, b}$$

$$0 < \theta_p < 1: \qquad R_n(x_m) = \sum_{p,q=1}^{M} x_p\, x_q \left.\frac{\partial^2 F_n}{\partial x_p\, \partial x_q}\right|_{x_p = \theta_p \varepsilon}. \tag{9.150c, d}$$

where: (i) the first term on the r.h.s. of (9.150a) is zero because the origin is an equilibrium point (9.149d); (ii) the first-order term specifies a linear system with constant coefficients in (9.150a) determined by the first-order partial derivatives of the forcing vector evaluated at the equilibrium point (9.150b); and (iii) the remainder (9.150d) consists of second-order partial derivatives of the forcing vector evaluated in the neighborhood (9.150c) of the equilibrium point. By the mathematical definition (subsection 9.2.1) stability concerns only a small neighborhood of the equilibrium point, suggesting that the last term in (9.150a) could be neglected.

This leads to the **third Lyapunov theorem**: *the stability of the autonomous differential system (9.149a, b) with forcing vector having continuous second-order derivatives (9.149c) and an equilibrium point at the origin (9.149d) is (standard CCXXXVIII) the same as that of the linearized system (9.150a) with coefficients determined (9.150b) by the partial derivatives of the forcing vector evaluated at the equilibrium point (9.149d). Thus if the eigenvalues are ordered by non-increasing real part (9.151a):*

$$\operatorname{Re}(a_1) \ge \operatorname{Re}(a_2) \ge \ldots \ge \operatorname{Re}(a_N): \quad \begin{cases} \operatorname{Re}(a_1) < 0: & \textit{stable}, \\ \operatorname{Re}(a_1) > 0: & \textit{unstable}, \\ \operatorname{Re}(a_1) = 0; a_1 \ne a_2: & \textit{indifferent}, \\ \operatorname{Re}(a_1) = 0, a_1 = a_2: & \textit{unstable}, \end{cases} \tag{9.151a–e}$$

it follows from (9.146a, b; 9.147a–c; 9.147a–c; 9.148a–c) that four cases can arise: (i) if the largest real part of an eigenvalue is negative (9.151b) all terms in (9.146b; 9.147c) decay to the equilibrium position that is stable; (ii) if the largest real part of an eigenvalue is positive (9.151c) at least one exponential term in (9.146b; 9.147c) diverges and the equilibrium is unstable; (iii) if the largest real part of an eigenvalue is zero, and that eigenvalue is single (9.151d), then all terms in (9.146b; 9.147c) are exponentially decaying or constant in modulus and the equilibrium is indifferent; or (iv) if the largest real part of an eigenvalues is zero and it is a multiple eigenvalue, then (9.147c) contains decaying exponentials and a polynomial of time at least of degree one and the equilibrium is unstable. In the stable case the solution (9.149a–c) satisfying the initial condition (9.152a) has (standard CCXXXIX) the asymptotic bound (9.152b) with positive coefficients (9.152c, d):

$$\bar{x}_0 = \bar{x}(0): \qquad \left|\bar{x}(t;\bar{x}_0)\right| \le A\left|\bar{x}_0\right| e^{-at}, \qquad a > 0 < A. \tag{9.152a–c}$$

The latter (9.152b–d) corresponds to the exponential growth found before for linear systems with constant (9.126a–c) or non-constant bounded coefficients (9.133a–c) as stated in the second Lyapunov theorem (subsection 9.2.11). These results are proved in the third Lyapunov theorem (subsections 9.2.17–9.2.21).

9.2.17 Fundamental Solution of an Autonomous Differential System

The proof is based on a positive-definite stability function (subsection 9.2.17) with negative-definite derivative along the differential system (subsection 9.2.16), as specified in the part (i) of the first Lyapunov theorem [(9.93a–c; 9.94c) in the subsection 9.2.4]; this leads to inequalities (subsection 9.2.19) similar to those [(9.131a–e; 9.132a–e) in the subsection 9.2.12] in the second Lyapunov theorem which establish the asymptotic behavior as in the second Lyapunov theorem. The asymptotic behavior corresponds to asymptotic stability, instability, or unconditional instability (subsections 9.2.20–9.2.21). The Lyapunov or stability function is defined (9.153a) as the integral over time of the square of the modulus of the solution $\bar{x}(t;\bar{x}_0)$ with initial condition (9.152a):

$$H(\bar{x}_0) \equiv \int_0^\infty \left|\bar{x}(t;x_0)\right|^2 dt > 0; \qquad \dot{H}_0 \equiv \lim_{t\to 0} \frac{dH}{dt} = -\left|\bar{x}_0\right|^2 < 0. \tag{9.153a, b}$$

its time derivative evaluated at initial time $t \to 0$ is (9.153b) negative-definite. It also proves that the Lyapunov function depends (9.153a) only on the initial position (9.152a).

Denote by (9.154a) the set of N **fundamental solutions** of the linear autonomous system (9.143a) satisfying the initial conditions (9.154b) specified by the identity matrix (9.154c):

$$x_n(t): \qquad x_n^{(m)}(0) = \delta_{nm} = \begin{cases} 1 & \text{if} \quad n = m, \\ 0 & \text{if} \quad n \ne m. \end{cases} \tag{9.154a–c}$$

or explicitly (9.155a, b):

$$x_n^{(n)}(0)=1, \quad 0=x_n(0)=\dot{x}_n(0)=....=x_n^{(n-1)}(0)=x_n^{(n+1)}(0)=...=x_n^{(N-1)}(0)=x_n^{(N)}(0). \tag{9.155a, b}$$

The functions (9.154a) are linearly independent as follows from the initial conditions (9.154b, c) ≡ (9.155a, b). Thus the general integral is their linear combination (9.156a):

$$\vec{x}(t;\vec{x}_0)=\sum_{m=0}^{N} C_m\,\vec{x}_m(t), \qquad \vec{x}(0)=\sum_{m=0}^{N} C_m\,\vec{x}_m(0)=\sum_{m=0}^{N} C_m\,\delta_{nm}=C_n. \tag{9.156a–d}$$

with the constants of integration given by (9.156b–d) where (9.154b, c) was used. Substituting (9.156d) in (9.156a) it follows that:

$$\dot{x}_n=\sum_{m=1}^{n} A_{nm}(t)\,x_m: \qquad \vec{x}(t;\vec{x}_0)=\sum_{n=0}^{\infty} x_n(0)\,\vec{x}_n(t), \tag{9.157a, b}$$

the linear autonomous system of differential equations (9.157a) has (standard CCXL) general integral (9.157b) as a linear combination of the fundamental solutions (9.154a–c) with the initial values as coefficients.

The Lyapunov function (9.153a) may be calculated by (9.158a) leading by (9.157b) to (9.158b):

$$H(\vec{x}_0)=\int_0^{\infty}\left[\vec{x}(t;\vec{x}_0).\vec{x}(t;\vec{x}_0)\right]dt=\sum_{m,n=1}^{0} x_m(0)x_n(0)\int_0^t\left(\vec{x}_m(t).\vec{x}_m(t)\right)dt, \tag{9.158a, b}$$

involving (9.158b) ≡ (9.159b) the initial condition with coefficients (9.159a):

$$B_{mn}\equiv\int_0^t\left(\vec{x}_m(t).\vec{x}_n(t)\right)dt: \qquad H(\vec{x}_0)=\sum_{m,n=1}^{N} B_{mn}\,x_m(0)\,x_n(0). \tag{9.159a, b}$$

It follows that the *Lyapunov function (9.153a) is (standard CCXLI) a positive-definite quadratic form (9.159a, b),* and some generic properties are proved next (subsection 9.2.18).

9.2.18 Properties of Positive-Definite Quadratic Forms

The following theorem will be used in the sequel: *given a positive-definite (9.153a) quadratic form (9.159b) there are (standard CCXLII) real positive numbers (9.160a) such that the form lies between (9.160b) their product by the norm of the vectors:*

$$\exists_{\bar{b}>\underline{b}>0}: \qquad \underline{b}\,|\vec{x}_0|^2 \le H(\vec{x}_0) \equiv \sum_{n,m=1}^{M} B_{nm}\, x_{0n}\, x_{0m} \le \bar{b}\,|\vec{x}_0|^2 \equiv \bar{b}\sum_{n=1}^{M}(x_{0n})^2. \qquad (9.160\text{a, b})$$

The proof is made in two steps: (i) if $\vec{c}$ is a unit vector (9.161a), that is, lies on the unit sphere, the positive definite function H specified by the quadratic form (9.161c) must have a maximum (minimum) on the unit sphere (9.161a), hence the values $\bar{b}\,(\underline{b})$ in (9.161b, d):

$$\vec{c}\,.\vec{c} = 1: \qquad \underline{b} \le H(\vec{c}) = \sum_{n,m=1}^{M} B_{nm}\, c_n\, c_m \le \bar{b}; \qquad (9.161\text{a–d})$$

and (ii) if $\vec{x}_0$ is an arbitrary vector it is of the form (9.162b) where λ is a real number (9.162a) implying (9.162c–e):

$$\lambda \in |R,\ \vec{x}_0 = \lambda\vec{c}: \qquad |\vec{x}_0| = \lambda, \quad H(\vec{x}_0) = \lambda^2 H(\vec{c}):$$

$$\underline{b}|\vec{x}_0|^2 = \underline{b}\lambda^2 \le \lambda^2 H(\vec{c}) = H(\vec{x}_0) \le \lambda^2\bar{b} = \bar{b}|\vec{x}_0|^2. \qquad (9.162\text{a–e})$$

where (9.162e) ≡ (9.160b). QED.

A consequence of the theorem (9.160a, b) is (9.163a–c):

$$\left|\frac{\partial H}{\partial x_n}\right| = \left|\frac{\partial H}{\partial \vec{x}}\right| \le 2\bar{b}\,|\vec{x}| < \frac{2\bar{b}}{\sqrt{\underline{b}}}\left|H(\vec{x})\right|^{1/2}, \qquad (9.163\text{a–c})$$

implying (9.163c) ≡ (9.164b, c) for (9.164a):

$$b \equiv \frac{2\bar{b}}{\sqrt{\underline{b}}}: \qquad \exists_{b>0}:\ |\nabla H| < b\left|H(\vec{x})\right|^{1/2}, \qquad (9.164\text{a–c})$$

thus *given a positive-definite (9.153a) quadratic form (9.159b), its partial derivatives (standard CCXLIII) form a vector whose modulus does not exceed (9.164c) where (9.164b) is a positive real number.* The properties (9.160a, b) and (9.164b, c) of quadratic forms are used to obtain an upper bound for the derivative of the stability function following the differential system (subsection 9.2.19).

9.2.19 Stability Function and Its Derivative Following the Differential System

The time derivative of the stability function (9.153a) may be calculated along the dynamical system (9.149c) ≡ (9.150a) by:

$$\frac{dH}{dt} = \sum_{n=1}^{N} \frac{\partial H}{\partial x_{0n}} \lim_{t\to 0} \frac{dx_n}{dt}$$
$$= \sum_{n,m=1}^{N} \frac{\partial H}{\partial x_{0n}} \lim_{t\to 0} A_{nm} x_m + \sum_{n=1}^{N} \frac{\partial H}{\partial x_{0n}} R_n = \lim_{t\to 0} \sum_{n=1}^{N} \frac{\partial H}{\partial x_{0n}} \dot{x}_{0n} + \nabla H.\vec{R}. \tag{9.165a–d}$$

The first term on the r.h.s. of (9.165d) is evaluated by (9.159b) and (9.153b):

$$\lim_{t\to 0} \sum_{n=1}^{N} B_{mn}\, x_{0m}\, \dot{x}_{0n} = \frac{1}{2} \lim_{t\to 0} \frac{d}{dt}\left(\sum_{n,m=1}^{N} B_{mn}\, x_n\, x_m \right) = \frac{1}{2} \dot{H}_0 ; \tag{9.166a, b}$$

from (9.150d) follows (9.167a, b) leading to the upper bound (9.167c) for the second term on the r.h.s. of (9.165d):

$$\varepsilon > 0: \qquad \left|\vec{R}\right| < \varepsilon \left|\vec{x}\right|^2 : \qquad \left|\vec{R}.\nabla H\right| \le \left|\vec{R}\right| \left|\nabla H\right| < \varepsilon \left|\vec{x}\right|^2 b \left|H\right|^{1/2}, \tag{9.167a–d}$$

implying (9.167d) by (9.164c). Substitution of (9.166b; 9.167d) in (9.165d) leads to (9.168a):

$$\frac{dH}{dt} \le \frac{\dot{H}_0}{2} + \varepsilon b \left|\vec{x}\right|^2 \left|H\right|^{1/2} \le -\frac{\left|\vec{x}_0\right|^2}{2} + \frac{\varepsilon b}{\underline{b}} \left|H\right|^{3/2}$$
$$\le -\frac{H}{2\underline{b}} + \frac{2\varepsilon}{\sqrt{\underline{b}}} \left|H\right|^{3/2} \le -\frac{H}{2\underline{b}}\left[1 - 4\varepsilon\sqrt{\underline{b}}\left|H\right|\right] \le -\frac{H}{2\underline{b}}, \tag{9.168a–e}$$

using (9.153b, 9.160b, 9.164a) to obtain (9.168b–e). The integration of (9.168e) leads to (9.169a, b):

$$\frac{d}{dt}(\log H) \le -\frac{1}{2\underline{b}}, \qquad H(t) \le H(0) \exp\left(-\frac{t}{2\underline{b}}\right), \tag{9.169a, b}$$

proving that the stability function decays with time and leading to the third Lyapunov theorem on the stability [subsection 9.2.20 (9.2.21)] of autonomous differential systems (autonomous differential equations of any order).

9.2.20 Third Lyapunov Theorem on Autonomous Systems

The result (9.169b) proves the stability theorem because: (i) as $t \to \infty$ then $H \to 0$ so (9.153a) implies that $\vec{x}(t;\vec{x}_0) \to 0$ and the system tends to the equilibrium point, ensuring asymptotic stability; using (9.160b) in (9.169b) implies (9.170a–d):

$$0 \le t < \infty: \qquad \left|\vec{x}(t;\vec{x}_0)\right|^2 \le \frac{H(\vec{x})}{\underline{b}} \le \frac{H(0)}{\underline{b}} \exp\left(-\frac{t}{2\bar{b}}\right) \le \frac{\bar{b}}{\underline{b}}\left|\vec{x}_0\right|^2 \exp\left(-\frac{t}{2\bar{b}}\right). \tag{9.170a–d}$$

Thus follows the **third Lyapunov theorem on asymptotic stability:** *the solution of the autonomous differential system (9.149a–d) has (standard CCXLIV) an upper bound (9.171a, b):*

$$0 \le t < \infty: \qquad \left|\vec{x}(t;\vec{x}_0)\right| \le \left|\vec{x}_0\right| \sqrt{\bar{b}/\underline{b}} \exp\left(-\frac{t}{4\bar{b}}\right), \tag{9.171a, b}$$

where $\underline{b}\left(\bar{b}\right)$ is an lower (upper) bound (9.160a, b) for the stability function (9.153a), that is, a positive-definite quadratic form (9.159a, b). This case corresponds to the stable matrix (9.150b) for which all eigenvalues have negative real parts (9.151b). If at least one eigenvalue has a positive real part (9.151c), the corresponding natural integral diverges at infinity, and since there is at least one such solution, the system is unstable. If all eigenvalues have positive real parts (9.172a), the solution is the same as for (9.151b) reversing the signs of: (i) of F_n in the autonomous system (9.149b); (ii) of the matrix (9.150b) so that the quadratic form (9.159b) is negative definite instead of positive definite; (iii) of $\bar{b}$ in (9.169a, b) which is replaced by (9.172b–d):

$$\mathrm{Re}(a_N) > 0: \qquad \frac{dH}{dt} \ge \frac{H}{2\bar{b}}, \quad \frac{d}{dt}(\log H) \ge \frac{1}{2\underline{b}}, \qquad H(t) \ge H(0)\exp\left(\frac{t}{2\underline{b}}\right). \tag{9.172a–d}$$

It follows that for every solution $H \to \infty$ as $t \to \infty$ so the system is unconditionally unstable. For any sphere $|\vec{x}| = r$ the system will leave the sphere after a finite time $t \ge t_1$ such that $\left|\vec{x}(t_1)\right| = r$; the system cannot return at any later time, because this would imply $\dot{H} < 0$ that contradicts (9.172b). The third Lyapunov theorem applies both to autonomous differential systems (equations) because in both cases [subsection 9.2.19 (9.2.20)] the independent variable does not appear explicitly.

9.2.21 Stability of Solutions of an Autonomous Differential Equation

An **autonomous differential equation** of order N does not explicitly involve the independent variable (9.173a):

$$y^{(n)}(x) = F\left(y, y', \dots, y^{(N-1)}\right) \in C^2\left(|R^N\right); \quad s = 0, \dots, N-1:$$
$$y_s(x) = y^{(s)}(x), \quad y'_{N-1} = F\left(y, y_1, \dots, y_s\right), \tag{9.173a–d}$$

so that the corresponding system (9.173b–d) of first-order equations (9.174a–d) is also autonomous:

$$s = 0, \dots, N-1: \quad y_0(x) = y(x), \quad y'_{s-1}(x) = y_s(x), \quad y'_{N-1}(x) = F\left(y_0, y_1, \dots, y_{N-1}\right). \tag{9.174a–d}$$

Since the $(N - 1)$ equations (9.174a–c) are already linear, the linearization applies only to (9.174d), leading to (9.175a):

$$y'_{N-1} = \sum_{s=0}^{N-1} A_s \, y_s, \qquad A_s \equiv \frac{\partial F}{\partial y_s} = \frac{\partial F}{\partial y^{(s)}}, \tag{9.175a, b}$$

with the coefficients (9.175b) evaluated at the equilibrium point. It has been shown that *the stability of an autonomous ordinary differential equation of order N where (9.173a) the function F does not depend on the independent variable (9.176a) and has continuous second-order derivatives (9.173b), and has an equilibrium position (9.176b, c), is specified (standard CCXLV) by the linearized equation (9.175a) with constant coefficients (9.175b) evaluated at the equilibrium point:*

$$\frac{\partial F}{\partial x} = 0: \qquad s = 0, \dots, N-1: \qquad y^{(n)}(0) = 0; \quad P_N(a) = a^N + \sum_{s=0}^{N-1} A_s \, a^s; \tag{9.176a–d}$$

to be more precise, the eigenvalues, that are the roots (9.124a–c) of the characteristic polynomial (9.176d), specify the stability according to (9.151a–e). An autonomous differential equation (9.173a) that is linear (9.136a) has coefficients that cannot depend on the independent variable, and hence are constant (9.122a); in this case the preceding theorem is a trivial identity (9.122b) ≡ (9.176d). The first three (four) Lyapunov theorems concern linear or non-linear (linear) differential systems or equations with non-uniform bounded (periodic) coefficients [section 9.2 (9.3)].

9.3 Linear Differential Equations with Periodic Coefficients (Floquet 1883; Lyapunov 1907)

The linear differential equations (simultaneous systems) with constant [sections 1.3–1.5 (7.4–7.5)] and power [sections 1.6–1.7 (7.6–7.7)] coefficients all have eigenvalues, corresponding to natural integrals, that satisfy decoupled first-order equations; the general integral is a linear combination of the natural integrals. The natural integrals lead to a diagonal matrix if the eigenvalues are distinct, and to double-banded blocks for multiple eigenvalues; the double-banded blocks can be chosen in more than one alternate form, including Jordan blocks (subsections 7.4.11, 7.6.8, 9.3.4). The linear ordinary differential equations of order N with periodic coefficients allow for the existence periodic solutions (subsection 9.3.1) specified by natural integrals (subsection 9.3.3) associated with single (multiple) eigenvalues (subsection 9.3.2) whose eigenfunctions lead (subsection 9.3.4) to diagonal (diagonal Jordan block) matrices. The natural integrals may be asymptotically (i) stable, (ii) unstable, or (iii) oscillatory. In the case of a linear second-order differential equation in invariant form with periodic coefficient (subsection 9.3.5), it can be shown that all three types of (i) growing, (ii) decaying, and (iii-1) monotonic or (iii-2) oscillatory solutions can exist (subsection 9.3.6). Using a fundamental system of solutions (subsection 9.3.7) of the linear second-order differential equation in invariant form can be proved the fourth Lyapunov theorem on asymptotic stability (subsection 9.3.9), based on a calculation of eigenvalues (subsection 9.3.8).

9.3.1 Conditions for the Existence of Periodic Solutions (Floquet 1883)

Consider a linear ordinary differential equation (9.177b) of order N with period coefficients (9.177c, d) with period τ, where q is any integer (9.177a):

$$q \in |Z: \qquad \sum_{n=0}^{N} A_n(t) \frac{d^n x}{dt^n} = 0, \qquad A_n(t) = A_n(t+\tau) = A_n(t+q\tau). \tag{9.177a–c}$$

It does not follow that all solutions have to be periodic. Let the general integral be represented as a linear combination of N linearly independent solutions that form a fundamental system (9.178a), where C_n are arbitrary constants of integration:

$$x(t) = \sum_{n=1}^{N} C_n \, x_n(t); \qquad x_m(t+\tau) = \sum_{n=1}^{N} B_{mn} \, x_n(t), \tag{9.178a, b}$$

after one period the differential equation (9.177b) is the same, so each function of the new fundamental system is a linear combination (9.178b) of the old. If it is required to have periodic solutions (9.179a) then must hold (9.179b) leading to (9.179c):

$$x_m(t+\tau) = a\,x_m(t) = \sum_{n=1}^{N} B_{mn}\,x_n(t); \qquad \sum_{N=1}^{N}\left(B_{mn} - \lambda\,\delta_{mn}\right)x_n(t) = 0. \qquad (9.179\text{a–c})$$

The existence of non-trivial solution (9.180a):

$$\{x_1(t), x_2(t), \ldots, x_N(t)\} \neq \{0,0,\ldots,0\}: \qquad P_N(a) \equiv Det\left(B_{mn} - a\,\delta_{mn}\right) = 0, \qquad (9.180\text{a–c})$$

leads to a characteristic polynomial (9.180b), whose roots (9.180c) are the **eigenvalues**. The eigenvalues may be single (9.181a–c):

$$P_N(a_n) = 0 \neq P_N'(a_n): \qquad P_N(a) = \prod_{n=1}^{N}(a - a_n), \qquad (9.181\text{a–c})$$

or multiple (9.124a–c) roots of the characteristic polynomial, leading to distinct forms of the natural integrals (subsection 9.3.2).

9.3.2 Distinct and Coincident Eigenvalues and Exponents

Consider one eigenvalue a to which corresponds the periodic solution (9.182a), that implies (9.182b):

$$x(t+\tau) = a\,x(t): \qquad e^{-\gamma(t+\tau)}\,x(t+\tau) = a\,e^{-\gamma t}e^{-\gamma\tau}x(t); \qquad (9.182\text{a, b})$$

the function (9.183a) satisfies (9.183b):

$$\phi(t) \equiv e^{-\gamma t}\,x(t): \qquad \phi(t+\tau) = a\,e^{-\gamma\tau}\,\phi(t); \qquad (9.183\text{a, b})$$

thus the function is periodic (9.184a) if the eigenvalue a is related (9.184b) to the **period** τ through the **exponent** γ:

$$\phi(t+\tau) = \phi(t): \qquad a = e^{\gamma\tau}. \qquad (9.184\text{a, b})$$

Thus a single eigenvalue (9.181a, b) ≡ (9.185a, b) leads to a solution (9.183a) ≡ (9.185c) where ϕ is a periodic function (9.185d):

$$P_N(a) = 0 \neq P_N'(a): \qquad x(t) = e^{\gamma t}\,\phi(t), \qquad \phi(t) = \phi(t+\tau); \qquad (9.185\text{a–d})$$

an eigenvalue with multiplicity S in (9.186a) leads to S solutions (9.186b, c) obtained by parametric differentiation:

$$P_N(a) = \dots = P'_N(a) = \dots = P_N^{(S-1)}(a) = 0 \neq P_N^{(S)}(a);$$

$$s = 0, \dots, S-1: \qquad x_S(t) = \frac{\partial^s}{\partial \gamma^s}\left[e^{\gamma t}\,\phi(t)\right] = t^s\, e^{\gamma t}\,\phi(t). \tag{9.186a–c}$$

This proves the Floquet theorem stated next (subsection 9.3.3).

9.3.3 Natural Integrals and Asymptotic Stability

The preceding results may be summarized in the **Floquet theorem**: *a linear ordinary differential equation (9.177b) of order N with periodic coefficients (9.177a, c), has (standard CCXLVI) characteristic polynomial (9.178a, b; 9.180b) whose roots (9.124a–c) determine the eigenvalues a_m and exponents γ_m in (9.187a) with multiplicity α_m:*

$$a_m = e^{\gamma_m \tau}; \qquad \alpha_m = 1: \qquad x_m(t) = e^{\gamma_m t}\,\phi_m(t), \qquad \phi_m(t) = \phi_m(t+\tau), \tag{9.187a–d}$$

such that: (i) single eigenvalues (9.187b) correspond to the natural integrals (9.187c) involving a period function (9.187d); and (ii) an eigenvalue of multiplicity α_m in (9.188a) leads to the same number of natural integrals (9.188b):

$$\beta_m = 0, \dots, \alpha_m - 1: \qquad x_{m,\beta_m}(t) = t^{\beta_m}\, e^{\gamma_m t}\,\phi_m(t). \tag{9.188a, b}$$

The general integral is a linear combination (9.189c) [(9.190c)] of natural integrals (9.187c) [(9.188b)] in the case of single (multiple) eigenvalues (9.189a) [(9.190a)] where $C_n\left(C_{m,\beta_s}\right)$ are arbitrary constants:

$$\alpha_m = 1: \qquad x(t) = \sum_{n=1}^{N} C_n\, x_n(t) = \sum_{n=1}^{N} C_n\,(a_m)^{t/\tau}\,\phi_n(t), \tag{9.189a–c}$$

$$\alpha_m = 2, \dots, 3: \quad x(t) = \sum_{n=1}^{M}\sum_{\beta_m=0}^{\alpha_m-1} C_{m,\beta_m}\, x_{m,\beta_m}(t) = \sum_{m=1}^{M}(a_m)^{t/\tau}\,\phi_n(t)\sum_{\beta_m=0}^{\alpha_m-1} t^{\beta_m}\, C_n\,\phi_n(t). \tag{9.190a–c}$$

In (9.187c) [(9.188b)] and (9.189c) [(9.190c)] are used respectively the exponents γ_m and eigenvalues a_m, that are related by (9.187a) implying (9.191a, b):

$$\exp(\gamma_m t) = \left[\exp(\gamma_m \tau)\right]^{t/\tau} = (a_m)^{t/\tau}. \tag{9.191a, b}$$

The ordering of the eigenvalues by non-increasing modulus (9.192a), corresponds (9.148a–c) to the ordering of the exponents by non-increasing real part (9.192b):

$$|a_1| \geq |a_2| \geq \ldots \geq |a_N| \quad \Leftrightarrow \quad \mathrm{Re}(\gamma_1) \geq \mathrm{Re}(\gamma_2) \geq \ldots \geq \mathrm{Re}(\gamma_N); \qquad \text{(9.192a, b)}$$

$$\text{asymtotically} \begin{cases} \textit{stable:} & |a_1| < 1, \quad \Leftrightarrow \quad \mathrm{Re}(\gamma_1) < 0, \\ \textit{unstable:} & |a_1| > 1, \quad \Leftrightarrow \quad \mathrm{Re}(\gamma_1) > 0, \\ \textit{indifferent:} & |a_1| = 1, \quad a_1 \neq a_2 \quad \Leftrightarrow \quad \mathrm{Re}(\gamma_1) = 0, \quad \gamma_1 \neq \gamma_2 \\ \textit{unstable:} & |a_1| = 1, \quad a_1 = a_2 \quad \Leftrightarrow \quad \mathrm{Re}(\gamma_1) = 0, \quad \gamma_1 = \gamma_2. \end{cases}$$

(9.192c–f)

and leads (standard CCXLVII) by (9.189a–c; 9.190a–c) to four cases, namely: (i) stability (9.192c) if all eigenvalues (exponents) are less than unity in modulus (have negative real parts); (ii) unstable (9.192d) if at least one eigenvalue (exponent) is larger than unity in modulus (has positive real part); (iii) indifferent (9.192e) if the largest modulus (real part) of an eigenvalue (exponent) is unity (zero) and it does not coincide with another eigenvalue (exponent); and (iv) if it is a multiple eigenvalue (exponent) with unit modulus (zero real part) then there is instability. Also the real (complex) exponents leads to monotonic (oscillatory) solutions. The comparison of (9.151a–e) with respectively (9.192a–f) shows that the asymptotic stability is the same in terms of eigenvalues a_m (exponents γ_m) of linear ordinary differential equations (9.136a) [≡ (9.177b)] with bounded (9.136b) [periodic (9.177a, c)] coefficients. The single (multiple) eigenvalues correspond to normal integrals that lead diagonal (7.96a–c) [double-banded diagonal (7.97a–d)] matrices; the double-banded diagonal matrices can be written in alternative forms consisting of Jordan blocks (subsection 9.4.4).

9.3.4 Diagonal Matrices and Jordan Blocks

A consequence of the preceding results (subsection 9.3.3) is that *the natural integrals (9.187c) [(9.188b)] corresponding to single (9.187b) [multiple (9.188a)] eigenvalues of a linear differential equation (9.177b) with periodic coefficients (9.177a, c) are (standard CCXLVIII) of the form (9.193a, b) [(9.193c, d)]:*

$$\alpha_m = 1: \quad x_m(t) = q_m(t)\phi_m(t); \qquad \beta_m = 1, \ldots, \alpha_m - 1: \quad x_{m,\beta_m}(t) = q_{m,\beta_m}(t)\,\phi_m(t), \qquad \text{(9.193a–d)}$$

where the coefficients (9.194a) [(9.195a)] of the periodic functions:

$$q_m(t) = e^{\gamma_m t}: \qquad \dot{q}_m = \gamma_m q_m; \qquad \text{(9.194a, b)}$$

$$q_{m,\beta_m}(t) = t^{\beta_m} e^{\gamma_m t}: \qquad \dot{q}_{m,\beta_m} = \gamma_m q_{m,\beta_m} + \beta_m q_{m,\beta_m - 1}, \qquad \text{(9.195a, b)}$$

satisfy totally (9.194b) [partially (9.195b)] decoupled first-order differential equations, leading for the exponents γ_m to diagonal (double-banded diagonal) matrices like (7.76c) [(7.97d)].

The double-banded diagonal matrix with the multiple exponent γ_0 or eigenvalue a_0 in the diagonal and integers $1,...,\alpha$ up to the multiplicity in the parallel line (7.97d) can be replaced by a **Jordan matrix** *with the digit unity along the parallel line (9.196):*

$$\begin{bmatrix} \dot{\bar{q}}_1 \\ \dot{\bar{q}}_2 \\ \dot{\bar{q}}_3 \\ \vdots \\ \dot{\bar{q}}_{m-1} \\ \dot{\bar{q}}_m \end{bmatrix} = \begin{bmatrix} a & 0 & 0 & \cdots & 0 & 0 & 0 \\ 1 & a & 0 & \cdots & 0 & 0 & 0 \\ 0 & 1 & a & \cdots & 0 & 0 & 0 \\ \vdots & \vdots & \vdots & \ddots & \vdots & \vdots & \vdots \\ 0 & 0 & 0 & \cdots & 0 & a & 0 \\ 0 & 0 & 0 & \cdots & 0 & 1 & a \end{bmatrix} \begin{bmatrix} \bar{q}_1 \\ \bar{q}_2 \\ \bar{q}_3 \\ \vdots \\ \bar{q}_{m-1} \\ \bar{q}_m \end{bmatrix}, \tag{9.196}$$

by (standard CCXLIX) considering the **alternate natural integrals** *(9.197a–c):*

$$s = 1,....,m: \qquad \bar{q}_s(t) = \frac{1}{s!} q_s(t) = \frac{t^s}{s!} e^{at}, \tag{9.197a–c}$$

that are linear combinations of the preceding (9.195a, b) and thus satisfy the same differential equations.

The proof consists in showing that the change of dependent variables (9.197a, b) transforms the differential system (9.195a, b) ≡ (9.79a–d) to (9.196). From (9.197a–c) follows (9.193a–d):

$$\dot{\bar{q}}_{s+1}(t) = \frac{\dot{q}_{s+1}(t)}{(s+1)!} = \frac{1}{(s+1)!}\left[q_{s+1}(t) + s q_s(t)\right] = \frac{q_{s+1}(t)}{(s+1)!} + \frac{q_s(t)}{s!} = \bar{q}_{s+1}(t) + \bar{q}_s(t); \tag{9.198a–d}$$

the relation (9.198d) ≡ (9.196) coincides with the Jordan matrix. QED. The Jordan blocks (9.196) are traditional in eigenvalue theory, and can be used also for simultaneous systems of linear ordinary differential equations with constant (7.79a–d) [homogenous (7.185a–d)] coefficients. Additional results on linear differential equations with periodic coefficients (subsections 9.3.1–9.3.4) can be obtained in the case of second order (subsections 9.3.5–9.3.9), starting with the cases of two equal (unequal) eigenvalues [subsection 9.3.5 (9.3.6)].

9.3.5 Invariant Second-Order Differential Equation

The nature of the solutions of a linear ordinary differential equation with periodic coefficients (9.177a–c) will be investigated further for order $N = 2$ when the equation (5.220b) always (note 5.8) via the change of dependent variable (5.242a) can be put into the invariant form (5.242b) ≡ (9.199a) without first-order derivative, leading to only one (5.243a) coefficient that is taken to be periodic (9.199b):

$$\ddot{x}(t)+I(t)x(t)=0, \qquad I(t+\tau)=I(t). \qquad (9.199\text{a, b})$$

If the invariant (9.199b) is a positive (5.251b) [non-positive (5.251d, e)] constant (9.199b), the solution of (9.194a) ≡ (5.251b) is (i) oscillatory [monotonic (ii) growing or (iii) decaying]; it will be shown next that the same linear second-order differential equation in invariant form (9.199a) can also have only the three types of solutions (i–iii) when the invariant is a periodic function of time. The characteristic polynomial is quadratic for a second-order linear differential equation, and in the case of (9.200a) of a double eigenvalue a [or (9.200b) exponent γ] the solution (9.200d) [(9.200e)] with arbitrary constants$\left(C_1, C_2\right)$ and periodic function (9.200c):

$$P_2(a)=P_2'(a)=0\neq P_2''(a), \quad a\equiv e^{\gamma\tau}, \phi(t)=\phi(t+\tau): \qquad (9.200\text{a–c})$$

$$x(t)=\left(C_1+C_2\,t\right)e^{\gamma\tau}\phi(t)=\left(C_1+C_2\,t\right)a^{t/\tau}\,\phi(t), \qquad (9.200\text{d, e})$$

is: (i) stable for the modulus of the eigenvalue (9.201a) [real part of the exponent (9.201b)] smaller than unity (negative); (ii) unstable (9.201c) [(9.201d)] otherwise:

$$x(t)\begin{cases} |a|<1 \quad \Leftrightarrow \quad \operatorname{Re}(\gamma)<0: \quad \textit{stable}, & (9.201\text{a, b}) \\ |a|\geq 1 \quad \Leftrightarrow \quad \operatorname{Re}(\gamma)\geq 0: \quad \textit{unstable}. & (9.201\text{c, d}) \end{cases}$$

The stable (unstable) solution is monotonic (oscillatory) for real (9.202a) [complex (9.202b)] eigenvalue:

$$x(t): \quad \begin{cases} a\in |R: \quad \textit{monotonic}, & (9.202\text{a}) \\ a\in C-|R: \quad \textit{oscillatory}. & (9.202\text{b}) \end{cases}$$

Thus the stable (unstable) oscillatory solution is a decaying (growing) oscillation, corresponding to oscillatory decay (overstability). It remains to prove that the possible solutions are also (i) oscillatory or monotonic (ii) increasing or (iii) decreasing in the case of distinct eigenvalues.

9.3.6 Growing/Decaying and Monotonic/Oscillatory Solutions

In the case of distinct (9.203a) eigenvalues (9.203b, c), there exist two linearly independent periodic solutions (9.203d) implying (9.185c; 9.191b) ≡ (9.203e), and involving a periodic function (9.203f):

$$a_1 \neq a_2\,,\; P_2(a_1) = 0 \neq P_2'(a_1)\,,\; P_2(a_2) = 0 \neq P_2'(a_2): \tag{9.203a–c}$$

$$x_{1,2}(t+\tau) = a_{1,2}\, x_{1,2}(t), \quad x_{1,2}(t) = (a_{1,2})^{t/\tau}\, \phi_{1,2}(t), \quad \phi_{1,2}(t+\tau) = \phi_{1,2}(t); \tag{9.203d–f}$$

both solutions satisfy (9.199a) ≡ (9.204a, b), that imply (9.204c):

$$\ddot{x}_1 + x_1 I = 0 = \ddot{x}_2 + x_2 I: \qquad 0 = \ddot{x}_1 x_2 - x_1 \ddot{x}_2 = \frac{d}{dt}(\dot{x}_1 x_2 - x_1 \dot{x}_2). \tag{9.204a–c}$$

The identity (9.204c) ≡ (9.205a) remains valid if t is replaced by $t+\tau$, and by (9.203d) is equivalent to multiplication by a_1, a_2, so the product of the two eigenvalues must be unity (9.205b):

$$\dot{x}_1 x_2 - x_1 \dot{x}_2 = const: \quad a_1 a_2 = 1; \qquad a_1 = a_2^* = \frac{1}{a_2} \quad or \quad a_{1,2} = a_{1,2}^*, \tag{9.205a–d}$$

since the equations (9.199a) ≡ (9.204a, b) are real, the complex conjugates (x_1^*, x_2^*) of the solutions (x_1, x_2) are also solutions, and the eigenvalues (a_1, a_2) must coincide with (a_1^*, a_2^*), leading to two possibilities (9.205c, d). In the first case (9.205c), the eigenvalues have modulus unity (9.206a, b) and opposite phases (9.206c) and the solutions are oscillatory and bounded (9.206d):

$$|a_1| = 1 = |a_2|, \qquad a_{1,2} = \exp(\pm i\theta\tau): \qquad x_{1,2}(t) = \exp(\pm i\theta t)\,\phi(t); \tag{9.206a–d}$$

$$a_1 > 1 > a_2 = \frac{1}{a_1}: \quad \lim_{t\to\infty} x_1(t) = \lim_{t\to\infty} (a_1)^{t/\tau}\,\phi(t) = \infty, \quad \lim_{t\to\infty} x_2(t) = \lim_{t\to\infty} (a_2)^{t/\tau}\,\phi(t) = 0, \tag{9.207a–d}$$

in the second case (9.205d) the eigenvalues are real and inverse (9.207a, b) and that larger (smaller) than unity leads to an asymptotically divergent (9.207c) [decaying (9.207d)] solution. Collecting the preceding results (9.200a–e; 9.203a–f; 9.206a–d; 9.207a–d) it follows that *the asymptotic solution of the linear second-order ordinary differential equation (9.199a) with periodic invariant (9.199b) to within the product by a periodic function (9.185d), leads (standard CCL) to two cases and four sub-cases. In case I of a double eigenvalue (9.200a–e) it is: (Ii) stable if the modulus of the eigenvalue is less than unity (9.201a) or equivalently the real part of the exponent is negative (9.201b); (Iii) unstable otherwise (9.201c, d), and in both cases monotonic (oscillatory) if the eigenvalue is real (9.202a) [complex (9.202b)].*

In case II of distinct eigenvalues (9.203a–f) the solutions are: (Ii) oscillatory with constant amplitude (9.206d) if the eigenvalues have unit modulus (9.206a, b) or imaginary conjugate exponents (9.206c); (IIii) growing (9.207c) [decaying (9.207d)] in time for the real eigenvalue larger (9.207a) [smaller (9.207b)] than unity. The assessment of stability thus depends on the eigenvalues, whose calculation is the subject of the fourth Lyapunov theorem (subsection 9.4.8), that uses the set of fundamental solutions of the differential equation (subsection 9.4.7).

9.3.7 Fundamental Solution of a Linear Differential Equation

Consider a linear differential equation (9.208b) of order N corresponding to the linear differential operator (9.208a) with N single-point boundary conditions (9.208c, d):

$$L\{y(x)\} \equiv \sum_{n=0}^{N} A_n(x)\frac{d^n y}{dx^n} = 0; \qquad s = 0,\dots,N-1: \qquad y^{(s)}(0) = y_{0,s}. \tag{9.208a–d}$$

The set of N **fundamental solutions** satisfy the differential equation (9.209a, b) with boundary conditions (9.204c–e):

$$m = 1,\dots,N: \qquad L\{y_m(x)\} = 0; \qquad y_m^{(s)}(0) = \delta_m^s = \begin{cases} 1 & \text{if} \quad m = s-1, \\ 0 & \text{if} \quad m \neq s-1. \end{cases} \tag{9.209a–e}$$

The fundamental solutions are linearly independent because each of them has a boundary condition unity where all the others are zero. Thus the general integral must be a linear combination (9.210a) of fundamental solutions:

$$y(x) = \sum_{n=1}^{N} C_n y_n(x); \qquad y^{(s)}(0) - \sum_{n=1}^{N} C_n y_n^{(s)}(0) = \sum_{n=1}^{N} C_n \delta_n^s = C_s; \tag{9.210a–d}$$

the arbitrary constants C_n in the general integral (9.210a) are given by (9.210b–d) where was used (9.209c–e). There is an analogy between the theorems on fundamental solutions (9.154a–c; 9.156a–d)[(9.209a–e; 9.210a–d)] of linear autonomous system (9.143a) [differential equation (9.208a, b)] of order N with initial conditions (9.156b–d) [(9.210b–d)]. Substituting (9.210d) in (9.210a) it follows that *the general integral of an ordinary unforced linear differential equation (9.208a, b) of order N with N single-point boundary conditions, is given (standard CCLI) by the linear combination (9.211):*

$$y(x) = \sum_{n=1}^{N} y^{(n-1)}(0)\, y_n(x), \tag{9.211}$$

of fundamental solutions (9.209a–e) with the boundary conditions (9.208c, d) as the coefficients (9.210b, d). In the case of the ordinary unforced linear second-order differential equation invariant form (9.199a) ≡ (9.212a) with two single-point boundary conditions (9.212b, c):

$$\ddot{x} + I x = 0; \qquad x(0) = x_0, \qquad \dot{x}(0) = \dot{x}_0, \tag{9.212a–c}$$

(i) the two fundamental solutions satisfy (9.213a, c) and (9.213b, d):

$$x_{1,2}(t) = \{1,0\}, \qquad \dot{x}_{1,2}(t) = \{0,1\}: \qquad x(t) = x_0\, x_1(t) + \dot{x}_0\, x_2(t), \tag{9.213a–e}$$

and (ii) the general integral is (9.213e). This result (subsection 9.3.7) is used together with the eigenvalues (subsection 9.3.8) of the differential equation (9.199a, b) in the proof of the fourth Lyapunov theorem (subsection 9.3.9).

9.3.8 Eigenvalues of the Invariant Second Order Equation

The solution of the ordinary unforced linear differential equation (9.199a) ≡ (5.251b) in the case of constant invariant (5.251a) is bounded (5.251c) [unbounded (5.251d, e)] asymptotically $t \to \infty$ if the invariant is positive (negative). This suggests the asymptotic stability (instability) of (9.199a) when the invariant is a positive (negative) function, leading to the fourth Lyapunov stability theorem that is proved next. Since differential equation (9.199a) has periodic coefficient with period τ, the fundamental solutions at the time $t+\tau$ are a linear combination of the solutions at the time t:

$$\begin{bmatrix} x_1(t+\tau) \\ x_2(t+\tau) \end{bmatrix} = \begin{bmatrix} B_{11} & B_{12} \\ B_{21} & B_{22} \end{bmatrix} \begin{bmatrix} x_1(t) \\ x_2(t) \end{bmatrix}. \tag{9.214}$$

Setting (9.215a) leads by (9.213a–d) to (9.215b, c):

$$t = 0: \quad x_1(\tau) = B_{11}, \qquad \dot{x}_2(\tau) = B_{22}: \quad B_{11} + B_{22} = x_1(\tau) + \dot{x}_2(\tau), \tag{9.215a–d}$$

and hence to (9.215d). The eigenvalues of the matrix in (9.214) ≡ (9.179a–c) are the roots of (9.178c) the quadratic characteristic polynomial (9.216a, b):

$$0 = P_2(a) = \begin{vmatrix} B_{11} - a & B_{21} \\ B_{21} & B_{22} - a \end{vmatrix} = a^2 - 2Ea + D, \tag{9.216a, b}$$

where the coefficients are the determinant (9.217a, b) [trace (9.217c, d)] of the matrix:

$$D \equiv B_{11}B_{22} - B_{12}B_{21} \equiv Det(B_{mn}), \quad 2E = B_{11} + B_{22} = Tr(B_{mn}) = x_1(\tau) + \dot{x}_2(\tau). \tag{9.217a–e}$$

$$P_2(a) = (a - a_1)(a - a_2) = a^2 - (a_1 + a_2)\, a + a_1 a_2, \tag{9.218a, b}$$

the comparison of (9.216b) ≡ (9.218b) implies (9.219a, c):

$$D = a_1 a_2 = 1, \qquad 2E = a_1 + a_2, \qquad \text{(9.219a–c)}$$

where: (i) the determinant (9.217a) is (9.219a) equal to unity (9.219b) by (9.205b); and (ii) the form of the invariant (9.199b) in the differential equation (9.199a) affects only the trace (9.219c) ≡ (9.217c–e). The characteristic polynomial (9.218b; 9.219a, c) ≡ (9.220a):

$$0 = a^2 - 2Ea + 1: \qquad a_\pm = E \pm \sqrt{E^2 - 1}, \qquad \text{(9.220a, b)}$$

has eigenvalues (9.220b) that depend only on (9.219c) ≡ (9.217c–e). It has been shown *that the eigenvalues (9.220b) of the unforced linear ordinary second-order differential equation (9.199a) with periodic invariant (9.199b) depend (standard CCLII) only on alternatively: (i) the trace (9.217c–e) of the matrix relating the fundamental solutions differing by one period (9.214); or (ii) the combination (9.215d) specified by the fundamental solutions (9.204a, b; 9.213a–d) at one period.* The proof of the fourth Lyapunov theorem (subsection 9.4.9) uses the preceding results (subsection 9.4.8) together with an iterative solution of the differential equation (9.199a) similar to the Picard method (subsection 9.1.2).

9.3.9 Proof of the Fourth Lyapunov (1907) Theorem

The invariant second-order differential equation (9.199a) is replaced by (9.221a) and the solution is sought as a power series (9.221b, c) in λ with leading terms satisfying (9.213a–d):

$$\ddot{x} + \lambda I(t) x = 0: \qquad x_{1,2}(t) = \{1, t\} + \sum_{n=1}^{\infty} \lambda^n \left\{ x_n^1(t),\, x_n^2(t) \right\}. \qquad \text{(9.221a–c)}$$

Substitution of (9.221b, c) in (9.221a) leads to the differential-difference equations (9.222a, b):

$$\ddot{x}_n^{1,2} + I(t) x_{n-1}^{1,2} = 0: \quad x_n^{1,2}(t) = -\int_0^s ds \int_0^t dr\, I(r) x_{n-1}^{1,2}(r), \quad x_0^{1,2}(t) = \{1, t\}, \qquad \text{(9.222a–f)}$$

that are equivalent to the integral-difference equations (9.222c, d) with initial conditions (9.222e–f). The differential equations (9.221a) ≡ (9.199a) coincide for (9.223a), in which case (9.217e), (9.221b, c) and (9.222e, f) imply (9.223b, c, d):

$$\lambda = 1: \quad 2E = x_1(\tau) + \dot{x}_2(\tau) = \sum_{n=0}^{\infty} \left[x_n^1(\tau) + \dot{x}_n^2(\tau) \right] = 2 + \sum_{n=1}^{\infty} \left[x_n^1(\tau) + \dot{x}_n^2(\tau) \right]. \qquad \text{(9.223a–d)}$$

If the invariant in (9.199a) is negative (9.224a), it follows: (i) from (9.222c, d) that (9.224b–d) are positive; (ii) then (9.223b) implies (9.224e); (iii) thus the larger eigenvalue in (9.220b) is real and larger than unity (9.224f); and (iv) by (9.201c) follows that there instability (9.224g):

$$I(t)<0: \qquad x_n^1(t), \quad x_n^2(t), \quad \dot{x}_n^2(t)>0, \quad E>1, \quad a_+>1, \quad x_{1,2}(t)\sim(a_+)^{t/\tau}. \tag{9.224a–g}$$

This proves the **fourth Lyapunov theorem**: *the linear ordinary differential equation of second-order in invariant form (9.199a) with periodic (9.199b) negative (9.224a) coefficient has (standard CCLIII) unstable solutions (9.224f, g); hence stable solutions are possible only if the invariant (9.199b) is positive for some values of t.* In the case the parametric resonance (4.88) ≡ (9.225b):

$$2h<1: \qquad \ddot{x}+I(t)x=0, \quad I(t)=\frac{k(t)}{m}=\omega_0^2\left[1+2h\left(\cos\omega_e t\right)\right]>0, \tag{9.225a–e}$$

corresponds to the periodic invariant (9.225c) with period $\tau_e=2\pi/\omega_e$ in (9.225d) that for excitation with small amplitude (9.225a) is positive (9.225e), implying that instability is possible (section 4.3). This qualitative result (subsection 9.3.9) agrees with: (i) the prediction of instability (9.121) from the first Lyapunov theorem (subsection 9.2.10); and (ii) the exact and approximate solutions for parametric resonance (section 4.3) that allow for stability and instability in certain excitation bands. The quantitative approaches to differential equations can be quite different. This is an instance of the difference between the methods to prove general properties (obtain general solutions) of differential equations [section 9.1–9.3 (9.4–9.9)], implying that for example an existence theorem may or may not give a hint of the form of the solution.

9.4 Analytic Coefficients and Generalized Circular/Hyperbolic Functions

The solution of differential equations may involve: (i) singularities of single-valued functions (subsection 9.4.1), namely simple or multiple poles and essential singularities (subsection 9.4.2); or (ii) multi-valued functions (subsection 9.4.3) and associated branch-points and branch-cuts in the complex plane, for example for the root of order N, the logarithm, or the power with non-integer exponent (subsection 9.4.4). The classification of linear ordinary differential equations (subsection 9.4.5) and of the corresponding integrals (subsection 9.4.6) is indicated by the simplest case of an unforced linear first-order differential equation considering its solution [subsection 9.4.6 (9.4.7)] in the neighborhood of a point in the finite plane (the point at infinity). The classification of singularities and solutions can be extended [subsection 9.4.8 (9.4.9)] to linear autonomous systems of differential equations (ordinary differential equations of any order). There are three cases: (I) a linear differential equation with analytic coefficients has analytic solutions (section 9.4), that are expressible as a series of positive integral powers; (II) the series may be multiplied by non-integral powers and/or logarithms leading to regular integrals (section 9.5) if the coefficients of the linear differential equation have poles up to a certain order; and (III) if the condition (II) is not met there are normal (or other irregular) integrals [section 9.6 (9.7)] with an essential singularity that involves an unending series of negative integral powers. The case (I) of linear second-order differential equations with analytic coefficients (subsections 9.4.10–9.4.11) is illustrated by the generalized hyperbolic (circular) differential equation [subsection 9.4.12 (9.4.16)] and cosine and sine functions [subsection 9.4.13 (9.4.15)] that involve a parameter; the Airy differential equation and functions (original circular and hyperbolic cosine and sine) are the particular cases [subsection 9.4.14 (9.4.12–9.4.13, 9.4.15–9.4.16)] with parameter unity (zero). The parameter can take in general complex values (subsection 9.4.17). The analytic power series expansions for the generalized hyperbolic and circular cosine and sine (subsections 9.4.12–9.4.17) can be used to (i) obtain differentiation formulas (inequalities) for complex (real) variable and parameter [subsection 9.4.18 (9.4.19)]; and (ii) define the generalized hyperbolic and circular secant, cosecant, tangent, and cotangent (subsection 9.4.20).

9.4.1 Singularities of Single-Valued Complex Functions

The solution of differential equations (simultaneous systems) will generally be considered in the complex plane for the independent x and dependent $y(y_m)$ variables in order to benefit from the theory of complex functions of complex variables (volumes I and II of this series). A **single-valued function** (I.9.1a) assigns (Figure 9.8a) to each point of the **domain** (9.226a) one point of the **range** (9.226b):

$$\mathcal{V}_1: \qquad \forall_{x\in D}\ \exists^1_{y\in E}: \qquad x\in D \ \Rightarrow\ y(x)\in E. \tag{9.226a, b}$$

A function is **differentiable** at a point if the limit of incremental ratio (I.11.6) is independent (9.227) of the direction in which that point is approached:

$$\mathcal{D}(D)\equiv\left\{f:\ \lim_{\Delta x\to 0}\frac{f(x+\Delta x)-f(x)}{\Delta x}\equiv f'(x)\right\}. \tag{9.227}$$

A point where the function is not differentiable is a **singularity** of that function; the singularity is **isolated** if there is at least one $\varepsilon>0$ so that the neighborhood of order ε does not contain any other singularity. It has been

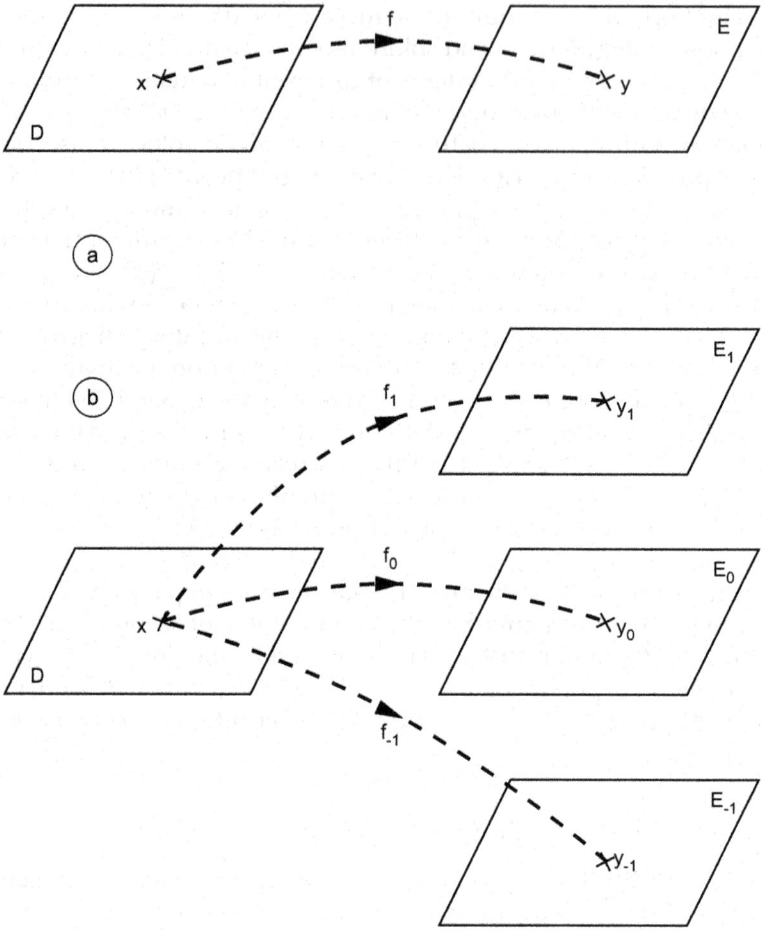

FIGURE 9.8
A complex single (multi)-valued function maps the domain in the x-plane to the range consisting of (a) one [(b) several] sheets of an ordinary (Riemann) surface.

shown (chapter I.25) that a *function differentiable in an annulus (9.228a) around an isolated singularity taken to be at the origin is represented by (standard CCLIV) a* **Laurent series** *of ascending and descending powers (9.228b–e):*

$$y \in \mathcal{D}\left(0<|x|<R\right): \quad y(x) = \sum_{n=-\infty}^{+\infty} c_n\, x^n = c_0 + \sum_{m=1}^{\infty}\left(c_m\, x^m + \frac{c_{-m}}{x^m}\right)$$

$$= \ldots + \frac{c_{-n}}{x^n} + \ldots + \frac{c_{-2}}{x^2} + \frac{c_{-1}}{x} + c_0 + c_1 x + c_2 x + \ldots + c_n x^n + \ldots$$

$$= c_0 + c_1\, x + \frac{c_{-1}}{x} + c_2 x^2 + \frac{c_{-2}}{x^2} + \ldots + c_n x^n + \frac{c_{-n}}{x^n} + \ldots \quad \text{(9.228a–e)}$$

where the coefficient c_{-1} *of* $1/x$ *is the* **residue** *in (9.228c). The Laurent series (9.228b, c) converges (Figure 9.9a): (i) absolutely, that is, the series of moduli converges (9.229b) in the open annulus (9.228a) ≡ (9.229a); (ii) uniformly (section I.21.4), that is, independently of the point (9.229d) in a closed sub-annulus (9.229c):*

$$0<|x|<R: \quad \sum_{n=-\infty}^{+\infty} |c_n|\,|x|^n \, C.; \qquad 0<\varepsilon \le |x| \le R-\delta: \quad \sum_{n=-\infty}^{+\infty} c_n\, x^n \, U.C. \tag{9.229a–d}$$

Thus in the open annulus (9.228a) ≡ (9.229a) [closed sub-annulus (9.229c)] the Laurent series can be deranged that is the order of the terms can be changed (the limit, differentiation, and integration can be taken under the integral sign) without changing the sum of the series as proved in the sections *I.21.1–I.21.4 (I.21.5–I.21.7)* of chapter *I.21*.

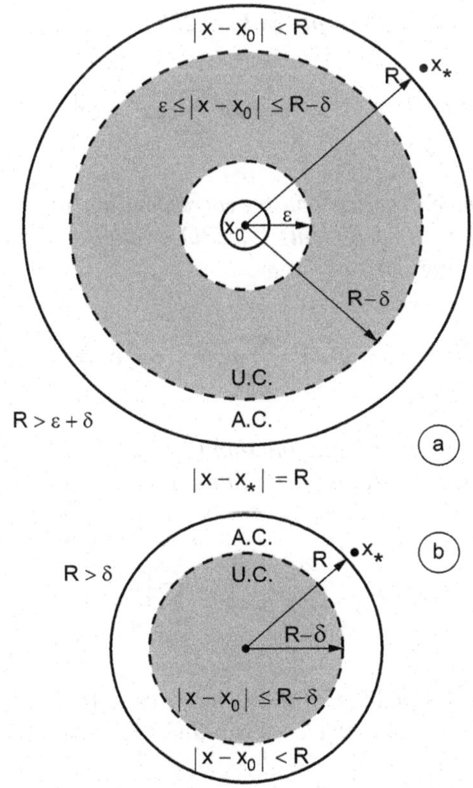

FIGURE 9.9
An isolated singularity x_0 can be surrounded by an annulus with infinitesimal inner radius ε and outer radius R limited by the nearest singularity x_*, so that the function is analytic in the annulus, and has an absolutely (and uniformly) convergent Laurent series in the open ring $0<|x-x_0|<R$ (closed sub-ring $\varepsilon<|x-x_0|<R-\delta$). If x_0 is a regular point the annulus (a) becomes a disk (b) with $\varepsilon = 0$ and the Laurent series is replaced by a Taylor series.

Four cases arise (chapter I.27) dependent (standard CCLV) on whether the Laurent series (9.228b, c): (case I) has (9.230a) an unending sequence of powers with negative exponents (9.230b) corresponding (subsection I.27.3.2) to an ***essential singularity:***

$$x = 0 \quad \text{is} \quad \text{an essential singularity:} \qquad \forall_{n \in |N} : \exists_{m \in |N} : \quad m > n \text{ and } c_{-m} \neq 0; \tag{9.230a, b}$$

(case II) terminates (subsection I.27.4.2) with the power –M corresponding (9.231b) to a ***multiple pole of order M*** *(9.231a):*

$$x = 0 \quad \text{is} \quad \text{a pole of order } M: \qquad y(x) = \sum_{n=-M}^{\infty} c_n\, x^n \sim O\left(\frac{1}{x^M}\right); \tag{9.231a, b}$$

(case III) terminates with the power –1 corresponding (9.232b) to a pole of order M = 1 in (9.231a, b), that is a ***simple pole*** *(9.232a):*

$$x = 0 \quad \text{is} \quad \text{a simple pole:} \qquad y(x) = \sum_{n=-1}^{\infty} c_n x^n = O\left(\frac{1}{x}\right); \tag{9.232a, b}$$

(case IV) does not have negative powers corresponding to the ***Maclaurin series*** *(I.23.24b) ≡ (9.233a) with coefficients (9.233b) around a* ***regular point*** *(standard CCLVI) that is not a singularity:*

$$x = 0 \quad \text{is} \quad \text{a regular point:} \qquad y(x) = \sum_{b=0}^{\infty} c_n\, x^n, \qquad c_n \equiv \frac{y^{(n)}(0)}{n!}. \tag{9.233a, b}$$

Since the corresponding analytic function (9.233a, b) is bounded in its neighborhood in the case of a regular point the annulus (Figure 9.9a) is replaced by a simply-connected region (Figure 9.9b) and:

$$|x| < \delta: \quad \sum_{n=0}^{\infty} \frac{|x|^n}{n!} \left| y^{(n)}(0) \right| \text{ C.}; \quad |x| \leq \delta - \varepsilon: \quad \sum_{n=0}^{\infty} \frac{|x|^n}{n!} y^{(n)}(0) \quad \text{U.C.}, \tag{9.234a–d}$$

and the Maclaurin series (9.233a, b) is absolutely (9.234b) [uniformly (9.234d)] convergent in the open disk (9.234a) [closed sub-disk (9.234c)].

9.4.2 Regular Points, Poles, and Essential Singularities

As examples of the four distinct types of points, four functions are given, namely: (i) the circular sine (II.7.15b) divided by the independent variable (9.235a) that is an analytic function (9.235b) with value unity (9.235c) at the origin, that is, a regular point; (ii) the circular cosine (II.7.14b) divided by its variable (9.236a) has a simple pole at the origin (9.236b) with residue unity (9.236c); (iii) the hyperbolic cosine (II.7.14c) divided by the cube of the independent variable (9.237a) has a triple pole at the origin (9.237b) with residue one-half (9.237c):

$$\frac{\sin x}{x} = \sum_{n=0}^{\infty} (-)^n \frac{x^{2n}}{(2n+1)!} = 1 - \frac{x^2}{6} + \frac{x^4}{120} + \ldots, \qquad \lim_{x\to 0} \frac{\sin x}{x} = 1; \tag{9.235a–c}$$

$$\frac{\cos x}{x} = \sum_{n=0}^{\infty} (-)^n \frac{x^{2n-1}}{(2n)!} = \frac{1}{x} - \frac{x}{2} + \frac{x^3}{24} + \ldots, \qquad c_{-1} = 1; \tag{9.236a–c}$$

$$\frac{\cosh x}{x^3} = \sum_{n=0}^{\infty} \frac{x^{2n-3}}{(2n)!} = \frac{1}{x^3} + \frac{1}{2x} + \frac{x}{24} + \ldots, \qquad c_{-1} = \frac{1}{2}; \tag{9.237a–c}$$

$$\exp\left(-\frac{1}{x}\right) = \sum_{n=0}^{\infty} (-)^n \frac{x^{-n}}{n!} = 1 - \frac{1}{x} + \frac{1}{2x^2} + \ldots, \qquad c_{-1} = -1, \tag{9.238a–c}$$

and (iv) the exponential (9.7b) of minus the inverse of the independent variable (9.238a) has an essential singularity (9.238b) at the origin with residue minus unity (9.238c).

The residue at a simple pole (9.232a, b) ≡ (9.239a) [pole of order M (9.231a, b) ≡ (9.240a)] is given (standard CCLVII) by (9.239b) [(9.240b)]:

$$y(x) = \frac{c_{-1}}{x} + \sum_{n=0}^{\infty} c_n\, x^n: \qquad c_{-1} = \lim_{x\to 0} x\, y(x); \tag{9.239a, b}$$

$$y(x) = \frac{c_{-M}}{x^M} + \ldots. + \frac{c_{-1}}{x} + \sum_{n=0}^{\infty} b_n\, x^n: \qquad c_{-1} = \frac{1}{(M-1)!} \lim_{x\to 0} \frac{d^{M-1}}{dx^{M-1}}\left[x^M\, y(x)\right]. \tag{9.240a, b}$$

The residue at a simple pole (9.239b) follows immediately from (9.239a); the residue at a pole of order M in (9.240b) ≡ (I.15.33b) includes the case (9.239b) of the simple pole for $M = 1$. The proof of (9.240b) is made in three steps: (i) multiplication of the function (9.240a) by the M-th power eliminates the pole and leads to an analytic function (9.241a):

$$x^M y(x) = c_{-M} + \ldots + c_{-1} x^{M-1} + \sum_{n=0}^{\infty} c_n\, x^{n+M}; \tag{9.241a}$$

$$\frac{d^{M-1}}{dx^{N-1}}\left[x^M\, y(x)\right] = (M-1)!\, c_{-1} + \sum_{n=0}^{\infty} \frac{(n+M)!}{n!} c_n\, x^{n+1}, \tag{9.241b}$$

(ii) differentiating $(M - 1)$ times puts the residue c_{-1} multiplied by $(M - 1)!$ as the leading term in (9.241b); and (iii) the limit $x \to 0$ eliminates all the remaining terms proving (9.240b). QED. *The two types of isolated singularities of a single-valued function have (standard CCLVIII) distinct properties: (i) a pole (9.231a, b) is eliminated by multiplication (9.241a) by the M-th power leading to a regular point (9.233a, b); (ii) an essential singularity (9.230a, b) cannot be removed by multiplication by any integral power.* The calculation of the residue at a simple or multiple pole of a complex single-valued function applies in particular to a rational function (sections I.38.1–I.38.2) in which case it leads to partial fraction decompositions (subsections 1.5.3–1.5.4) and the extended residue rule. The main singularities of single(multi)-valued complex functions [subsection 9.4.1 (9.4.3)] are poles and essential singularities (subsection 9.4.2) [branch-points (subsection 9.4.4)].

9.4.3 Sheets of the Riemann Surface of a Multi-Valued Function

A multi-valued function (Figure 9.8b) assigns to a single point (9.242a) in the domain (9.242b) at least two distinct point (9.242c) in the range:

$$\mathcal{V}_2: \qquad \exists_{x \in D} \ \exists_{y_1; y_2 \in E}: \qquad y_1(x) \neq y_2(x), \tag{9.242a–c}$$

each corresponding to a different **branch** of the function and represented in a different plane or sheet. The sheets may be connected, forming a **Riemann surface** (chapter I.7) as briefly explained next. The independent variable is a complex number in the Cartesian (9.243a) [polar (9.243b)] representation consisting of a real (9.243c) and an imaginary (9.243d) part [a modulus (9.243e) and an argument (9.243f)]:

$$x = \zeta + i\eta = re^{i\phi}: \qquad \zeta = \mathrm{Re}(x), \quad \eta = \mathrm{Im}(x), \tag{9.243a–d}$$

$$r \equiv |x| = \left|\zeta^2 + \eta^2\right|^{1/2}, \quad \phi \equiv \arg(x) = arc\tan\left(\frac{\eta}{\zeta}\right). \tag{9.243e, f}$$

The multiplication (9.244c) by unity (9.244a) any number of times (9.244b): (i) is equivalent to a rotation around the origin; (ii) does not change the point in the domain (9.244d):

$$e^{i2\pi} = 1; \qquad \forall_{n \in Z}: \qquad 1 = \left(e^{i2\pi}\right)^n = e^{i2\pi n}, \qquad x = xe^{i2\pi n}; \tag{9.244a–d}$$

and (iii) could change the branch in the range, implying that the sheets of the Riemann surface are connected.

As an example, consider the N-th root (9.245b) that (9.244d) is given by (9.245c–e):

$$n = 0,\ldots,N-1: \qquad \sqrt[N]{x} \equiv x^{1/N} = \left(x\,e^{i2\pi n}\right)^{1/N} = \left(\left|x\right| e^{i\phi+i2\pi n}\right)^{1/N} = \left|x\right|^{1/N} e^{i\phi/N+i2\pi n/N}, \tag{9.245a–e}$$

implying that there are N distinct roots (9.245a). Multiplying by (9.244a) does not change the variable x in (9.244d) but changes its N-th root to the next branch in (9.245e). Thus the N sheets of the Riemann surface for the N-th root are connected (Figure 9.10a) and multiplying (dividing) by (9.244a) in the domain passes to the next (preceding) sheet in the range. All branches of the function coincide at the origin; that is, a **branch-point**; making a

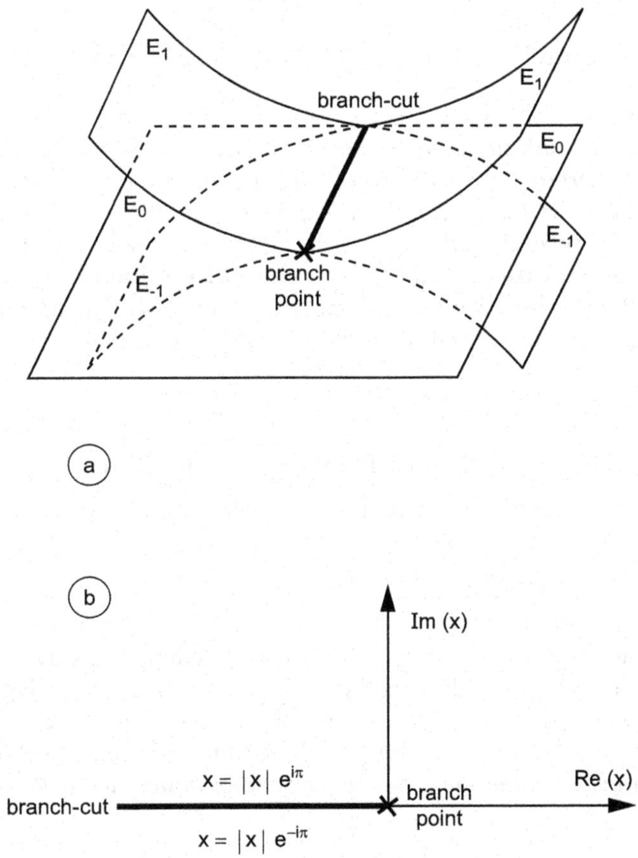

FIGURE 9.10
The range of a multi-valued function (Figure 9.8b) consists of several sheets joined (Figure 9.9a) at a branch-cut in the domain (Figure 9.9b) that should not be crossed in order to avoid passing to another sheet of the Riemann surface in the range.

semi-infinite **branch-cut** joining the origin to infinity, say along the negative x-axis (Figure 9.10b), prevents passage from one branch to another; thus the N-th root can be made **single-valued** choosing the principal branch (9.246b) in the complex-x **cut-plane**:

$$x \notin (-\infty, 0): \qquad x^{1/N} = |x|^{1/N} \exp\left(i\frac{\phi}{N}\right). \tag{9.246a, b}$$

The principal branch (9.246b) of the N-th root (9.245a–e) takes (standard CCLIX) distinct values (9.247a, b) above and below (Figure 9.10b) the branch-cut (9.247a):

$$\left(-|x| \pm i0\right)^{1/N} = \left(|x| e^{\pm i\pi}\right)^{1/N} = |x|^{1/N} e^{\pm i\pi/N}, \tag{9.247a, b}$$

$$\left(|x| e^{i\pi}\right)^{1/N} - \left(|x| e^{-i\pi}\right)^{1/N} = |x|^{1/N}\left(e^{i\pi/N} - e^{-i\pi/N}\right) = 2\, i|x|^{1/N} \sin\left(\frac{\pi}{N}\right), \tag{9.247c}$$

and thus: (i) is discontinuous across the branch-cut (9.247c); (ii) the discontinuity of $2\pi/N$ in the argument corresponds to changing to the next branch; and (iii) the branch-cut along the negative real axis does not include the origin (9.246a) because all roots take the same value zero there. The N-th root (logarithm) is an example of a **multi-valued (many-valued) function** with N branches (a denumerably infinite number of branches) and both can be made single-valued choosing the principal branch in the complex cut plane [subsection 9.4.3 (9.4.4)].

9.4.4 Principal Branch, Branch-Point, and Branch-Cut

The logarithm applied to (9.244a–d) leads to (9.248b):

$$n \in |N: \qquad \log x = \log\left(|x| e^{i\phi + i2\pi n}\right) = \log|x| + i\phi + i2\pi n, \tag{9.248a–c}$$

implying that it is a many-valued function with a denumerably infinite number of branches (9.248a) differing by multiples of 2π in the imaginary part. *The logarithm (9.248a–c) can be made (standard CCLX) single-valued choosing the principal branch (9.249b) in the complex-x cut-plane with the branch-cut (9.249a) joining the branch-point at the origin to the point at infinity along the negative real axis (Figure 9.10b):*

$$x \notin (-\infty, 0): \qquad \log x = \log|x| + i\phi. \tag{9.249a, b}$$

The branch-cut (9.246a) [(9.249a)] for the N-th root (9.246b) [logarithm (9.249b)] differ in that it includes $x = 0$ (excludes $x \neq 0$) the branch-point, because the function *is (is not) defined there. The principal branch of the logarithm (9.249b) takes different values (9.250a, b) above and below the branch-cut:*

$$\log\left(x e^{\pm i\pi}\right) = \log|x| \pm i\pi, \qquad \log\left(x e^{\pm i\pi}\right) - \log\left(x e^{-i\pi}\right) = 2\pi i, \qquad \text{(9.250a–c)}$$

and thus is discontinuous across the branch-cut with a jump (9.243c) equal to the passage (9.249a–c) to the next branch. A single (multi)-valued function [subsection 9.4.1 (9.4.3)] can have several poles or essential singularities (branch-points) at $x = x_1, x_2, \ldots$ that can be translated to the origin [subsection 9.4.2 (9.4.4)] replacing x by $x - x_1, x - x_2, \ldots$

The power with complex base (9.246a) and exponent (9.251a) is (standard CCLXI) defined (9.251b) using the exponential and logarithm leading to the principal branch (9.251c) ≡ (9.251d):

$$a = \alpha + i\beta: \quad x^a \equiv \exp\left[\log\left(x^a\right)\right] = \exp\left(a \log x\right) = \exp\left\{(\alpha + i\beta)\left[\log|x| + i\phi\right]\right\}$$

$$= \exp\left[\alpha \log|x| - \beta\phi + i\beta \log|x| + i\alpha\phi\right] = |x|^\alpha e^{-\beta\phi} \exp\left\{i\left[\beta \log|x| + \alpha\phi\right]\right\}. \qquad \text{(9.251a–d)}$$

and therefore has modulus (9.252a) and argument (9.252b):

$$\left|x^a\right| = |x|^\alpha e^{-\beta\phi}, \qquad \arg\left(x^a\right) = \beta \log|x| + \alpha\,\phi. \qquad \text{(9.252a, b)}$$

In particular *the power with complex base and real exponent leads (standard CCLXII) to five cases:*

$$x^a \begin{cases} a \in |N: & \textit{zero of order } a, & \text{(9.253a)} \\ a = 0: & \textit{finite value unity: } x^0 = 1, & \text{(9.253b)} \\ -a \in |N: & \textit{pole of order } a, & \text{(9.253c)} \\ a = \dfrac{n}{m} \in |Q: & m\textit{-valued function} & \text{(9.253d)} \\ a \in |R - |Q: & \textit{many-valued function} & \text{(9.253e)} \end{cases}$$

namely: (i) an **ordinary point** *for non-negative integer exponent corresponding to the finite value unity (9.253b) [**zero of order N** (9.253a)] for zero (positive) integer exponent; (ii) a pole of order m (9.253c) for exponent a negative integer; (iii) a multi-valued function with m branches (9.253d) if the exponent is a rational number n/m in its lowest terms; (iv) a many-valued function with an infinite number of branches (9.253e) if the exponent is an irrational number.* Thus an ordinary point is a regular point that is not a zero; a branch-point may correspond to a multi-(many-) valued function with a finite (denumerably infinite) number of branches and a single principal branch in all cases. The singularities of single(multi)-valued functions [subsections 9.4.1–9.4.2 (9.4.3–9.4.4)] play a fundamental role in the classification and solution of linear differential equations with variable coefficients (subsection 9.4.5).

9.4.5 Regular Points and Regular/Irregular Singularities

The simplest linear unforced ordinary differential equation is of first order (3.19a) ≡ (9.254a) with integrable coefficient (9.254b) and has solution or integral (3.20a, b) ≡ (9.254c):

$$P \in \mathcal{E}(|C): \; y' + P(x)y = 0: \; y(x) = C\exp\left\{ -\int^{x} P(\xi)\,d\xi \right\}; \; P \in \mathcal{A}(|C) \Rightarrow y \in A\,(|C), \tag{9.254a–d}$$

where C is an arbitrary constant, leading to three cases (Table 9.3). Case I, when $x = 0$, is a **analytic point** of the differential equation; the coefficient $P(x)$ is an analytic function (9.254d) and the solution (9.254c) is also (9.254e) an **analytic integral.** Case II of a **regular singularity** of the differential equation corresponds to: (i) the coefficient with a simple pole (9.255a, b) with residue $-a$:

$$p \in \mathcal{A}(|C); \; P(x) = -\frac{a}{x} + p(x): \tag{9.255a, b}$$

$$\begin{aligned} y(x) &= C\exp\left\{ \int^{x} \left[\frac{a}{\xi} - p(\xi) \right] d\xi \right\} = C\exp\left\{ a\log x - \int^{x} p(\xi)\,d\xi \right\} \\ &= C x^{a} \exp\left\{ -\int^{x} p(\xi)\,d\xi \right\}, \end{aligned} \tag{9.255c–e}$$

TABLE 9.3

First-Order Linear Differential Equation: Classification of Points and Integrals

	Differential Equation			Solution or Integral		
Case	**Point**	**Coefficient**	**Equation**	**Integral**	**Equation**	**To be Determined**
I	regular	analytic (9.254c) ≡ (9.258a)	(9.254b)	analytic (9.254d)	(9.258b)	coefficients $c_o\, c_1, \ldots, c_n \ldots$
II	regular singularity	Simple pole (9.255a, b)	(9.259a)	regular integral	(9.259b)	index a plus coefficients $c_o(a),\, c_1(a), \ldots,\, c_n(a), \ldots$
III	pole of order M or essential singularity $M = \infty$	(9.256a, b)	(9.260a)	irregular integral	(9.260b)	index a plus coefficients $c_o(a), c_{\pm 1}(a), \ldots,\, c_{\pm n}(a), \ldots$

* to be determined as part of the solution

(ii) the solution (9.255c, d) is a **regular integral of the first kind** (9.255e) multiplying an analytic function by a power that may have a branch-point. The remaining case III of an **irregular singularity** of the differential equation corresponds to: (i) a coefficient (9.256a, b) that has a pole of order $\infty > M \geq 2$ or an essential singularity $M = \infty$; (ii) a solution (9.256c, d) that multiplies the power and analytic function as before:

$$p(x) \in \mathcal{A}(|C); \qquad P(x) = \sum_{m=2}^{M} p_{-m}\, x^{-m} - \frac{a}{x} + p(x): \tag{9.256a, b}$$

$$y(x) = C\exp\left\{\int\left(\frac{a}{\xi} - p(\xi) - \sum_{m=2}^{M} p_{-m}\xi^{-n}\right)d\xi\right\} = C\,x^{a}\exp\left\{-\int^{x} p(\xi)\,d\xi\right\}X(x), \tag{9.256c, d}$$

by an extra factor (9.257a, b):

$$\begin{aligned} X(x) &= \exp\left\{-\sum_{m=2}^{M}\int^{x} p_{-m}\xi^{-m}\,d\xi\right\} = \exp\left[\sum_{m=2}^{M}\frac{p_{-m}}{m-1}x^{1-m}\right] \\ &= \sum_{k=0}^{\infty}\frac{1}{k!}\left(\sum_{m=2}^{M}\frac{p_{-m}}{m-1}x^{1-m}\right)^{k} = \sum_{n=1}^{\infty} q_n\, x^{-n}, \end{aligned} \tag{9.257a–d}$$

that leads (9.7b) = (9.257c) to an essential singularity (9.257d) with coefficients q_n; thus (iii) the **irregular integral of the first kind** consists of the product of an analytic function by a power (9.256c) by an essential singularity (9.257d). Thus the classification of regular points (regular/irregular singularities) of a differential equation (subsection 9.4.5) leads the identification of the corresponding solutions (subsection 9.4.6) as analytic (regular/irregular) integrals.

9.4.6 Analytic, Regular, and Irregular Integrals

It has been shown that *the unforced linear first-order differential equation (9.254b) with integrable coefficient (9.254a) can (standard CCLXIII) have three types of solutions (9.254c), namely (Table 9.3): (case I) near a regular point of the differential equation (9.254b) the coefficient is an analytic function (9.258a):*

$$P(x) = \sum_{k=0}^{\infty} p_k x^k: \qquad y(x) = \sum_{n=0}^{\infty} c_n\, x^n, \tag{9.258a, b}$$

and the solution is (9.254c) an analytic integral (9.258b) with ***coefficients*** c_n *of the power series expansion to be determined; (case II) near a regular singularity* *of the differential equation (9.254b) the coefficient has a simple pole (9.259a) with residue −a:*

$$P(x) = -\frac{a}{x} + \sum_{k=0}^{\infty} p_k x^k: \qquad y(x) = x^a \sum_{n=0}^{\infty} c_n x^n, \tag{9.259a, b}$$

and the solution is a regular integral (9.259b) including multiplication by a power whose exponent is the ***index*** *a; (case III) in the remaining case, that is near an irregular singularity of the differential equation (9.254b), the coefficient (9.260a) has a pole of order M or an essential singularity M = ∞:*

$$P(x) = \sum_{m=2}^{M} p_{-m} x^{-m} - \frac{a}{x} + \sum_{k=0}^{\infty} p_k x^k: \qquad y(x) = x^a \sum_{\substack{n=-\infty \\ n \neq -1}}^{\infty} c_n x^n, \tag{9.260a, b}$$

and the solution is an irregular integral (9.260b) multiplying a power by a Laurent series of ascending and descending powers.

In all cases I to III, the radius of convergence of the series solutions around the point x_1 is the circle with center at x_1 and radius $R < |x_2 - x_1|$ excluding the nearest singularity (Figure 9.11a). If there are several singularities $x_1, x_2\,(x_3)$ and the respective ***circles of convergence*** *overlap, the solutions must coincide in the overlapping regions and are thus extended by* ***analytic continuation*** *(section I.31.1) outside the original radius of convergence [Figure 9.11a (b)].* The three types of integrals possible for a linear first-order differential equation also apply to autonomous system and differential equations of higher orders, with several indices; if the indices coincide the powers x^a also coincide and linearly independent integrals require logarithmic factors; the logarithmic factor may also occur if the indices differ by an integer (sections 9.5 and 9.7). A simple example is a linear second-order differential equation with homogenous coefficients (9.261a) with exponents (9.261b) corresponding to the indices (9.261c, d):

$$x^2 y'' - (\alpha + \beta - 1)\, x y' + \alpha\beta y = 0: \quad y(x) = x^a,$$

$$0 = a^2 - (\alpha + \beta)\, a + \alpha\beta = (a - \alpha)(a - \beta). \tag{9.261a–d}$$

If the indices are distinct (9.262a) [coincide (9.262c)], the general integral is [subsection 1.6.2 (1.6.3)] a linear combination of powers (9.262b) [involves a logarithmic factor (9.262d)]:

$$\alpha \neq \beta: \quad y(x) = A x^\alpha + B x^\beta; \qquad \alpha = \beta: \quad y(x) = x^\alpha (A + B \log x), \tag{9.262a–d}$$

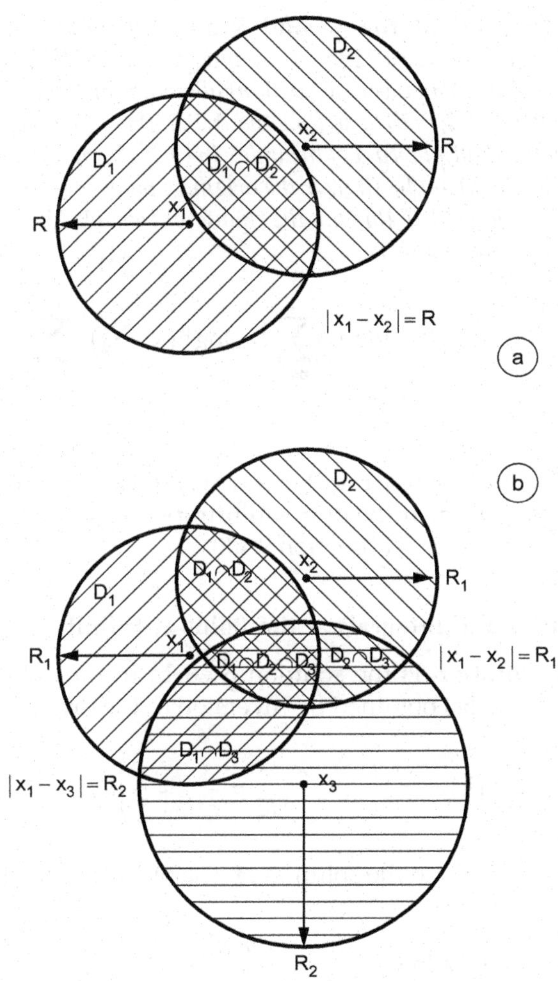

FIGURE 9.11
The Laurent series (Figure 9.10a) around two isolated singularities x_1 and x_2, both have radius of convergence $|x_2 - x_1| = R$ and their coincidence in the overlapping region $D_1 \cap D_2$ allows (a) analytic continuation between the annuli $D_{1,2} \equiv \left\{ |x - x_{1,2}| < R \right\}$. If there are several isolated singularities $x_1, x_2, x_3, \ldots$ the analytic continuation can be performed (b) along a sequence of overlapping annuli, specifying a monogenic function.

where (A, B) are arbitrary constants. This suggests that *the most general form of a particular solution of a linear differential equation of order N with variable coefficients near an isolated singularity (9.263a):*

$$\sum_{n=0}^{N} A_n(x) \frac{d^n y}{dx^n} = 0: \qquad y(x) = x^a \sum_{\beta=0}^{\alpha-1} b_\beta \log^\beta x \sum_{\substack{n=-M \\ n\neq -1}}^{+\infty} c_{n,\beta}\, x^n, \qquad (9.263\text{a, b})$$

is a **irregular integral of the second kind** *(9.263b) multiplying (standard CCLXIV): (i) a Laurent series (9.228a–c) allowing for a pole of order M (an essential singularity M = ∞): (ii/iii) a power (logarithm) allowing for the power (logarithmic) of branch-points (9.251a–d; 9.252a, b) [(9.249a, b; 9.250a–c)] with exponent specified by the index a [by the multiplicity α of the index in (9.263b, c)]. The integrals (9.258b; 9.259b; 9.260b; 9.263a, b) apply: (i) near the origin as power series in x; (ii) near any point x_0 in the finite plane (9.264b) with the change of variable (9.264a) leading to the expansion (9.264d) near (9.264c):*

$$\bar{x} = x - x_0: \quad |x_0| < \infty \Rightarrow \bar{x} = 0: \quad y(x) = \sum_{\beta=0}^{\alpha-1} g_\beta \log^\beta (x - x_0) \sum_{\substack{n=-\infty \\ n\neq -1}}^{+\infty} c_{n,\beta} (x - x_0)^{a+n}. \tag{9.264a–d}$$

The case M = 0 in (9.263b) is a **regular integral of the second kind.** The singularities and integrals near the point-at-infinity are not included in (9.264a–d) and are considered next (subsection 9.4.7).

9.4.7 Singularities and Integrals at the Point-at-Infinity

The **asymptotic solution** is the solution (9.265b) in a neighborhood of the **point-at-infinity** (9.265c) obtained by inversion of the origin (9.265a):

$$\xi \equiv \frac{1}{x}: \qquad y(x) \equiv w(\xi) = w\left(\frac{1}{x}\right), \qquad \frac{dw}{d\xi} = \frac{1}{\xi^2} P\left(\frac{1}{\xi}\right) w, \tag{9.265a–c}$$

and corresponds (9.265b) to the solution of (9.266) ≡ (9.265c) for large x:

$$P\left(\frac{1}{\xi}\right) w(\xi) = P(x) y(x) = -\frac{dy}{dx} = -\frac{dw}{d\xi}\frac{d\xi}{dx} = \frac{1}{x^2}\frac{dw}{d\xi} = \xi^2 \frac{dw}{d\xi}. \tag{9.266}$$

The point at infinity (9.267a) for x corresponds to the origin (9.267b) for ξ and to the **asymptotic coefficient** (9.267c) in (9.267d):

$$x \to \infty, \qquad \xi \to 0: \qquad P_1(\xi) = -\frac{1}{\xi^2} P\left(\frac{1}{\xi}\right), \qquad \frac{dw}{d\xi} + P_1(\xi)\, w = 0, \tag{9.267a–d}$$

leading to three cases. Case I of (9.258a) an **analytic asymptotic integral** (9.268c) corresponds to the asymptotic coefficient (9.268a) ≡ (9.268b) decaying like x^{-2}:

$$P(x) = -\frac{1}{x^2} P_1\left(\frac{1}{x}\right) = -\sum_{k=0}^{\infty} p_k\, x^{-k-2} \sim O\left(\frac{1}{x^2}\right): \qquad y(x) = \sum_{n=0}^{\infty} c_n\, x^{-n}. \tag{9.268a–c}$$

Case II of (9.259a) a **regular asymptotic integral** (9.269b) corresponds to a asymptotic coefficient (9.269a) decaying like x^{-1}:

$$P(x) = \frac{a}{x} - \sum_{k=0}^{\infty} p_k x^{-k-2} \sim O\left(\frac{1}{x}\right): \qquad y(x) = x^{-a} \sum_{n=0}^{\infty} c_n x^{-n}. \tag{9.269a, b}$$

Case III of (9.260a) an **irregular asymptotic integral** corresponds to a coefficient (9.206a) not decaying at infinity:

$$P(x) = -\sum_{m=2}^{M} p_{-m} x^{m-2} + \frac{a}{x} - \sum_{k=0}^{\infty} p_k x^{-k-2}: \qquad y(x) = x^{-a} \sum_{n=-\infty}^{+\infty} c_n x^{n}. \tag{9.270a, b}$$

Thus *an unforced linear differential equation of the first order (9.254b) ≡ (9.265b, c) has asymptotic solution (9.265a; 9.267c, d) for (9.265a; 9.267a, b) large x that can be (standard CCLXV) of three types: (I) an asymptotic analytic integral (9.268c) if the coefficient decays (9.268a, b) like x^{-2}; (II) an asymptotic regular integral (9.269b) if the coefficient decays (9.269a) like x^{-1}; (III) an asymptotic irregular integral (9.270b) if the coefficient (9.270a) does not decay at infinity.* The classification of singularities and integrals of an unforced linear differential equation of first-order (subsections 9.4.5–9.4.7) can be extended to linear autonomous systems of differential equations (subsections 9.4.8–9.4.9).

9.4.8 Linear Autonomous System with Analytic Coefficients

The linear autonomous system of ordinary differential equations (9.271a, b) with integrable matrix of coefficients (9.271c) has general integral (9.271d):

$$m, n = 1, \dots, N: \qquad \frac{dy_m}{dx} + \sum_{n=1}^{N} P_{n,m}(x) y_n(x) = 0, \tag{9.271a, b}$$

$$P_{m,n} \in \mathcal{E}(|C): \qquad y_m(x) = \sum_{n=1}^{N} C_n \exp\left\{-\int^x P_{n,m}(\xi)\, d\xi\right\}, \tag{9.271c, d}$$

with C_n arbitrary constants, because differentiation of (9.271d) leads back to (9.272a, b) ≡ (9.271a, b):

$$\begin{aligned} k, m, n = 1, \dots, N: \qquad \frac{dy_m}{dx} &= \frac{d}{dx}\left[\sum_{k=1}^{N} C_k \exp\left\{-\int^x P_{k,m}(\xi)\, d\xi\right\}\right] \\ &= -\sum_{k,n=1}^{N} C_k \exp\left\{-\int^x P_{k,n}(\xi)\, d\xi\right\} P_{n,m}(x) \\ &= -\sum_{n=1}^{N} P_{n,m}(x) y_n(x). \end{aligned} \tag{9.272a, b}$$

The exponential of a matrix (9.273a) in (9.271d) is interpreted as the exponential series (9.7b) of matrices (9.273b):

$$A_{mn}(x) = -\int^{x} P_{mn}(\xi)\, d\xi: \qquad \exp(A_{mn}) = \sum_{k=0}^{\infty} \frac{(A_{mn})^k}{k!}, \tag{9.273a, b}$$

where: (i) the power with exponent zero is the identity matrix (9.274a); (ii) the exponent unity corresponds to the matrix itself (9.274b); (iii) the square is the product of the matrix by itself (9.274c):

$$(A_{ij})^0 \equiv \delta_{ij}, \; (A_{ij})^1 \equiv A_{ij}, \qquad (A_{ij})^2 \equiv \sum_{k=1}^{N} A_{ik} A_{kj}, \; (A_{ij})^{n+1} \equiv \sum_{k=1}^{N} (A_{ik})^n (A_{kj}), \tag{9.274a–d}$$

and (iv) the $(n + 1)$-th power is defined (9.274d) by recurrence as the n-th power multiplied by the matrix.

Substituting (9.274a–d) in (9.273b) it follows that the exponential of a matrix is given by (9.275):

$$\exp(A_{ij}) = \delta_{ij} + A_{ij} + \frac{1}{2!}\sum_{k=1}^{N} A_{ik} A_{kj} + \frac{1}{3!}\sum_{k,\ell=1}^{N} A_{ik} A_{k\ell} A_{\ell j} + \ldots. \tag{9.275}$$

where a repeated index implies a summation from 1 to N, for example $k = 1, 2, \ldots, N = \ell$. If the matrix is bounded (9.276a) then: (i) its square is bounded by (9.276b) because it consists of the sum of N terms with bound B^2; and (ii) each extra power adds N terms multiplied by B leading to (9.276c):

$$|A_{mn}| < B: \qquad \left|(A_{mn})^2\right| \le N B^2, \qquad \left|(A_{mn})^k\right| \le N^{k-1} B^k; \tag{9.276a–c}$$

thus the exponential series (9.273b) of a bounded matrix (9.276a) is bounded in modulus by (9.277a–c):

$$|\exp(A_{mn})| \le \sum_{k=0}^{\infty} \frac{\left|(A_{mn})^k\right|}{k!} \le \frac{1}{N}\sum_{k=0}^{\infty} \frac{(NB)^k}{k!} = \frac{e^{NB}}{N}. \tag{9.277a–c}$$

It has been shown that *the exponential (9.273b; 9.274a–d) ≡ (9.275) of a bounded matrix (9.276a) has (standard CCLXVI) the upper bound (9.277c) for its modulus.* Thus *the linear autonomous system of differential equations (9.271a, b) with integrable coefficients (9.271c) ≡ (9.278a) has (standard CCLXVII) general integral (9.271d) specified by an exponential (9.273b; 9.274a–d) ≡ (9.275) of bounded functions (9.273a; 9.276a) ≡ (9.278b) that is bounded in modulus by (9.277c):*

$$P_{mn} \in \mathcal{E}(|C) \Rightarrow A_{mn} \in \mathcal{B}(|C); \qquad P_{mn} \in \mathcal{A}(|C) \Rightarrow y_n \in \mathcal{A}(|C). \tag{9.278a–d}$$

In addition, *if the linear autonomous system of differential equations (9.271a, b) has (standard CCLXVIII) coefficients that: (i) are analytic the integrals are analytic; (ii) have simple poles the integrals are regular; and (iii) have multiple poles or essential singularities the integrals are irregular.* The last result (9.278c, d) applies to linear differential equations of any order (subsection 9.4) because they are reducible to a linear autonomous system (subsections 7.1.1 and 9.1.18).

9.4.9 Linear Differential Equation with Analytic Coefficients

The linear differential equation (9.279c) of order N with analytic coefficients (9.279a, b):

$$s = 0,\dots,N-1: \qquad P_s \in \mathcal{A}(|C): \qquad \frac{d^N y}{dx^N} + \sum_{s=0}^{N-1} P_s(x)\frac{d^s y}{dx^s} = 0, \tag{9.279a–c}$$

is equivalent to the linear autonomous system of differential equations (9.280a, b) with analytic coefficients:

$$y_s(x) \equiv y^{(s)}(x) = y'_{s-1}(x), \qquad \frac{dy_N}{dx} = -\sum_{s=0}^{N-1} P_s(x)\, y_s(x): \quad y(x) = \sum_{n=0}^{\infty} c_n x^n, \tag{9.280a–c}$$

and thus has analytic solutions (9.280c). In particular, the linear second-order differential equation (5.220b) ≡ (9.281a) is reducible via a change of dependent variable (5.241c) ≡ (9.281b):

$$z'' + P(x)\, z' + Q(x) z = 0: \qquad z(x) = y(x)\exp\left\{-\frac{1}{2}\int^x P(\xi)\, d\xi\right\}, \tag{9.281a, b}$$

to the invariant (5.245c) ≡ (9.282b) form omitting the first-order derivative (5.242b) = (9.282a):

$$y'' + I(x) y = 0, \qquad I(x) = Q(x) - \frac{P'(x)}{2} - \frac{[P(x)]^2}{4}. \tag{9.282a, b}$$

If the coefficients in the general form (9.281a) are analytic (9.283a, b), then the coefficient (9.282b) in the invariant form (9.282a) is also analytic (9.283c) and has Maclaurin series (9.283d):

$$P, Q \in \mathcal{A}(|C) \;\Rightarrow\; I \in \mathcal{A}(|C) \;\Rightarrow\; I(x) = \sum_{n=0}^{\infty} I_n x^n. \tag{9.283a–d}$$

It has been shown *that a linear ordinary differential equation (9.279c) of any order N with analytic coefficients (9.279a, b) has (standard CCLIX) analytic solutions (9.280c). In particular, for N = 2 the linear second-order differential equation (9.281a) with analytic coefficients (9.283a, b) has (standard CCLX) an analytic transformation (9.281b) to the invariant form (9.282a) with analytic (9.283d) coefficient (9.282b).* These results hold for a neighborhood of the origin, or by translation $y = x - a$ to a neighborhood of any point $x = a$ in the finite real line or complex plane. The method of explicit calculation of the analytic solution is illustrated next (subsection 9.4.10) for the linear second-order differential equation (9.282a).

9.4.10 Calculation of the Coefficients of the Analytic Solution

It has been shown (subsection 9.4.9) that the linear second-order differential equation (9.282a) with analytic coefficient (9.282b) has a Maclaurin series solution (9.280c) ≡ (9.284c), where the first two coefficients (9.284a, b) are arbitrary constants determined by two single-point boundary conditions:

$$c_0 = y(0) \equiv y_0, \qquad c_1 = y'(0) \equiv y_0' : \qquad y(x) = c_0 + c_1 x + \sum_{n=2}^{\infty} c_n x^n; \qquad (9.284\text{a–c})$$

to obtain the general integral all the remaining coefficients in (9.284c) must be expressed (9.285b, c) as linear functions of (c_0, c_1) involving only the coefficients in the invariant (9.283d; 9.285a):

$$n = 0,\ldots,\infty,\ k = 2,\ldots,\infty: \qquad c_k = c_0\, d_k(I_n) + c_1\, e_k(I_n). \qquad (9.285\text{a–c})$$

The coefficients (d_k, e_k) in (9.285c) can be determined by two equivalent methods. Method I has three steps: (i) the differential equation (9.282a) is differentiated n-times (9.286a) using the Leibnitz chain rule (I.13.31) = (9.286b):

$$y^{(n+2)}(x) = -\frac{d^n}{dx^n}\left[I(x)y(x)\right] = -\sum_{k=0}^{n}\binom{n}{k} I^{(k)}(x)\, y^{(n-k)}(x); \qquad (9.286\text{a, b})$$

(ii) the Maclaurin series (9.233a, b) for the analytic integral (9.280c) [invariant (9.283d)] have coefficients (9.287a) [(9.287b)] related by (9.287c):

$$n!\{c_n, I_n\} = \left\{y^{(n)}(0), \quad I^{(n)}(0)\right\}:$$

$$(n+2)!\,c_{n+2} = y^{(n+2)}(0) = -\sum_{k=0}^{n}\frac{n!}{k!(n-k)!} I^{(k)}(0)\, y^{n-k}(0) = -n!\sum_{k=0}^{n} I_k c_{n-k}; \qquad (9.287\text{a–d})$$

(ii) substitution of (9.287a–c) in (9.286b) with $x = 0$ leads to (9.287d) ≡ (9.288):

$$c_{n+2} = -\frac{1}{(n+2)(n+1)} \sum_{k=0}^{n} I_k \, c_{n-k} \,. \tag{9.287e}$$

Thus all coefficients can be determined iteratively (1.288a–n):

$n = 0$:
$$c_2 = -\frac{1}{2.1} \sum_{k=0}^{0} I_k \, c_{-k} = -\frac{1}{2} I_0 \, c_0 \,, \tag{9.288a–c}$$

$n = 1$:
$$c_3 = -\frac{1}{3.2} \sum_{k=0}^{1} I_k \, c_{1-k} = -\frac{1}{6}\left(I_0 \, c_1 + I_1 \, c_0\right), \tag{9.288d–f}$$

$n = 2$:
$$\begin{aligned} c_4 &= -\frac{1}{4.3} \sum_{k=0}^{2} I_k \, c_{2-k} = -\frac{1}{12}\left(I_0 \, c_2 + I_1 \, c_1 + I_2 \, c_0\right) \\ &= \left(\frac{1}{24} I_0^2 - \frac{1}{12} I_2\right) c_0 - \frac{1}{12} I_1 \, c_1 \,, \end{aligned} \tag{9.288g–j}$$

$n = 3$:
$$\begin{aligned} c_5 &= -\frac{1}{5.4} \sum_{k=0}^{3} I_k \, c_{3-k} = -\frac{1}{20}\left(I_0 \, c_3 + I_1 \, c_2 + I_2 \, c_1 + I_3 \, c_0\right) \\ &= \left(\frac{1}{30} I_0 I_1 - \frac{1}{20} I_3\right) c_0 + \left(\frac{1}{120} I_0^2 - \frac{1}{20} I_2\right) c_1 \,; \end{aligned} \tag{9.288k–n}$$

the substitution of (9.288c, f) in (9.288i) [(9.288m)] leads to (9.288j) [(9.288n)] as linear combinations of (c_0, c_1), with coefficients depending on I_k as stated in (9.285a–c). Thus *the recurrence formula (standard CCLXI) specifies the coefficients* c_{n+2} *of the analytic integral (9.284c) of the linear second-order differential equation (9.282a) with analytic coefficient (9.283d) as linear functions of the preceding coefficients* $c_n, c_{n-1}, \ldots, c_1, c_0$ *involving* $I_0, \ldots, I_n$*; applying (9.287e) by recurrence n-times leads to (9.285a–c) involving the two single-point boundary conditions (9.284a, b).* The same results can be obtained by another method II of direct substitution of the series into differential equation (subsection 9.4.11). Method II does not depend on the coefficients and solution being integral functions and applies also to regular (irregular) singularities and integrals [section(s) 9.5 (9.6–9.7)].

9.4.11 Two Methods to Obtain the Recurrence Relation for the Coefficients

Substituting in the linear second-order differential equation (9.282a) both the analytic solution (9.280c) and coefficient (9.283d) leads to (9.289):

$$0=\sum_{m=2}^{\infty} c_m\, x^{m-2} m(m-1)+\sum_{q,k=0}^{\infty} I_k\, c_q\, x^{k+q}. \tag{9.289}$$

The changes in variables of summation (9.290a, b) led to (9.290c):

$$n=m-2, \quad k+q=n: \qquad 0=\sum_{n=0}^{\infty} x^n\left[(n+1)(n+2)c_{n+2}+\sum_{k=0}^{\infty} I_k\, c_{n-k}\right]. \tag{9.290a–c}$$

The coefficients of all powers of x must vanish in (9.290c) leading to the recurrence formula for the coefficients (9.291a):

$$(n+1)(n+2)c_{n+2}=-\sum_{k=0}^{n} I_k\, c_{n-k}=-I_0\, c_n-I_1\, c_{n-1}\ldots-I_{n-1}\, c_1-I_n\, c_0, \tag{9.291a, b}$$

that: (i) coincides with (9.287e) ≡ (9.291a) obtained by method I; (ii) can be written explicitly (9.291b) with particular cases (9.288a–n); (iii) when applied n-times by recurrence leads to a linear combination (9.285a–c) of the arbitrary constants (c_0, c_1); and (iv) can be used to confirm (c_0, c_1) are arbitrary.

The latter point (iv) follows setting (9.292b, c) in (9.291a, b) leading to (9.292d, e) because (9.292a) do not exist in the analytic solution (9.280c):

$$0=c_{-1}=c_{-2}=\ldots: \qquad n=-2,-1 \quad \Rightarrow \quad 0.c_0=0=0.c_1; \tag{9.292a–e}$$

from (9.292d, e) it follows that (c_0, c_1) are arbitrary constants determined by the boundary conditions (9.284a, b). Also, all other coefficients are linear functions (9.285a–c) of (c_0, c_1), and substitution in (9.280c) leads to (9.293a):

$$y(x)=c_0+c_1\, x+\sum_{k=2}^{\infty} x^k\left(c_0\, d_k+c_1\, e_k\right)=c_0\, y_1(x)+c_1\, y_2(x); \tag{9.293a, b}$$

the general integral (9.293b) is a linear combination with arbitrary constants (c_0, c_1) of two particular integrals (9.294a) [(9.294c)]:

$$y_1(x)=1+\sum_{k=2}^{\infty} d_k\, x^k \sim O(1), \qquad y_2(x)=x+\sum_{k=2}^{\infty} e_k\, x^k \sim O(x), \tag{9.294a–d}$$

that are linearly independent because they have different orders (9.294b) [(9.294d)]. It has been shown that *the linear second-order differential equation in invariant form (9.282a) with analytic coefficient (9.283d) has (standard CCLXII) general integral (9.293a, b) where: (i) the arbitrary constants are determined by single-point boundary conditions (9.284a, b); and (ii) the coefficients (9.285a–c) of the first (second) linearly independent particular integrals (9.294a, b) [(9.294c, d)] follow from the recurrence formula (9.288) ≡ (9.291a) ≡ (9.291b).* The same method applies to a linear differential equation in the general form (9.281a, b). It is illustrated next for the generalized circular (hyperbolic) differential equations [subsections 9.4.12–9.4.15 (9.4.16–9.4.17)].

9.4.12 Generalized Hyperbolic Differential Equation

The **generalized hyperbolic differential equation** is defined as the linear second-order differential equation in invariant form (9.295a) with the **parameter** m:

$$y'' - x^m y = 0 \quad \Leftrightarrow \quad y(x) = c_0 \cosh(x;m) + c_1 \sinh(x;m). \qquad (9.295\text{a, b})$$

The case of order zero (9.296a) leads to the ordinary differential equation (9.296b) whose even (odd) solution is proportional to the hyperbolic cosine (9.296c) [sine (9.296d)]. This suggests the definition of **generalized circular cosine (sine)** as the solution (9.295b) of the generalized hyperbolic differential equation (9.295a) with parameter m, that reduces (9.296b) to the ordinary hyperbolic cosine (9.296c) [sine (9.296d)] for zero parameter (9.296a):

$$m = 0: \qquad y'' - y = 0, \quad \cosh(x;0) = \cosh x, \qquad \sinh(x;0) = \sinh x. \quad (9.296\text{a–d})$$

The constant coefficient –1 in (9.296b) is replaced by the power x^m in (9.295a). In the case of a non-negative integral power (9.297a), the differential equation (9.295a) has analytic coefficient and its solution is an analytic function (9.297c) in the finite complex x-plane of the independent variable (9.297b); that is, (subsection I.27.9.1) an integral function:

$$m \in |N_0; \qquad |x| < \infty: \qquad y(x) = \sum_{n=0}^{\infty} c_n x^n. \qquad (9.297\text{a–c})$$

Substituting (9.297c) in (9.295a) leads to (9.298c), and hence to (9.298d) with the changes of summation variables (9.298a, b):

$$p - 2 = n = k + m: \qquad 0 = \sum_{p=2}^{\infty} c_p\, p(p-1) x^{p-2} - \sum_{k=0}^{\infty} c_k\, x^{k+m}$$
$$= \sum_{n=0}^{\infty} x^n \left[c_{n+2} (n+1)(n+2) - c_{n-m} \right]. \qquad (9.298\text{a–d})$$

The coefficients of powers of x must vanish, leading to the recurrence formula for the coefficients (9.299b):

$$0 = c_{-1} = c_{-2} = \ldots : \qquad c_{n+2} = \frac{c_{n-m}}{(n+1)(n+2)}, \tag{9.299a, b}$$

where the coefficients (9.299a) vanish because they do not exist in the analytic solution (9.297c). The recurrence formula for the coefficients leads to the generalized hyperbolic cosine and sine functions (subsection 9.4.13).

9.4.13 Generalized Hyperbolic Cosine and Sine

Setting (9.300a) in (9.299b) leads to (9.300b):

$$n = m: \qquad c_{m+2} = \frac{c_0}{(m+1)(m+2)}, \tag{9.300a, b}$$

from which follows (9.301b, c) using (9.301a):

$$n = 2m+2: \qquad c_{2m+4} = \frac{c_{m+2}}{(2m+3)(2m+4)} = \frac{c_0}{(m+1)(m+2)(2m+3)(2m+4)}; \tag{9.301a–c}$$

by recurrence it follows that all coefficients of even order are proportional (9.302a, b) to c_0 that is arbitrary:

$$\begin{aligned} c_{pm+2p} &= \frac{c_0}{(m+1)(m+2)(2m+3)(2m+4)\cdots(pm+2p-1)(pm+2p)} \\ &= c_0 \prod_{k=1}^{p} \frac{1}{(km+2k-1)(km+2k)}; \end{aligned} \tag{9.302a, b}$$

$$\begin{aligned} c_{pm+2p+1} &= \frac{c_1}{(m+2)(m+3)(2m+4)(2m+5)\cdots(pm+2p)(pm+2p+1)} \\ &= c_1 \prod_{k=1}^{p} \frac{1}{(km+2k)(km+2k+1)}, \end{aligned} \tag{9.303a, b}$$

likewise the coefficients of odd order (9.303a) are all proportional (9.303b) to c_1 that is arbitrary. From (9.299a, b) it follows that all coefficients other than

(9.302a, b; 9.303a, b) are zero; thus substituting (9.302b; 9.303b) in (9.297c) leads to the general integral:

$$y(x)=\sum_{n=0}^{\infty} c_n\, x^n=\sum_{p=0}^{\infty} c_{pm+2p}\, x^{mp+2p}+\sum_{n=0}^{\infty} c_{nm+2n+1}\, x^{mp+2p+1}, \tag{9.304}$$

that is of the form (9.295b) with:

$$\cosh(x;m)=1+\sum_{n=1}^{\infty} x^{mn+2n}\prod_{k=1}^{n}\frac{1}{(mk+2k-1)(mk+2k)}, \tag{9.305}$$

$$\sinh(x;m)=x+\sum_{n=1}^{\infty} x^{mn+2n+1}\sum_{k=1}^{n}\frac{1}{(mk+2k)(mk+2k+1)}, \tag{9.306}$$

where only the non-zero coefficients were retained.

It has been shown that *the general integral (9.295b) of the second-order linear ordinary differential equation (9.295a) with analytic non-negative integral power coefficient (9.297a) is (standard CCLXIII) a linear combination with arbitrary constants* $c_0\,(c_1)$ *of the (9.305) [(9.306)]* ***generalized hyperbolic cosine (sine)*** *with parameter m. The generalized hyperbolic cosine (sine) are most conveniently calculated using the recurrence relations (9.307a–c) [(9.308a–c)]:*

$$\cosh(x;m)=\sum_{n=0}^{\infty} u_n(x;m):\qquad u_0(x;m)=1,\ u_n(x;m)=u_{n-1}(x;m)\frac{x^{m+2}}{(nm+2n-1)(nm+2n)}, \tag{9.307a–c}$$

$$\sinh(x;m)=\sum_{n=0}^{\infty} v_n(x;m):\qquad v_0(x;m)=x,\ v_n(x;m)=v_{n-1}(x;m)\frac{x^{m+2}}{(nm+2n)(nm+2n+1)}. \tag{9.308a–c}$$

The particular case of zero parameter (9.309a) leads in (9.305) [(9.306)] to the original hyperbolic cosine (9.309b) ≡ (II.7.6b) [sine (9.309c) ≡ (II.7.7b)] that are solutions of (9.296b):

$$m=0:\quad \cosh(x;0)=\sum_{n=0}^{\infty}\frac{x^{2n}}{(2n)!}\equiv\cosh x,\quad \sinh(x;0)=\sum_{n=0}^{\infty}\frac{x^{2n+1}}{(2n+1)!}=\sinh x. \tag{9.309a–c}$$

The Airy (1838) differential equation is a particular case (subsection 9.4.14) of the generalized hyperbolic differential equation (subsection 9.4.12) with parameter unity and thus the Airy functions of the first and second type coincide respectively with the generalized hyperbolic cosine and sine with parameter unity.

9.4.14 Airy (1838) Differential Equation and Functions

The generalized hyperbolic differential equation (9.295a) with parameter unity (9.310a) coincides with the **Airy (1838) differential equation** (9.310b):

$$m=1: \qquad y''-xy=0, \qquad y(x)=c_0\,Ai(x)+c_1\,Bi(x), \tag{9.310a–c}$$

and thus its solution is (standard CCLXIV) a linear combination (9.310c) of Airy first (9.311a–d) [second (9.312a–d)] functions that coincide with the generalized hyperbolic cosine (9.305) [sine (9.306)] with parameter unity:

$$\begin{aligned} Ai(x)&=\cosh(x;1)=1+\sum_{n=1}^{\infty}x^{3n}\prod_{k=1}^{n}\frac{1}{(3k-1)3k} \\ &=1+\frac{x^3}{2.3}+\frac{x^6}{2.3.5.6}+\frac{x^9}{2.3.5.6.8.9}+\ldots=1+\frac{x^3}{3!}+\frac{4}{6!}x^6+\frac{4.7}{9!}x^9+\ldots. \end{aligned} \tag{9.311a–d}$$

$$\begin{aligned} Bi(x)&=\sinh(x;1)=x+\sum_{n=1}^{\infty}x^{3n+1}\prod_{k=1}^{n}\frac{1}{3k(3k+1)} \\ &=x+\frac{x^4}{3.4}+\frac{x^7}{3.4.6.7}+\frac{x^{10}}{3.4.6.7.9.10}+\ldots=x+\frac{2}{4!}x^4+\frac{2.5}{7!}x^7+\frac{2.5.8}{10!}x^{10}+\ldots. \end{aligned} \tag{9.312a–d}$$

The generalized hyperbolic cosine (9.305) and sine (9.306) with parameters m may be considered as generalizations of respectively the hyperbolic cosine (9.309b) and sine (9.309c) [Airy first (9.311a–d) and second (9.312a–d)] functions that are the particular cases of parameter zero (unity).

9.4.15 Generalized Circular Cosine and Sine

A change of sign in the generalized hyperbolic differential equation (9.295a) leads to the **generalized circular differential equation** (9.313a) with parameter m:

$$y''+x^m y=0 \quad \Leftrightarrow \quad y(x)=b_0\cos(x;m)+b_1\sin(x;m), \tag{9.313a, b}$$

whose general integral (9.313b) is a linear combination with arbitrary constants (b_0,b_1) of the **generalized circular cosine and sine**, that reduce

(9.314b) to the original cosine (9.314c) and sine (9.314d) for zero parameter (9.314a):

$$m = 0: \qquad y'' + y = 0, \qquad \cos(x;0) = \cos x, \qquad \sin(x;0) = \sin x. \qquad \text{(9.314a–d)}$$

In the case of a non-negative integral power (9.297a), the solution is an analytic (9.297c) integral (9.297b) function (9.297b) and substitution in (9.313a) leads to (9.298a–d) with the – sign replaced by + sign. This leads to a – sign in (9.299b) and hence to alternating signs $(-)^n$ in (9.302a, b; 9.303a, b). It follows that *the general integral of the generalized circular differential equation (9.313a) with non-negative integral power coefficient (9.297a) is (standard CCLXV) a linear combination (9.313b) with arbitrary constants* (b_0, b_1) *of the generalized circular cosine (9.315) [sine (9.316)]:*

$$\cos(x;m) = 1 + \sum_{n=1}^{\infty} (-)^n x^{mn+2n} \prod_{k=1}^{n} \frac{1}{(km+2k-1)(km+2k)}, \qquad \text{(9.315)}$$

$$\sin(x;m) = x + \sum_{n=1}^{\infty} (-)^n x^{mn+2n+1} \prod_{k=1}^{n} \frac{1}{(km+2k)(km+2k+1)}, \qquad \text{(9.316)}$$

that are most conveniently calculated using the recurrence relations (9.317a–c) [(9.318a–c)]:

$$\cos(x;m) = \sum_{n=0}^{\infty} r_n(x;m); \; r_0(x;m) = 1, \; r_n(x;m) = -r_{n-1}(x;m) \frac{x^{m+2}}{(nm+2n-1)(nm+2n)}, \qquad \text{(9.317a–c)}$$

$$\sin(x;m) = \sum_{n=0}^{\infty} s_n(x;m); \; s_0(x;m) = 1, \; s_n(x;m) = -s_{n-1}(x;m) \frac{x^{m+2}}{(nm+2n)(nm+2n+1)}. \qquad \text{(9.318a–c)}$$

The generalized hyperbolic (circular cosine (9.305) [(9.315)] and sine (9.306) [(9.316)] are analytic functions in the finite complex x-plane (9.319a–d) hence integral functions:

$$\cosh(x;m), \cos(x;m), \sinh(x;m), \sin(x;m) \in \mathcal{A}(|x| < \infty); \quad m \neq -2, -2 \pm 1/p, \; p \in |N, \qquad \text{(9.319a–g)}$$

and are also analytic functions of the parameter in the complex m-plane excluding the poles (9.319e, g) [(9.319f, g)]; the residues at the poles are obtained starting the series at $n = p$ *and omitting the zero term in the denominator.* The solution of the generalized hyperbolic (9.295a) [circular (9.313a)] differential equation can also be extended to complex values (subsections 9.4.16).

9.4.16 Generalized Circular Differential Equation

If in the generalized hyperbolic (9.295a) [circular (9.313a)] differential equation the parameter m is (i) a non-negative integer (9.297a) the coefficient is an analytic function. Otherwise (9.320a) if the parameter is: (ii) a negative integer the coefficient has a pole of order $-|m|$; or (iii) real non-integer or complex in (9.320b) [(9.320c)]:

$$x \in |C - |N_0: \qquad y'' - x^m\, y = 0 = y'' + x^m\, y. \qquad (9.320\text{a–c})$$

In case (iii) of (9.320a–c) the coefficient has a branch-point (9.321a, b):

$$n \in |N: \quad x^m = x^m\, e^{i2\pi n}: \quad x^m \equiv \exp\left(\log x^m\right) = \exp\left(m \log x + i\, 2\pi\, n\right), \qquad (9.321\text{a–c})$$

leading (subsection 9.4.4) to an infinity of branches (9.321c). In (9.320a) both cases (i) and (ii) the coefficient of the differential equations (9.320b, c) is not an analytic function, and there is no solution as an analytic function (9.297c). It can be checked that substitution of (9.297c) in the first (second) term in (9.320b, c) leads to integral (9.322a) [non-integral (9.322b)] powers for m, not an integer:

$$y'' = \sum_{n=2}^{\infty} c_n\, n(n-1)\, x^n, \qquad x^m\, y = \sum_{n=0}^{\infty} c_n\, x^{n+m}, \qquad (9.322\text{a, b})$$

so that the equality is impossible (9.322a) ≠ (9.322b) with either plus + or minus – sign; the equality would also be impossible for m a negative integer smaller than –2, that is $m = -3, -4, \ldots$. The generalized hyperbolic (circular) differential equation (9.295a) ≡ (9.320b) [(9.313a) ≡ (9.320c)] is solved next (subsection 9.4.17) for all complex values of the parameter m, except negative integer values (that are considered in Example 10.20).

9.4.17 Complex Non-Integer Values of the Parameter

For complex values of the parameter other than integers (9.323a), the coefficient in the differential equations (9.420b, c) has a branch-point and the solution is sought (subsection 9.5.5) as a regular integral (9.323b) ≡ (9.377b):

$$m \in |C - |Z: \qquad y_a(x) = x^a \sum_{n=0}^{\infty} x^n\, e_n(a), \qquad (9.323\text{a, b})$$

with index a and coefficients e_n to be determined. Substitution of (9.323b) in (9.320b, c) leads to (9.324a):

$$0=\sum_{p=0}^{\infty} x^{a+p-2}\, e_p(a)(p+a)(p+a-1)\mp\sum_{k=0}^{\infty} x^{a+k+m}\, e_k(a), \tag{9.324a}$$

that is equivalent to (9.324b) with the changes of summation variable (9.298a, b):

$$0=\sum_{n=0}^{\infty} x^n\left[(n+a+1)(n+a+2)\, e_{n+2}(a)\mp e_{n-m}(a)\right]. \tag{9.324b}$$

The vanishing of the coefficients of powers in (9.324b) leads to (9.325):

$$(n+a+1)(n+a+2)\, e_{n+2}(a)=\pm\, e_{n-m}(a). \tag{9.325}$$

Setting (9.326a) and noting (9.326c) otherwise trivial solution results:

$$n=-2: \qquad a(a-1)e_0(a)=0, \qquad e_0(a)\neq 0: \qquad a=0,1, \tag{9.326a–e}$$

leads (9.326b) to the values (9.326d, e) for the index.

Substitution of the first value (9.326d) in (9.325) leads to the recurrence formula for the coefficients (9.327a):

$$e_{n+2}(0)=\pm\frac{e_{n-m}(0)}{(n+1)(n+2)}; \qquad n=m: \qquad e_{m+2}(0)=\pm\frac{e_0(0)}{(m+1)(m+2)}, \tag{9.327a–c}$$

and in particular (9.327b, c). Comparing (9.327c) with the upper + sign with (9.300b) follows (9.328a):

$$e_{m+2}(0)=c_{m+2}: \qquad y(x)=\sum_{n=0}^{\infty} x^n\, e_n(0)=\sum_{n=0}^{\infty} x^n\, c_n=\cosh(x;m), \tag{9.328a–d}$$

and thus the solution (9.323b) is (9.328b) the generalized hyperbolic cosine (9.305); the lower minus – sign in (9.327c) would lead to the generalized circular cosine (9.315). The higher index (9.326e) in (9.325) would have led with the upper + (lower –) sign to the generalized hyperbolic (9.306) [circular (9.316)] sine.

It has been shown that *the general integral (9.295b) [(9.313b)] of the generalized hyperbolic (circular) differential equation (9.295a) [(9.313a)] is (standard CCLXVI) a linear combination of generalized hyperbolic (circular) cosine (9.305) [(9.315)] and sine (9.317) [(9.316)] for: (i) all finite (9.329b) complex values (9.329a) of the variable:*

$$x \in |C, \qquad |x| < \infty; \qquad m \in |C, \qquad m \neq -1, -2, \ldots. \tag{9.329a–d}$$

and (ii) all complex values (9.329c) of the parameter except negative integers (9.329d) and the values (9.319e–g). The exceptional values of the parameter are considered in Example E10.20; the fractional values lead to logarithmic terms, as in the subsections 9.5.9–9.5.11. The series expansions for the generalized hyperbolic and circular cosine and sine can be used to derive properties such as differentiation relations (subsection 9.4.18) and inequalities (subsection 9.4.19).

9.4.18 Differentiation of the Generalized Cosine and Sine Functions

From (9.306) [(9.316)] follows *the derivative (9.330a) [(9.330b)] of the (standard CCLXVII) generalized hyperbolic (circular) sine of variable x and parameter m:*

$$\frac{d}{dx}\left[\sinh(x;m)\right] = 1 + \sum_{n=1}^{\infty} \frac{x^{mn+2n}}{(m+2)(m+3)(2m+4)(2m+5)\ldots(nm+2n)}, \tag{9.330a}$$

$$\frac{d}{dx}\left[\sinh(x;m)\right] = 1 + \sum_{n=1}^{\infty} \frac{(-)^n\, x^{mn+2n}}{(m+2)(m+3)(2m+4)(2m+5)\ldots(nm+2n)}, \tag{9.330b}$$

that includes for (9.331a) the derivative (9.331b) [(9.331c)] of the original hyperbolic (circular) sine:

$$m = 0: \qquad \frac{d}{dx}(\sinh x) = \cosh x, \qquad \frac{d}{dx}(\sin x) = \cos x; \tag{9.331a–c}$$

the derivative (9.332b) of (standard CCLXVIII) the second Airy function (9.312a–d):

$$m = 1: \qquad \frac{d}{dx}\left[Bi(x)\right] = 1 + \frac{x^3}{3} + \frac{x^6}{3.4.6} + \frac{x^9}{3.4.6.7.9} + \ldots \tag{9.332a, b}$$

coincides with (9.330a) for (9.332a).

From (9.305) [(9.315)] follows *the derivative (9.333a) [(9.333b)] of (standard CCLXIX) the generalized hyperbolic (circular) cosine with variable x and parameter m:*

$$\frac{d}{dx}\left[\cosh(x;m)\right] = \sum_{n=0}^{\infty} \frac{x^{mn+2n-1}}{(m+1)(m+2)\ldots.(mn+2n-1)}. \tag{9.333a}$$

$$\frac{d}{dx}\left[\cos(x;m)\right]=x^m\sum_{n=0}^{\infty}\frac{(-)^n\,x^{mn+2n-1}}{(m+1)(m+2)(2m+3)(2m+4)....(mn+2n-1)},\tag{9.333b}$$

that includes for (9.334a) the derivative (9.334b) [(9.334c)] of the original hyperbolic (circular) cosine:

$$m=0:\qquad \frac{d}{dx}(\cosh x)=\sinh x,\qquad \frac{d}{dx}(\cos x)=\sin x;\tag{9.334a–c}$$

the derivative (9.335b) of standard CCLXVIII) the first Airy function (9.311a–d):

$$m=1:\qquad \frac{d}{dx}\left[(Ai(x))\right]=\sum_{n=1}^{\infty}\frac{(-)^n\,x^{3n}}{2.3.5.6...(3n-1)}.\tag{9.335a, b}$$

coincides with (9.333a) for (9.335a). Besides the **differentiation formulas** *for the generalized hyperbolic and circular sine (9.330a, b; 9.332a, b) [cosine (9.333a, b; 9.335a, b)]* some inequalities are obtained next (subsection 9.4.19).

9.4.19 Inequalities for Generalized Cosines and Sines

For positive real values of the variable (9.336a) and of the parameter (9.336b) the (standard CCLXX) hyperbolic cosine and sine are: (i) increasing functions of the variable (9.336c, d); (ii) decreasing functions of the parameter (9.336e, f) if the variable is less than unity:

$$m>0<x:\qquad \frac{\partial}{\partial x}\left[\cosh(x;m)\right]>0<\frac{\partial}{\partial x}\left[\sinh(x;m)\right],\tag{9.336a–c}$$

$$m>0<x<1:\qquad \frac{\partial}{\partial m}\left[\cosh(x;m)\right]<0>\frac{\partial}{\partial m}\left[\sinh(x;m)\right],\tag{9.336d–f}$$

because in (9.305, 9.306): (i) all terms are positive for (9.336a, b); (ii) all terms increase with increasing x in the numerator; and (iii) for increasing m the denominator increases and (iv) the numerator decreases for (9.336d) so that the fractions in each term decrease. Since for real positive x, m all terms in (9.305, 9.306) are positive, it follows that *for positive variable (9.337a) and parameter (9.337b) the generalized (standard CCLXXI) hyperbolic cosine (9.305) [sine (9.306)] larger than unity (9.327c) [the variable (9.327d)]:*

$$x>0<m:\qquad \cosh(x;m)>1,\qquad \sinh(x;m)>x,\tag{9.337a–d}$$

$$1>x>0<m:\qquad \cos(x;m)<1,\qquad \sin(x;m)<x,\tag{9.338a–e}$$

the generalized circular cosine (9.315) [sine (9.316)] is less than unity (9.338d) [less than the variable (9.338e)] for positive parameter (9.325c) and positive variable (9.325b) less than unity (9.325a).

The latter results (9.338a–e) follow noting that the series for the generalized circular cosine (9.315) [sine (9.316)] is a sum (9.339) [(9.340)] over odd n:

$$\cos(x;m) = 1 - \sum_{n}^{odd} x^{mn+2n} \prod_{m+2}^{n} \frac{1}{(km+2k-1)(km+2k)} \left[1 - \frac{x^{m+2}}{(nm+2n+m+1)(nm+2n+m+2)}\right], \tag{9.339}$$

$$\sin(x;m) = x - \sum_{n}^{odd} x^{mn+2n+1} \prod_{k=1}^{n} \frac{1}{(km+2k)(km+2k+1)} \left[1 - \frac{x^{m+2}}{(nm+2n+m+3)}\right], \tag{9.340}$$

where: (i) the terms in square brackets are positive for (9.338a); (ii) hence all terms are negative beyond the first term, that is the upper bound in (9.338d) [(9.338e)]. Also for real positive x, m the series for the hyperbolic (circular) cosine (9.305) [(9.315)] and sine (9.306) [(9.316)] have all terms positive (some terms negative), so the sum is larger (smaller), that is *for positive variable (9.341a) and parameter (9.341b) the generalized hyperbolic cosine (sine) is (standard CCLXXII) larger (9.341c) [(9.341d)] than the generalized circular cosine (sine):*

$$x > 0 < m: \qquad \cosh(x;m) > \cos(x;m), \qquad \sinh(x;m) > \sin(x;m). \tag{9.341a–d}$$

The differentiation formulas (inequalities) for the generalized hyperbolic and circular cosine and sine [subsection 9.4.18 (9.4.19)] can be extended to the generalized hyperbolic and circular secant, cosecant, tangent, and cotangent (subsection 9.4.20).

9.4.20 Generalized Secant, Cosecant, Tangent, and Cotangent

The generalized hyperbolic (circular) **secant** (9.342a) [(9.342e)], **cosecant** (9.342b) [(9.342f)], **tangent** (9.342c) [(9.342g)], and **cotangent** (9.342d) [(9.342h)] are defined from the generalized hyperbolic (circular) cosine (9.305) [(9.315)] and sine (9.306) [(9.316)] as for (section II.5.2.1) the original functions:

$$\operatorname{sech}(x;m) = \frac{1}{\cosh(x;m)}, \quad \operatorname{csch}(x;m) = \frac{1}{\sinh(x;m)},$$
$$\tanh(x;m) = \frac{\sinh(x;m)}{\cosh(x;m)} = \frac{1}{\coth(x;m)}, \tag{9.342a–d}$$

$$\sec(x;m) = \frac{1}{\cos(x;m)}, \quad \csc(x;m) = \frac{1}{\sin(x;m)},$$
$$\tan(x;m) = \frac{\sin(x;m)}{\cos(x;m)} = \frac{1}{\cot(x;m)}. \tag{9.342e–h}$$

From the properties of the generalized cosine and sine (subsection 9.4.19) and the definitions (9.342a–h) follow corresponding properties for the generalized secant, cosecant, tangent, and cotangent, some of which are stated next. *For real positive variable (9.336a) [(9.343a)] and parameter (9.336b) [(9.343b)] the (standard CCLXXIII) hyperbolic cosine and sine (9.336c–f) [secant and cosecant (9.343c–f)] have opposite dependences:*

$$m > 0 < x: \qquad \frac{\partial}{\partial x}\left[\operatorname{sech}(x;m)\right] < 0 > \frac{\partial}{\partial x}\left[\operatorname{csch}(x;m)\right], \tag{9.343a–c}$$

$$m > 0 < x < 1: \qquad \frac{\partial}{\partial m}\left[\operatorname{sech}(x;m)\right] > 0 < \frac{\partial}{\partial m}\left[\operatorname{csch}(x;m)\right]. \tag{9.343d–f}$$

For real positive variable (9.344a) and parameter (9.344b) all generalized hyperbolic functions satisfy the inequalities (9.337c, d; 9.344c–f):

$$x > 0 < m: \qquad \operatorname{sech}(x;m) < 1, \quad \operatorname{csch}(x;m) > \frac{1}{x}, \qquad \tanh(x;m) > 0, \quad \coth(x;m) > 0, \tag{9.344a–f}$$

$$x > 0 < m: \qquad \sec(x;m) < 1, \csc(x;m) > \frac{1}{x}, \qquad \tanh(x;m) > 0, \quad \cot(x;m), \tag{9.345a–g}$$

and the inequalities (9.338d, e; 9.345d–g) apply to the generalized circular functions with (9.338a–c) ≡ (9.345a–c) variable less than unity. From (9.341a–d) it follows that *for real positive variable (9.346a) and parameter (9.346b) the generalized hyperbolic secant (cosecant) is (standard CCLXXIV) smaller (9.346c) [(9.346d)] than the generalized circular secant (cosecant):*

$$x > 0 < m: \qquad \operatorname{sech}(x;m) < \sec(x;m), \qquad \operatorname{csch}(x;m) < \csc(x;m). \tag{9.346a–d}$$

The ordinary differential equation for the generalized hyperbolic (9.295b) [circular (9.313a)] functions has a pole in the coefficient for m a negative integer, and thus (Example 10.20) is a singular differential equation; the extension from ordinary differential equations with analytic (section 9.4) to singular coefficients is considered next, both for regular (irregular) singularities leading to regular (irregular) integrals [section(s) 9.5 (9.6–9.7)].

9.5 Regular Singularities and Integrals of Two Kinds (Fuchs 1860, Frobenius 1873)

A generalized linear autonomous system will have all its integrals regular (subsection 9.4.6) if: (i) at least one coefficient has a simple pole; and (ii) none of the other coefficients has a singularity of higher order than a simple pole. In this case the natural integrals have: (i) indices that are the eigenvalues of the matrix of residues of the leading terms (subsection 9.5.1); and (ii) coefficients of the power series specified by a matrix recurrence formula (subsection 9.5.2). The general integral for each dependent variable is (subsection 9.5.3) a linear combination of natural integrals that satisfies initial and compatibility conditions (subsection 9.5.4). A linear differential equation of order N has all its integrals regular if (subsection 9.5.5) the coefficient of the n-th order derivative has at most a pole of order N–n. In this case: (i) the indices are (subsection 9.5.5) the roots of a characteristic polynomial of degree N; and (ii) the coefficients of the power series expansion are obtained from a recurrence relation (subsection 9.5.6).

The method of calculation of regular integrals (subsection 9.5.7) is presented in detail for a linear second-order differential equation (subsection 9.5.8) leading to three cases depending on the two indices: (i) if the indices are distinct and do not differ by an integer (subsection 9.5.8) they lead to two linearly independent regular integrals specifying functions of the first kind; (ii/iii) if the indices coincide (differ by a non-zero integer) the second linearly independent particular integral is [subsection 9.5.9 (9.5.10)]} of the second kind first (second) type. Thus the general integral is a linear combination of functions of the first kind (of functions of the first and second kinds) in the case(s) (i) [(ii, iii)]. The linear independence of the two particular integrals of a linear second-order differential equation can be established from the value at one point of their Wronskian (subsection 1.2.2) that can be calculated from the coefficient of the first-order derivative (subsection 9.5.12). Also it is proved that the series in the regular integrals converge absolutely (and uniformly) in an open annulus (closed sub-annulus) containing the singularity of the differential equation (subsection 9.5.11) and extending up to the nearest singularity; if the only other singularity is the point at infinity the convergence holds in the whole finite complex plane.

An important linear second-order differential equation is (subsection 9.5.22) the cylindrical Bessel differential equation of order ν; the method of regular integrals (subsections 9.5.5–9.5.12) is applied to a more general differential equation, namely (subsection 9.5.14) the generalized Bessel differential equation. There are three cases of solution of the generalized Bessel differential equation of order ν and degree μ, of which the original Bessel differential equation is the particular case of degree zero (subsection 9.5.22). The three cases of solution of the generalized Bessel differential equation are: (a) if the order is (subsection 9.5.14) not an integer the general integral is a linear combination of generalized Bessel functions of orders $\pm\nu$ and degree μ that are linearly independent functions of the first kind (subsection 9.5.15); (b) if the order of the generalized Bessel differential equation is an integer, then the generalized Bessel functions of orders $\pm n$ are linearly dependent (subsection 9.5.15), and one of them must be replaced (subsection 9.5.19) in the general integral by a function of the second kind, namely (subsections 9.5.17–9.5.18) the generalized Neumann function of integer order n and arbitrary complex degree μ; (c) the generalized Neumann function of arbitrary complex degree μ may be extended (subsection 9.5.20) from integer n to complex ν order, and thus the general integral of the generalized Bessel differential equation, without restriction on the order or degree, is (subsection 9.5.21) a linear combination of generalized Bessel (Neumann) functions, that are of the first (second) kind, that is are specified by a regular power series without (with) logarithmic term and involve gamma (digamma) functions [subsection 9.5.13 (9.5.16)].

The cylindrical Bessel differential equation (subsection 9.5.22) is the particular case of zero degree of the generalized Bessel differential equation and thus the general integral in the three cases (a) to (c) involve the original Bessel and Neumann functions. The spherical Bessel differential equation (subsection 9.5.23) can be transformed to a cylindrical Bessel differential equation of order integer plus one-half; the spherical Bessel differential equation can also be solved in terms of derivatives of elementary functions (subsection 9.5.26). Thus the spherical Bessel and Neumann functions of integer order can be expressed (subsection 9.5.24) alternatively and equivalently as: (α) cylindrical Bessel and Neumann functions of order integer plus one-half (subsection 9.5.23); (β) as derivatives involving powers and circular sines and cosines (subsection 9.5.26). Both the cylindrical (spherical) Bessel and Neumann functions [subsection(s) 9.5.22 (9.5.23–9.5.26)] are particular cases of the generalized Bessel and Neumann functions whose order and degree can be arbitrary complex numbers (subsections 9.5.13–9.5.21) and provide examples (subsection 9.5.25) of the six types of regular integrals (subsections 9.5.5–9.5.12).

9.5.1 Linear Autonomous System with a Regular Singularity

A generalized autonomous system of linear first-order differential equations (9.271a, b) ≡ (9.347a, b), whose coefficients have at most a simple pole:

$$m,n=1,\ldots,N: \qquad \frac{dy_m}{dx}=\sum_{n=1}^{N}\left[\frac{a_{m,n}}{x}+p_{m,n}(x)\right]y_n(x), \tag{9.347a, b}$$

will have all its natural integrals regular (9.348a):

$$y_m(x)=x^a\sum_{k=0}^{\infty}x^k\,c_{m,k}(a), \qquad p_{m,n}(x)=\sum_{\ell=0}^{\infty}p_{m,n,\ell}\,x^{\ell}, \tag{9.348a, b}$$

with indices a_n (coefficients $c_{n,k}$) determined by the residues $-a_{m,n}$ at the poles in (9.347b) [the coefficients $p_{m,n,\ell}$ of the analytic functions (9.348b)].

Substitution of the natural regular integrals (9.348a) in the generalized linear autonomous differential system (9.347b; 9.348b), leads to (9.349):

$$\sum_{u=0}^{\infty} x^{a+u-1}\left[(a+u)c_{m,u}(a)-\sum_{n=1}^{N} a_{m,n}\, c_{n,u}(a)\right]=\sum_{n=1}^{N}\sum_{\ell,v=0}^{\infty} x^{a+\ell+v}\, p_{m,n,\ell}\, c_{m,v}(a). \tag{9.349}$$

The lowest power in (9.349) is (9.350a) where $u=0$ and its coefficient in (9.349) must vanish leading to (9.350b):

$$x^{a-1}: \qquad 0=a\,c_{m,0}(a)-\sum_{n=1}^{N} a_{m,n}\, c_{n,0}(a)=-\sum_{n=1}^{N}\left(a_{m,n}-a\,\delta_{m,n}\right)c_{n,0}(a), \tag{9.350a–c}$$

using the unit matrix (6.305a–d) in (9.350c). The coefficients (9.351a) cannot all vanish, otherwise a trivial solution $y_n=0$ would result in (9.348a):

$$\left\{c_{0,0}, c_{1,0}, \ldots\right\}\neq\{0,0,\ldots.\}: \qquad 0=Det\left(a_{mn}-a\,\delta_{mn}\right)\equiv P_N(a), \tag{9.351a–c}$$

thus the determinant (9.351b) must vanish, specifying the characteristic polynomial (9.351c) of degree N whose roots are the indices. The indices and coefficients of the regular natural integrals (9.351a) are determined next (subsection 9.5.2).

9.5.2 Indices and Coefficients of the Regular Natural Integrals

If the roots of the characteristic polynomial (9.351b, c) are all distinct, then (9.352a) the corresponding N linearly independent particular integrals (9.352b):

$$P_N(a)=\prod_{n=1}^{N}(a-a_n): \qquad y_{m,n}(x)=x^{a_n}\sum_{k=0}^{\infty} c_{n,k}\, x^k, \tag{9.352a, b}$$

are **functions of the first kind** specified by power series; repeated roots of the characteristic polynomial, such as an index a of multiplicity α would lead to **functions of the second kind** (9.263b) multiplying the regular power series (9.352b) by powers $\beta=0,\ldots,\alpha-1$ of logarithms. Changing the indices of summation in (9.349) to (9.353a, b) leads to (9.353c):

$$u-1=k=\ell+v: \qquad \sum_{k=-1}^{\infty} x^k\left[(a+k+1)c_{m,k+1}(a)-\sum_{n=1}^{N} a_{m,n}\, c_{n,k+1}(a)\right]$$

$$=\sum_{k=1}^{\infty} x^k\sum_{n=1}^{N}\sum_{\ell=0}^{k} p_{m,n,\ell}\, c_{n,k-\ell}(a). \tag{9.353a–c}$$

Setting $k = -1$ in (9.353c) leads to the indicial equation (9.350a–c); concerning all remaining powers the vanishing of their coefficients in (9.353c) leads to (9.354):

$$(a+k+1)c_{m,k+1}(a) - \sum_{n=1}^{N} a_{m,n}\, c_{n,k+1}(a) = \sum_{n=1}^{N}\sum_{\ell=0}^{k} p_{m,n,\ell}\, c_{n,k-\ell}(a), \tag{9.354}$$

as the recurrence formula for the coefficients.

The preceding results (subsections 9.5.1–9.5.2) may be summarized as follows: *consider the generalized linear autonomous system of ordinary differential equations (9.347a, b) in which (standard CCXCI) the coefficients have a simple pole with residue* $-a_{m,n}$ *in addition to the analytic function (9.348b). The natural regular integrals (9.348a) are functions of the first kind (9.352b) with: (i) indices that are distinct roots (9.352a) of the characteristic polynomial (9.351c), that is the indices are (9.351b) the eigenvalues of the matrix of residues; and (ii) for each index the recurrence formula for the coefficients is (9.354). In the case of repeated indices of multiplicity* α*, the corresponding regular integrals are functions of the second kind like (9.263b) with finite M. The general integral for each dependent variable is a linear combination of natural regular integrals, such as (9.355a, b) for distinct indices:*

$$y_m(x) = \sum_{n=1}^{N} D_{m,n}\, y_{m,n}(x) = \sum_{n=1}^{N} D_{m,n} \sum_{k=0}^{\infty} x^{k+a_n}\, c_{n,k}(a_n), \tag{9.355a, b}$$

where: (i) the arbitrary constants $D_{1,n}$ *are determined by N initial conditions; and (ii) the remaining constants are related to the former by compatibility conditions obtained substituting the general integrals (9.355a, b) back in the differential system (9.347a, b).* The method of regular integrals applied to a generalized linear autonomous system of ordinary differential equations (subsections 9.5.1–9.5.2) is illustrated next by a case of two dependent variables (subsections 9.5.3–9.5.4).

9.5.3 Two Related Sets of Regular Natural Integrals

Consider the generalized linear autonomous system of coupled ordinary differential equations (9.356a, b) with the independent variable x and the two dependent variables y, z:

$$y' = \frac{y}{x} + z, \qquad z' = \frac{z}{2x} + \frac{y}{x}. \tag{9.356a, b}$$

The system is of the first-order and three coefficients have simple poles at the origin, and thus the solutions exist as regular natural integrals (9.357a, b):

$$y_a(x) = \sum_{n=0}^{\infty} x^{n+a}\, c_n(a), \qquad z_a(x) = \sum_{n=0}^{\infty} x^{n+a}\, d_n(a). \tag{9.357a, b}$$

Substitution of (9.357a, b) in (9.356b) [(9.356a)] leads to (9.357a, b) [(9.358a, b)]:

$$0 = z' - \frac{z}{2x} - \frac{y}{x} = \sum_{n=0}^{\infty} x^{n+a-1}\left[\left(n+a-\frac{1}{2}\right)d_n(a) - c_n(a)\right], \tag{9.358a, b}$$

$$0 = y' - \frac{y}{x} - z = \sum_{m=0}^{\infty}(m+a-1)x^{m+a-1}\, c_m(a) - \sum_{n=0}^{\infty} x^{n+a}\, d_n(a). \tag{9.359a, b}$$

The change of variable of summation (9.360a) leads from (9.359b) to (9.360b):

$$m = 1+n: \qquad 0 = \sum_{n=1}^{\infty} x^n\left[(n+a)\, c_{n+1}(a) - d_n(a)\right]; \tag{9.360a, b}$$

the vanishing of the coefficients of all powers in (9.360b) [(9.358b)] lead to the recurrence formulas (9.361a) [(9.361b)] for the coefficients:

$$c_{n+1}(a) = \frac{d_n(a)}{n+a}, \quad d_n(a) = \frac{c_n(a)}{n+a-1/2}: \qquad c_n(a) = \frac{c_{n-1}(a)}{(n+a-1)(n+a-3/2)}, \tag{9.361a–c}$$

that can be solved for either set of coefficients, for example c_n in (9.361c).

The lowest powers (9.362a) in (9.358b, 9.360b) lead to (9.362b):

$$x^{a-1}: \quad \begin{bmatrix} -1 & a-1/2 \\ a-1 & 0 \end{bmatrix}\begin{bmatrix} c_0 \\ d_0 \end{bmatrix} = 0; \quad \{c_0, d_0\} \neq \{0, 0\}: \quad (a-1)\left(a-\frac{1}{2}\right) \equiv P_2(a), \tag{9.362a–e}$$

the coefficients (9.362c) cannot be both zero, otherwise all coefficients in (9.361a, b) would be zero, leading to a trivial solution in (9.357a, b). Thus the determinant in (9.362b) must vanish (9.362d), specifying the quadratic characteristic polynomial (9.362e) with roots (9.363a; 9.364a):

$$a_1 = 1: \qquad y_1(x) = \sum_{n=0}^{\infty} c_n(a_1)\, x^{n+a_1} = \sum_{n=0}^{\infty} c_n(1)\, x^{n+1}, \tag{9.363a–c}$$

$$a_2 = 1/2: \qquad y_{1/2}(x) = \sum_{n=0}^{\infty} c_n(a_2)\, x^{n+a_2} = \sum_{n=0}^{\infty} c_n(1/2)\, x^{n+1/2}; \tag{9.364a–c}$$

each index (9.363a) [(9.364a)] leads to a regular natural integral (9.363b, c) [(9.364b, c)] with coefficients (9.365b, c) [(9.366b, c)]:

$$(2n-1)!! \equiv (2n-1)(2n-3)...3.1: \quad c_n(1) = \frac{2c_{n-1}(1)}{n(2n-1)} = \frac{2^n c_0(1)}{n!(2n-1)!!}, \tag{9.365a–c}$$

$$c_0(1/2) = 0: \qquad c_n(1/2) = \frac{2c_{n-1}(1/2)}{(2n-1)(n-1)} = \frac{2^{n-1} c_1(1/2)}{(2n-1)!!(n-1)!}, \tag{9.366a–c}$$

where: (i) the double factorial (9.365a) is used in (9.365c; 9.366c); (ii) the recurrence relation (9.365b) is applied $n-1$ times leading to (9.365c) because $c_0(1)$ is not zero for (9.363a) in (9.362b); (iii) the recurrence relation (9.366b) is applied n–2 times leading to (9.366c) to end at $c_1(1/2)$, short of $c_0(1/2) = 0$ for (9.364a) in (9.362b).

Introducing the arbitrary constants (9.367a, b) the general integral for $y(x)$ is (9.367c):

$$D_1 \equiv c_0(1), \qquad D_2 = c_1(1/2): \qquad y(x) = D_1\, y_1(x) + D_2\, y_{1/2}(x), \tag{9.367a–c}$$

where the natural regular integrals are given by (9.363c; 9.365c) ≡ (9.368a) [(9.364c; 9.366c) ≡ (9.368c)]:

$$y_1(x) = x + \sum_{n=1}^{\infty} \frac{2^n x^{n+1}}{n!(2n-1)!!} \sim O(x), \; y_{1/2}(x) = x^{3/2} + \sum_{n=2}^{\infty} \frac{2^{n-1} x^{n+1/2}}{(n-1)!(2n-1)!!} \sim O\left(x^{3/2}\right), \tag{9.368a–d}$$

and are linearly independent because they have different orders (9.368b) [≠ (9.368d)]. The other dependent variable $z(x)$ can be obtained substituting (9.367c; 9.368a, c) in (9.356a) ≡ (9.369a) leading to (9.369b):

$$z(x) = y'(x) - \frac{y(x)}{x} = D_1 \sum_{n=1}^{\infty} \frac{2^n x^n}{(n-1)!(2n-1)!!} + \frac{1}{2} D_2 \left[x^{1/2} + \sum_{n=2}^{\infty} \frac{2^{n-1} x^{n-1/2}}{(n-1)!\,(2n-3)!!} \right], \tag{9.369a, b}$$

as an alternative to the general method applied next (subsection 9.5.4) to z.

9.5.4 Application of Compatibility and Initial Conditions

The general method can also be applied to $z(x)$ using (9.361a, b) the coefficients (9.370a):

$$d_n(a) = \frac{d_{n-1}(a)}{(n+a-1/2)(n+a-1)}: \quad d_n(1) = \frac{2^n d_0(1)}{n!(2n+1)!!}, \; d_n\left(\frac{1}{2}\right) = \frac{2^n d_1\left(\frac{1}{2}\right)}{n!\,(2n-1)!!}, \tag{9.370a–c}$$

for the two indices (9.363a) [(9.364a)] leading to (9.370b) [(9.370c)]. The general integral for $z(x)$ is (9.371c) involving the arbitrary constants (9.371a, b):

$$E_1 = d_0(1), \qquad E_2 = d_0(1/2); \qquad z(x) = E_1\, z_1(x) + E_2\, z_{1/2}(x), \qquad (9.371\text{a–c})$$

in the linear combination (9.371c) of regular natural integrals (9.372a) [(9.372c)]:

$$z_1(x) = \sum_{m=0}^{\infty} d_m(1)\, x^{m+1} = \sum_{m=0}^{\infty} \frac{2^m x^{m+1}}{m!(2m+1)!!} \sim O(x), \qquad (9.372\text{a, b})$$

$$z_{1/2}(x) = x^{1/2} + \sum_{m=1}^{\infty} d_m(1/2)\, x^{m+1/2} = x^{1/2} + \sum_{m=1}^{\infty} \frac{2^m x^{m+1/2}}{m!(2m-1)!!} \sim O\left(x^{1/2}\right), \qquad (9.372\text{c, d})$$

that are linearly independent because they have different orders (9.372b) ≠ (9.372d).

The two expressions (9.369b) and (9.371c; 9.372a, c) for $z(x)$ coincide with: (i) the change of index of summation (9.359a); and (ii) the arbitrary constants (E_1, E_2) related to (B_1, B_2) by (9.373b, c):

$$n = m+1: \qquad E_1 = 2D_1, \qquad D_2 = 2E_2; \qquad (9.373\text{a–c})$$

$$1 = y'(0) = D_1, \qquad 1 = \lim_{x\to 0} x^{-1/2} z(x) = E_2; \quad E_1 = 2, \quad D_2 = 2, \qquad (9.373\text{d–g})$$

thus there are only two independent arbitrary constants as appropriate for a second-order system (9.356a, b). The two independent arbitrary constants are determined by two compatible and non-redundant initial conditions, such as (9.373d) [(9.373e)] that are evaluated from (9.367c; 9.368a, c) [(9.371c; 9.372a, c)]; from (9.373b, c) follow the two remaining constants (9.373f, g). Thus *(standard CCXCII) the generalized autonomous system of linear differential equations (9.356a, b) has general integrals (9.367c) [(9.371c)] as a linear combination of pairs of natural regular integrals (9.368a, c) [(9.372a, c)] that are linearly independent (9.368b, d) [(9.372b, d)]. The constants of integration are related by (9.373b, c); in the case of the initial conditions (9.373d, e) the constants (9.373f, g) lead to the general integrals (9.373h, i):*

$$y(x) = y_1(x) + 2\, y_2(x), \qquad z(x) = 2\, z_1(x) + z_2(x). \qquad (9.373\text{h, i})$$

of (9.356a, b) involving (9.368a–d; 9.372a–d).

The autonomous system of two linear coupled first-order differential equations (9.356a, b) can be eliminated for either of the dependent variables (y, z), leading to a linear second-order differential equation. The elimination for

y starts solving (9.356b) for y in (9.374a), and then substituting in (9.356a) leading to (9.374b) ≡ (9.374c):

$$y = x z' - \frac{z}{2}: \quad \left(x z' - \frac{z}{2} \right)' = z' - \frac{z}{2x} + z \to z'' - \frac{z'}{2x} + \left(\frac{1}{2} - x \right) \frac{z}{x^2} = 0; \qquad (9.374a–c)$$

$$z = y' - \frac{y}{2}: \quad \left(y' - \frac{y}{x} \right)' = \frac{y'}{2x} - \frac{y}{2x^2} + \frac{y}{x} \to y'' - \frac{3}{2}\frac{y'}{x} + \left(\frac{3}{2} - x \right) \frac{y}{x^2} = 0, \qquad (9.374d–f)$$

conversely, the elimination for z starts solving (9.356a) for z in (9.374d) and substituting in (9.356b) leading to (9.374e) ≡ (9.374f). Both dependent variables satisfy a linear second-order differential equation of the form (9.375a) where (9.375b, c) are analytic functions:

$$\{ y'', z'' \} + \frac{p(x)}{x} \{ y', z' \} + \frac{q(x)}{x^2} \{ y, z \} = 0:$$
$$p(x) = \left\{ -\frac{3}{2}, -\frac{1}{2} \right\}, \quad q(x) \equiv \left\{ \frac{3}{2} - x, \frac{1}{2} - x \right\}. \qquad (9.375a–c)$$

These examples suggest that a linear second-order differential equation (9.375a) has regular integrals (9.357a, b) when the coefficient of the first derivative (and the dependent variable) has at most a simple (double) pole. This result will be proved and extended by showing that the method of regular integrals also applies to a linear ordinary differential equation of order N for which (subsection 9.5.5) the coefficient of the n-th derivative has a pole of order no higher than $N - n$.

9.5.5 Linear Differential Equation with Regular Singularities (Fuchs 1868)

Consider the linear second-order ordinary regular differential equation (9.376e) where the coefficients of the dependent variable (its derivative) have at most a double (9.376c) [single (9.376d)] pole:

$$p(x), q(x) \in \mathcal{A}(|C); \quad P(x) = \frac{p(x)}{x}, \quad Q(x) = \frac{q(x)}{x^2}: \quad y'' + P(x)\, y' + Q(x) y = 0, \qquad (9.376a–e)$$

that is, the differential equation can be written in the form (9.377a) with (9.376a, b) analytic functions in the neighborhood of the origin:

$$x^2 y'' + x p(x)\, y' + q(x)\, y = 0: \qquad y_a(x) = x^a \sum_{n=0}^{\infty} x^n c_n(a). \qquad (9.377a, b)$$

It will be shown that the origin is a regular singularity and thus the solutions are regular integrals (9.377b) with index a and coefficients c_n. To prove this the linear second-order differential equation (9.377a) is written as a second-order generalized linear autonomous system (9.378a, b):

$$xy' = z, \qquad xz' = x(xy')' = xy' + x^2 y'' = z - xpy' - qy = (1-p)z - qy, \tag{9.378a–c}$$

where (9.377a) was used in (9.378b) leading to (9.378c). The coefficients of the linear generalized autonomous system (9.378a, c) ≡ (9.379a, b) have simple poles:

$$y' = \frac{z}{x}, \qquad z' = \frac{1-p}{x} z - \frac{q}{x} y: \qquad z = xy' = x^a \sum_{n=0}^{\infty} (a+n)\, x^n c_n(a), \tag{9.379a–c}$$

and thus both $y(z)$ have regular integrals (9.377b) [(9.379c)].

The preceding result can be generalized: consider *(standard CCXCIII) a linear* ***regular differential equation of N-th order*** *(9.380d) whose coefficients of derivatives of orders (9.380a) have at most poles (9.380b, c) of order $N-n$:*

$$m = 0, 1, \ldots, N-1:$$

$$p_m(x) \in \mathcal{A}(|C), \quad P_m(x) = x^{m-N} p_m(x), \quad x^N y^{(N)}(x) + \sum_{m=0}^{N-1} P_m(x) y^{(m)}(x) = 0; \tag{9.380a–d}$$

the differential equation (9.380d) can be written equivalently (9.380d) ≡ (9.381a) ≡ (9.381b) where (9.380b) are analytic functions:

$$0 = x^N y^{(N)}(x) + \sum_{m=0}^{N-1} x^m p_m(x)\, y^{(m)}(x), \tag{9.381a}$$

$$= x^N y^{(N)}(x) + x^{N-1} p_{N-1}(x)\, y^{(N-1)}(x) + \ldots + x\, p_1(x)\, y'(x) + p_0(x)\, y, \tag{9.381b}$$

and all its integrals are regular. The simplest case is when all the analytic coefficients (9.380b) are constants (9.382a) and the linear differential equation (9.381b) has (9.382b) constant coefficients and homogenous derivatives (1.291a):

$$p_m = const \equiv A_m: \qquad 0 = y^{(N)}(x) + \sum_{m=0}^{N-1} A_m x^m y^{(m)}(x); \tag{9.382a, b}$$

the solutions are powers (1.291b) ≡ (9.383a) whose exponents are the roots of the characteristic polynomial (1.292b, c) ≡ (9.383b, c):

$$y(x)=x^a:\quad 0=a(a-1)\dots(a-N+1)+\sum_{m=0}^{N-1}A_m\,a(a-1)(a-m+1)\equiv P_N(a). \tag{9.383a–c}$$

In this case, the simple (1.294a) [multiple (1.295a–c)] roots lead to particular integrals that are powers (1.291b) [multiplied by logarithms (1.296a, b)] leading to the general integrals (1.298) [(1.299a–c)]. It will be shown next (subsection 9.5.6) that by replacing the constants (9.382a) by analytic functions (9.380a, b) in the linear differential equation (9.380d), then: (i) the indices are the roots of the characteristic polynomial (9.383b, c) determined by the value (9.384a) of the analytic functions at the origin:

$$A_m=p_m(0);\quad \beta=0,1,\dots,\alpha-1:\quad y_s(x)=g_\beta\,x^a\,\log^\beta x\sum_{n=0}^{\infty}x^n\,c_{n,\beta}(a), \tag{9.384a–c}$$

and (ii) the single roots a (roots a of multiplicity α) lead to regular integrals of the first kind (9.377b) [second kind (9.384b, c)] with a power (plus logarithmic) branch-point. In the case of constant coefficients (9.382a), the power series in (9.377b) [(9.384b, c)] is suppressed, and only the leading factors (1.291b) [(1.296a, b)] remain.

9.5.6 Indicial Equation and Recurrence Formula for the Coefficients

The linear differential equation (9.380c, d) ≡ (9.381a) ≡ (9.381b) with analytic coefficients (9.380a, b) ≡ (9.385a) has a regular singularity at the origin, and the corresponding regular integral (9.377b) substituted in (9.381a) leads to (9.385b) where only the lowest power was written explicitly:

$$p_m(x)=\sum_{\ell=0}^{\infty}p_{m,\ell}\,x^\ell:$$
$$\left[a(a-1)\dots(a-N+1)+\sum_{m=0}^{N-1}p_{m,0}\,a(a-1)\dots(a-m+1)\right]x^a\,c_0(a)=0. \tag{9.385a, b}$$

The coefficient of the power x^a must vanish and $c_0(a)\neq 0$ otherwise a trivial solution (9.377b) results, so the term in square brackets must vanish, leading to the **indicial equation** (9.386c):

$$A_m=p_m(0)=p_{m,0}:\quad 0=(a-N+1)_N+\sum_{m=0}^{N-1}(a-m+1)_m\,p_{m,0}\equiv P_N(a), \tag{9.386a–c}$$

where: (i) the coefficients (9.386a) ≡ (9.384a) are the value (9.384a) of the analytic functions (9.380a, b) ≡ (9.385a) at the origin; (ii) the Pochhammer symbol (I.29.79a) ≡ (1.293a) ≡ (9.386b) was used; and (iii) the indices are the roots of the characteristic polynomial (9.383b, c) ≡ (9.386c).

In (9.385b), only the lowest power resulting from the substitution of the regular integral (9.377b) in the differential equation (9.380d; 9.385a) was written explicitly, and all powers appear in (9.387):

$$\begin{aligned} 0 &= \sum_{k=0}^{\infty} (a+k)\dots(a+k-N+1)\, x^{a+k} c_k(a) \\ &+ \sum_{m=0}^{N-1} \sum_{q,\ell=0}^{\infty} p_{m,\ell} (a+q)\dots(a+q-m+1)\, x^{a+q+\ell}\, c_q(a). \end{aligned} \tag{9.387}$$

The change of index of summation (9.388a) leads from (9.387) to (9.388b):

$$q+\ell=k: \qquad \begin{aligned} 0 &= \sum_{k=0}^{\infty} x^k \Big[(a+k)\dots(a+k-N+1) c_k(a) \\ &+ \sum_{m=0}^{N-1} \sum_{\ell=0}^{k} (a+k-\ell)\dots(a+k-\ell-m+1)\, p_{m,\ell}\, c_{k-\ell}(a)\Big]. \end{aligned} \tag{9.388a, b}$$

Setting $k=0=\ell$ in (9.388b) leads to the indicial equation (9.386a–c) ≡ (9.383a, b); the vanishing of the coefficients of all other powers in (9.388b) leads to (9.389):

$$\begin{aligned} &\left[(a+k)\dots(a+k-N+1) + \sum_{m=0}^{N-1} (a+k)\dots(a+k-m+1)\right] c_k(a) \\ &= -\sum_{\ell=1}^{k} c_{k-\ell}(a) \sum_{m=0}^{N-1} p_{m,\ell} (a+k-\ell)\dots(a+k-\ell-m+1), \end{aligned} \tag{9.389}$$

as the **recurrence formula for the coefficients**. The preceding results are summarized next (subsection 9.5.7).

9.5.7 Regular Integrals of the First and Second Kinds

It has been shown *that a linear ordinary differential equation (9.380d) of order N with the coefficients of (9.380a) the derivatives of order m up to $N-1$ having (9.380b) at most a pole (9.380c) of order $N-m$, has (standard CCXCIV) a regular singularity at the origin, implying that: (i) the indicial equation corresponds to the vanishing of the characteristic polynomial (9.386c) ≡ (9.383b) whose coefficients*

(9.386a, b) involve only the value (9.384a) of the analytic functions (9.380a, b) at the origin; (ii) a single root of the indicial equation or characteristic polynomial leads to a particular integral that is a regular integral of the first kind (9.377b) with recurrence formula for the coefficients (9.389) involving the coefficients (9.385a) of the analytic functions (9.380a, b); (iii) if all indices are single (9.390a), the general integral is a linear combination (9.390b) of regular integrals of the first kind (9.390c):

$$P_N(a) = \prod_{n=1}^{N}(a - a_n): \; y(x) = \sum_{n=1}^{N} C_n\, y_{a_n}(x) = \sum_{n=1}^{N} C_n\, x^{a_n} \sum_{k=0}^{\infty} x^k\, c_k(a_n), \quad (9.390a–c)$$

and only power-type branch points can appear; (iv) an index of multiplicity α leads to α particular integrals (9.263b) of which the first $\beta = 0$ (all the others $\beta = 1,...,\alpha - 1$) are regular integrals of the first (second) kind possibly involving a branch-point of power-type only (also of logarithmic type); (v) if the characteristic polynomial (9.391b) has multiple roots (9.391a), the general integral (9.391c) is a linear combination of (9.384c) regular integrals of two kinds (9.391d):

$$\sum_{m=1}^{M} \alpha_m = N, \quad P_N(a) = \prod_{m=1}^{M}(a - a_m)^{\alpha_m}:$$

$$y(x) = \sum_{m=1}^{M}\sum_{\beta_m=1}^{\alpha_m - 1} C_{m,\beta_m}\, y_{m,\beta_m}(x) = \sum_{m=1}^{M} x^{a_m} \sum_{\beta_m=1}^{\alpha_m-1} \log^{\beta_m} x \sum_{k=0}^{\infty} x^k\, C_{m,\beta_m}(a_m); \quad (9.391a–d)$$

and (vi) the N arbitrary constants of integration $C_n\left(C_{m,\beta_m}\right)$ in the case of single (9.390a–c) (multiple (9.391a–d)] indices are determined from N non-redundant and compatible initial conditions. Two is the lowest order of a linear differential equation with regular singularities for which regular integrals of two kinds exist, and is used to illustrate in more detail their calculation (subsection 9.5.8).

9.5.8 Second-Order Differential Equation with a Regular Singularity

In a second-order linear differential equation with a regular singularity at the origin (9.377a): (i) the coefficients (9.376a, b) are analytic functions with Maclaurin series (9.392a, b); (ii) the solutions are regular integrals (9.377b); and (iii) substitution of (i) and (ii) in the differential equation (9.377a) leads to (9.392c):

$$p(x) = \sum_{k=0}^{\infty} p_k\, x^k, \qquad q(x) = \sum_{k=0}^{\infty} q_k\, x^k:$$

$$\sum_{n=0}^{\infty}(a+n)(a+n-1)\, x^{a+n}\, c_n(a) + \sum_{k,\ell=0}^{\infty} x^{a+k+\ell}\, c_k(a)\left[(a+k)p_\ell + q_\ell\right] = 0. \quad (9.392a–c)$$

The change of index of summation (9.393a) in (9.392c) leads to (9.393b):

$$k+\ell=n: \quad 0=\sum_{n=0}^{\infty} x^n \left\{(a+n)(a+n-1)\, c_n(a)+\sum_{\ell=0}^{n} c_{n-\ell}(a)\left[(a+n-\ell)p_\ell+q_\ell\right]\right\}. \tag{9.393a, b}$$

The coefficients of all powers in (9.393b) must vanish leading to (9.394):

$$\left[(a+n)(a+n-1)+p_0(a+n)+q_0\right]c_n(a)=-\sum_{\ell=1}^{n} c_{n-\ell}(a)\left[(a+n-\ell)p_\ell+q_\ell\right], \tag{9.394}$$

where the $\ell=0$ term was brought to the l.h.s.

Bearing in mind (9.395a) because powers with negative exponents are not present in (9.377b), setting (9.395b) in (9.394) leads to (9.395c):

$$0=c_{-1}=c_{-2}=....;n=0: \qquad \left[a(a-1)+p_0\, a+q_0\right]c_0(a)=0. \tag{9.395a–c}$$

If $c_0(a)=0$, then (9.394) implies all coefficients vanish $0=c_1=c_2=....$ leading (9.377b) to a trivial solution $y=0$. Thus a non-trivial solution (9.396a) requires (9.396b) implying that the term in square brackets in (9.395c) must vanish (9.396c):

$$y_a(x)\neq 0 \Rightarrow c_0(a)\neq 0 \Rightarrow 0=a^2+(p_0-1)\,a+q_0=(a-a_+)(a-a_-)\equiv P_2(a); \tag{9.396a–e}$$

for a second-order differential equation $N=2$ in (9.381a), the characteristic polynomial coincides in (9.383b) ≡ (9.396c) and its vanishing specifies the indicial equation (9.396d) with roots (9.397a) ordered by their real parts:

$$\operatorname{Re}(a_+)\geq \operatorname{Re}(a_-): \qquad y_\pm(x)=x^{a_\pm}\sum_{n=0}^{\infty} x^n\, c_n(a_\pm). \tag{9.397a–c}$$

The corresponding regular integrals are (9.397b, c) where the coefficients satisfy (9.394) the recurrence formula (9.398b):

$$c_0(a_\pm)=1: \quad P_2(a_\pm+n)\, c_n(a_\pm)=-\sum_{\ell=1}^{n} c_{n-\ell}(a_\pm)\left[(a_\pm+n-\ell)p_\ell+q_\ell\right]. \tag{9.398a, b}$$

noting that: (i) the term multiplying c_n on the r.h.s. of (9.394) is the characteristic polynomial (9.396d) calculated for $a+n$:

$$P_2(a+n)=(a+n)(a+n-1)+p_0(a+n)+q_0; \tag{9.398d}$$

and (ii) the lowest order coefficient (9.398a) can be set to unity by incorporating it in the arbitrary constants $C_\pm$ in the general integral.

Thus *the general integral of the linear second-order regular differential equation of second-order (9.377a) with analytic coefficients (9.392a, b) is (standard CCXCV) a linear combination (9.399c) of regular integrals of the first kind (9.397b, c) with: (i) indices (9.397a) specified by the roots of the characteristic polynomial (9.396c–e); (ii) recurrence formula for the coefficients (9.398a–c); and (iii) arbitrary constants of integration (9.399b):*

$$a_+ - a_- \not\in |N_0: \qquad C_\pm \equiv C_0(a_\pm): \qquad y(x) = C_+\, y_+(x) + C_-\, y_-(x). \tag{9.399a–c}$$

The general integral (9.399c) involving only regular integrals of the first kind (9.397b, c) is valid if (9.399a) the indices do not differ by an integer. The two exceptions of coincident indices (indices differing by a non-zero integer) are considered next [subsection 9.5.9 (9.5.10)] and lead to a regular integral of the second kind first (second) type with one logarithmic singularity like (9.263b) with $\alpha = 2$ and $M = 0(1 \le M < \infty)$.

9.5.9 Regular Integral of Second Kind First Type

The need for the exclusion (9.399a) of indices differing by an integer may be explained by going back to the regular integral (9.377b), substituting in the differential equation (9.377a), and assuming that the recurrence formula for the coefficients (9.394) is satisfied, so that only one term (9.400c) involving the characteristic polynomial (9.396d, e) remains, forcing the differential equation (9.400b) with operator (9.400a):

$$\left\{L\left(\frac{d}{dx}\right)\right\} y_a(x) = \left\{x^2 \frac{d^2}{dx^2} + x p(x) \frac{d}{dx} + q(x)\right\} y_a(x) \\ = x^a c_0(a) P_2(a) = x^a c_0(a)(a - a_+)(a - a_-). \tag{9.400a, b}$$

Choosing the larger (9.397a) index $a = a_+$, the r.h.s. of (9.400b) vanishes, and thus $y_+(x)$ in (9.397b) is a regular integral whose coefficients $c_n(a_+)$ are always finite because (9.398b) they are multiplied by the characteristic polynomial of $n + a_+$ that is not zero (9.401a); thus $y_+(x)$ is always a valid solution:

$$P_2(n + a_+) \neq 0; \qquad a_+ = a_- + s \in |N_0: \qquad P_2(s + a_-) = P_2(a_+) = 0, \tag{9.401a–d}$$

suppose that the lower index (9.397a) differs from the higher by an integer (9.401b); then the coefficient (9.401c) of $c_s(a_-)$ is zero in (9.401d) leading (9.402a):

$$0.c_s(a_-) = -\sum_{\ell=1}^{s} c_{s-\ell}\left[p_\ell(a_- + \ell) + q_\ell\right] \begin{cases} \neq 0 \Rightarrow c_s(a_-) = \infty, \\ = 0 \Rightarrow 0.c_s(a_-) = 0, \end{cases} \tag{9.402a–c}$$

to two cases: (i) if the r.h.s. of (9.402a) is non-zero (9.402b) then $c_s(a_-)$ is infinite; or (ii) if the r.h.s. of (9.387a) is zero (9.387c) then $c_s(a_-)$ is indeterminate. In both cases (i) and (ii) the solution $y_-(x)$ breaks down for $a_+ - a_- = s$, a positive integer. The remaining case in (9.401b) is coincident indices $a_+ = a_-$ in which case $y_\pm(x)$ coincide in (9.397c), and (9.399c) involves only one arbitrary constant of integration $C_+ + C_-$ and cannot be the general integral of the second-order differential equation. Thus the **Frobenius-Fuchs method** (subsection 9.5.8) must be modified [subsection 9.5.9 (9.5.10)] if the indices coincide (differ by a non-zero integer).

Considering first the case of coincident indices (9.403a), the differential equation (9.400a) becomes (9.403b):

$$a_+ \equiv a_-: \quad \left\{L\left(\frac{d}{dx}\right)\right\} y_a(x) = x^a c_0(a)(a-a_+)^2: \quad y_+(x) = \lim_{a\to a_+} y_a(x), \qquad (9.403\text{a, b})$$

$$\left\{L\left(\frac{d}{dx}\right)\right\}\frac{\partial y_a(x)}{\partial a} = 2x^a c_0(a)(a-a_+): \qquad \bar{y}_+(x) = \lim_{a\to a_+}\frac{\partial}{\partial a}\left[y_a(x)\right], \qquad (9.403\text{c, d})$$

showing (9.403b) that two particular integrals are (9.403b, d). The first particular integral (9.403c) is a regular integral of the first kind (9.397b) that is always valid. In the case (9.403a) of coincident indices $y_-(x) = y_+(x)$ is replaced by the particular integral (9.403d) ≡ (9.404a):

$$\bar{y}_+(x) \equiv \lim_{a\to a_+}\frac{\partial}{\partial a}\left[x^a\sum_{n=0}^{\infty}x^n c_n(a)\right] = \log x\left[x^{a_+}\sum_{n=0}^{\infty}x^n c_n(a_+)\right] + x^{a_+}\sum_{n=0}^{\infty}x^n \lim_{a\to a_+}\frac{d}{da}\left[c_n(a)\right], \qquad (9.404\text{a, b})$$

that is (9.404b) linearly independent from $y_+(x)$ because it involves a logarithmic singularity in (9.405a, b):

$$d_n(a) \equiv \frac{d}{da}\left[c_n(a)\right]: \qquad \bar{y}_+(x) = y_+(x)\log x + x^{a_+}\sum_{n=0}^{\infty}x^n d_n(a_+). \qquad (9.405\text{a, b})$$

It has been shown that *the linear second-order differential equation (9.377a) with a regular singularity at the origin (9.392a, b) in the case (9.403b) (≡ 9.406a) of equal roots (9.403a) ≡ (9.406a) ≡ (9.406b) of the indicial equation (9.396d, e), has (standard CCXCVI) a general integral (9.406c):*

$$a_+ = a_- \quad \Leftrightarrow \quad (p_0-1)^2 = 4q_0: \qquad y(x) = C_+\, y_+(x) + C_-\, \bar{y}_+(x), \qquad (9.406\text{a–c})$$

specified by a linear combination with arbitrary constants $C_\pm$ of two linearly independent particular integrals, namely: (i) a regular integral of the first kind (9.397b) with recurrence formula (9.398b) for the coefficients that may have a power-type branch-point; (ii) a ***regular integral of the second kind first type*** *(9.405b)* *that may have both power-type and logarithmic branch-points because it is the sum of: (i) the regular integral of the first kind (9.397b) multiplied by a logarithm; (ii) a* ***complementary function of first type*** *that is similar to the regular integral of first kind (9.397b) with distinct coefficients (9.405a) and thus equals a power series multiplied by an analytic function.* It remains to consider (subsection 9.5.10) the: (i) third case of linear second-order differential equation (9.377a) with a regular singularity (9.392a, b) at the origin; and (ii) the second exception to (9.399a, b), that is, indices differing by a non-zero integer.

9.5.10 Regular Integral of the Second Kind Second Type

In the case when the indices (9.397a) that are the roots of the characteristic polynomial (9.396e) differ by a non-zero integer (9.407a), the failure of the coefficient $c_s(a_-)$ in (9.402a–c) is due to the zero of the characteristic polynomial for $a_- = a_+ - s$, and this can be resolved using the coefficients (9.407b) instead:

$$a_+ - a_- = s \in |N: \qquad \overline{c}_n(a) = (a - a_-)\, c_n(a), \tag{9.407a, b}$$

implying that: (i) the coefficients up to (9.408a) are zero (9.408b) and the first non-zero coefficient is the next (9.408c):

$$n = 0, \dots, s-1: \quad \overline{c}_n(a_-) = 0 \neq \overline{c}_s(a_-); \quad P_3(a) = (a - a_-) P_2(a) = (a - a_+)(a - a_-)^2, \tag{9.408a–e}$$

and (ii) the characteristic polynomial (9.396e) is multiplied (9.408d) by $(a - a_-)$ and becomes a cubic (9.408e). The coefficients (9.407b) satisfy the same recurrence relation (9.394) and the regular integral (9.377b) substituted in the differential equation (9.377a) leads (9.400a) by (9.408e) to (9.409a):

$$\left\{L\left(\frac{d}{dx}\right)\right\} y_a(x) = x^a\, c_0(a)(a - a_+)(a - a_-)^2 :$$
$$y_\pm(x) = \lim_{a \to a_\pm} y_a(x), \quad \overline{y}_-(x) = \lim_{a \to a_-} \frac{\partial}{\partial a}\left[(a - a_-) y_a(x)\right], \tag{9.409a–d}$$

that has three solutions (9.409b–d). Since the differential equation (9.377a) is of the second-order, one of the three particular integrals (9.409b–d) must be linearly dependent on the other two. The upper regular integral of the first kind (9.409b) is always valid (9.397b) and is unaffected by the factor $a_+ - a_- = s$. Concerning $y_-(x)$ in (9.409c) the multiplication of the coefficients (9.407b) leads to (9.410a):

$$y_-(x) = \lim_{a \to a_-} \sum_{n=0}^{\infty} \overline{c}_n(a) x^{n+a} = \sum_{n=s}^{\infty} \overline{c}_n(a_-) x^{n+a_-} = O\left(x^{s+a_-}\right) = O\left(x^{a_+}\right) = A\, x^{a_+}\left[1 + O(x)\right], \tag{9.410a–e}$$

where: (i) the first s terms vanish (9.408a, b) leading to (9.410b); and (ii) the leading term (9.410c) is of order (9.410d) hence of the form (9.410e); that is, the leading power is the same as for $y_+(x)$ in (9.397e). It follows that the linear combination (9.411a) must satisfy the differential equation (9.377a) even though its index is $1+a_+$:

$$A y_+(x) - y_-(x) \sim O\left(x^{1+a_+}\right); \qquad P_3(1+a_+) \neq 0 \quad \Rightarrow \quad y_+(x) = y_-(x), \qquad \text{(9.411a–c)}$$

this is impossible because $(1+a_+)$ is not (9.411b) a root of the characteristic polynomial on the r.h.s. of (9.409a). Thus $A=1$ and (9.409b) $\equiv$ (9.409c) must coincide (9.411c) leading only two particular integrals (9.409b, d).

The new particular integral (9.409d) is given by (9.412):

$$\bar{y}_-(x) = \lim_{a \to a_-} \frac{\partial}{\partial a}\left[x^a\,(a-a_-)\sum_{n=0}^{\infty} x^n\, c_n(a)\right], \qquad \text{(9.412)}$$

that can be evaluated as follows: (i) in the sum from $n=0$ to $n=s-1$ the coefficients (9.408a, b) vanish, unless the differentiation is applied to $a-a_-$, leading to the first term in the r.h.s. of (9.413):

$$\bar{y}_-(x) = x^{a_-}\sum_{n=0}^{s-1} x^n\, c_n(a_-) + x^{a_-}\sum_{n=s}^{\infty} e_n(a_-)\, x^n + b\log x\, x^{a_-}\sum_{n=s}^{\infty} x^n\, \bar{c}_n(a_-), \qquad \text{(9.413)}$$

(ii) in the sum from $n=s$ to $n=\infty$, if the power is not differentiated, then appears the series in the second term on the r.h.s. of (9.413) with coefficients:

$$m = n-s: \qquad e_m(a_-) = \lim_{a \to a_-} \frac{d}{da}\left[(a-a_-)c_{m+s}(a_-)\right]; \qquad \text{(9.414a, b)}$$

(iii) the remaining differentiation of the power x^a with regard to a leads to a constant b times a logarithmic factor $\log x$ multiplying the same series as in (9.410a–e) that coincides with the function of first kind (9.411c) and appears as the third term on the r.h.s. of (9.413).

Using (9.407a; 9.414a, b) it follows that *the general integral of the linear second-order differential equation (9.377a) with a regular singularity at the origin (9.392a, b) in the case (9.407a) ≡ (9.415a) when the indices (9.397a) that are the roots of the indicial equation (9.396d) differ by a positive integer is given (standard CCXCVII) by (9.415b):*

$$a_+ - a_- = s \in |N: \qquad y(x) = C_+\, y_+(x) + C_-\, \bar{y}_-(x), \qquad \text{(9.415a, b)}$$

as a linear combination with arbitrary constants $C_\pm$ of: (i) a regular integral of the first kind (9.397b) with recurrence formula for the coefficients (9.398b) involving the *index with larger real part; and (ii) a* **regular integral of the second kind second type** (9.413) ≡ (9.416):

$$\bar{y}_-(x) = b\, y_+(x)\log x + x^{a_-}\sum_{m=0}^{\infty} x^m\, e_m(a_-) + x^{a_+}\sum_{n=0}^{a_+-a_--1} x^n\, c_n(a_-), \tag{9.416}$$

consisting of the sum of three terms, namely: (ii-1) a constant b multiplying the function of the first kind; (ii-2) a **complementary function of the second type** *involving the coefficients (9.414b); and (ii-3) a* **preliminary function** *with coefficients (9.394) that is a finite sum and has a pole of order $M = a_-$ if $a_- = -1, -2, \ldots$.* The general integrals (9.399a, b; 9.406a–c; 9.415a, b) involve the power series (9.397b, c; 9.405b; 9.416) with coefficients (9.398a–c; 9.405a; 9.414b) whose convergence is proved next (subsection 9.5.11).

9.5.11 Convergence of the Series in the Regular Integrals

It is not necessary to prove the convergence of the series (chapter I.21) in the regular integrals in every particular case, because it is assured in general by the following **theorem of convergence of regular integrals**: *the linear differential equation of second-order with a regular singularity at the origin (9.377a) has coefficients (9.376a, b) analytic (9.417b) in an open circle of radius R:*

$$0 < \varepsilon < R:\quad p, q \in \mathcal{A}(|x| < R):\quad \sum_{n=0}^{\infty} x^{a+n}\, c_n(a) \begin{cases} \text{A.C.} & \text{if} \quad |x| < R, \\ \text{T.C.} & \text{if} \quad |x| \le R - \varepsilon. \end{cases} \tag{9.417a–e}$$

It follows that (standard CCXCVIII) the regular integrals of the first kind (9.397b, c) ≡ (9.417c) and of the second kind first (9.405b) [second (9.416)] type: (i) converge absolutely (9.417d) in the same circle, that is, the series of moduli converges (section I.21.3), and the sum of the series is unchanged by rearrangement of the order of the terms; (ii) converge totally (section I.21 .7), that is, absolutely and uniformly, in a closed sub-circle (9.417a, e), so that the convergence is independent of the variable (section I.21.5) and limits, differentiation, and integration can be applied to the series term-by-term (section I.21.6). The theorem is proved for the series in the regular integral of the first kind (9.377b) ≡ (9.417c); the proof extends to the series in the regular integrals of the second kind and first (9.405b) [second (9.416)] type because they are obtained from the totally convergent series that specify the functions of the first kind.

Since the functions (9.417b, c) are analytic in the circle of radius R, their Maclaurin power series around the origin (9.392a, b) have bounded coefficients (9.418a, b):

$$|p_k| \equiv \frac{\left|p^{(k)}(0)\right|}{k!} < B > |q_k| \equiv \frac{\left|q^{(k)}(0)\right|}{k!};$$

$$\left|c_n(a)\right| < \left|P_2(a+n)\right|^{-1} B\left[\,|a+n| + 1\right]\sum_{\ell=1}^{n}\left|c_{n-\ell}(a)\right| \equiv f_n(a), \tag{9.418a–c}$$

since the modulus of the sum cannot exceed the sum of the moduli the recurrence formula for the coefficients (9.398b) leads to (9.418c). From (9.418c) follows (9.419a):

$$\frac{|c_n(a)|}{|c_0(a)|+....+|c_{n-1}(a)|}\le B\frac{|a+n|+1}{|P_2(a+n)|}=O\left(\frac{1}{|a+n|}\right): \qquad \lim_{n\to\infty}\frac{|c_n(a)|}{\sum_{m=0}^{n-1}|c_m(a)|}=0, \tag{9.419a, b}$$

implying the limit (9.419b).

The ratio of (9.418c) for $n+1$ and n is given by (9.420a):

$$\frac{f_{n+1}(a)}{f_n(a)}=\left|\frac{P_2(a+n)}{P_2(a+n+1)}\right|\frac{|a+n+1|+1}{|a+n|+1}\frac{\sum_{\ell=1}^{n+1}|c_{n+1-\ell}(a)|}{\sum_{\ell=1}^{n}|c_{n-\ell}(a)|}, \tag{9.420a}$$

where both the first and second factors tend to unity (9.420b, c):

$$\lim_{n\to\infty}\left|\frac{P_2(a+n)}{P_2(a+n+1)}\right|=1=\lim_{n\to\infty}\frac{(a+n+1)+1}{|a+n|+1}; \tag{9.420b, c}$$

substitution of (9.420b, c) in (9.420a) leads to (9.421a):

$$\lim_{n\to\infty}\frac{f_{n+1}(a)}{f_n(a)}=\frac{\sum_{\ell=1}^{n+1}|c_{n+1-\ell}(a)|}{\sum_{\ell=1}^{n}|c_{n-\ell}(a)|}=1+\frac{|c_n(a)|}{\sum_{m=0}^{n-1}|c_m(a)|}=1. \tag{9.421a–c}$$

where the numerator is a sum over $|c_1|+...+|c_n|$ and in the denominator the sum is over $|c_1|+...+|c_{n-1}|$ leading to (9.421b); using (9.419b) shows that the limit is unity in (9.421c).

The series in (9.377b) specifying the regular integral (9.417c) has upper bound (9.422a) in modulus:

$$|x^{-a}||y_a(x)|\le\sum_{n=0}^{\infty}|x|^n|c_n(a)|<\sum_{n=0}^{\infty}R^n f_n(a), \quad \lim_{n\to\infty}\frac{f_{n+1}(a)\,R^{n+1}}{f_n(a)\,R^n}=R\lim_{n\to\infty}\frac{f_{n+1}(a)}{f_n(a)}=R, \tag{9.422a–c}$$

showing that its radius of convergence (I.29.31b) ≡ (9.422b) is (9.422c) where (9.421c) was used; the radius of convergence (9.422c) of the regular series solution (9.417c) is the same radius of convergence (9.417b, c) as the coefficients of the differential equation (9.377a). Since (9.422a) is a series of moduli, the absolute convergence (section I.21.3) of the regular integral (9.417c) is proved in (9.417d) the circle of radius R. Within a closed sub-circle (9.417a, e) the convergence is independent of x and hence (section I.21.5) uniform. QED. Before applying the theory of regular integrals to the generalized (original) Bessel differential equation [subsections 9.5.14–9.5.21 (9.5.22)], the Wronskian of a linear second-order differential equation is calculated (subsection 9.5.12).

9.5.12 Wronskian of a Linear Second-Order Differential Equation

Let y_1 and y_2 be two solutions (9.423a, b) of a linear second-order differential equation (9.376e), leading to (9.423c):

$$y_1''+Py_1'+Qy_1=0=y_2''+Py_2'+Qy_2: \quad y_2\left(y_1''+Py_1'\right)=-Q\,y_1\,y_2=y_1\left(y_2''+Py_2'\right). \tag{9.423a–c}$$

From (9.423c) follows (9.424a) ≡ (9.424b):

$$-P\left(y_1y_2'-y_2y_1'\right)=y_1\,y_2''-y_2\,y_1''=\left(y_1y_2'-y_2y_1'\right)', \tag{9.424a, b}$$

that is (9.424b) ≡ (9.425c) is a first order differential equation for the Wronskian (1.40c) ≡ (9.425a, b):

$$W\left(y_1,y_2\right)=\begin{vmatrix} y_1 & y_2 \\ y_1' & y_2' \end{vmatrix}=y_1\,y_2'-y_2\,y_1': \quad W'+PW=0, \quad W(x)=W(x_0)\exp\left\{-\int_{x_0}^{x}P(\xi)\,d\xi\right\}, \tag{9.425a–d}$$

whose solution (3.19a, b; 3.20a, b) is (9.425d). It follows that *the Wronskian (9.425a, b) of two solutions (9.423a, b) of a linear second-order differential equation (9.376e) is (standard CCXCIX) determined (9.425d) by the coefficient of the first derivative.* If the Wronskian (9.425b) of two functions is zero (9.426a), they are related by (9.426b) that is integrated (9.426c) and implies that the functions are proportional; that is, linearly dependent:

$$0=W\left(y_1(x),y_2(x)\right)\Rightarrow\frac{y_2'(x)}{y_2(x)}=\frac{y_1'(x)}{y_1(x)}\Rightarrow\log\left[y_2(x)\right]=\log C+\log\left[y_1(x)\right]\Rightarrow y_1(x)=C\,y_1(x); \tag{9.426a–d}$$

conversely, it was shown (subsection 1.2.3) that a sufficient condition for the linear independence of two functions (9.427a) is that the Wronskian (9.425a, b) is non-zero (9.427b); in the case of a linear second-order differential equation (9.423a, b) the Wronskian (9.425d) is not zero at all points (9.427b) provided that it is not zero at one point (9.427c):

$$\{y_1(x), y_2(x)\} \textit{linearly independent} \qquad W(x) = y_1(x)y_y'(x) - y_2(x)y_1'(x) \neq 0 \quad \Leftarrow \quad W(x_0) \neq 0. \tag{9.427a–c}$$

Thus *a sufficient condition for two particular integrals of a linear second-order differential equation (9.423a, b) to be linearly independent (9.427a) is (standard CCC) that their Wronskian (9.425a, b) is not zero at one point (9.427c),* because then it will be non-zero (9.425d) at all other points (9.427b).

The Wronskian is calculated next for the **generalized Bessel differential equation** (9.4282f) with **order** ν, **degree** μ and independent x and dependent y variables, (Campos et al. 2019) all generally complex (9.412a–d):

$$x, y, \mu, \nu \in |C; \ \mathrm{Re}(\nu) \geq 0: \qquad x^2 y'' + x\left(1 - \frac{\mu}{2}x^2\right)y' + \left(x^2 - \nu^2\right)y = 0; \tag{9.428a–f}$$

the differential equation (9.428f) is unchanged reversing the sign of the order $\nu \to -\nu$, and thus its solution is needed only for (9.428e). When the differential equation (9.428f) is written in the form (9.376e) the coefficient of the first derivative is (9.429a) and the Wronskian (9.425d) is given by (9.429b):

$$P(x) = \frac{1}{x} - \frac{\mu x}{2}: \ W(x) = W_0 \exp\left[-\int_0^x \left(\frac{1}{\xi} - \frac{\mu\xi}{2}\right)d\xi\right] = \frac{W_0}{x}\exp\left(\frac{\mu x^2}{4}\right), \tag{9.429a–c}$$

where W_0 is a constant. It has been shown that *(9.429c) is the Wronskian (standard CCCI) of the generalized Bessel differential equation (9.428f); in the particular case (9.430a) of the original Bessel differential equation (9.430b) the Wronskian is (9.430c):*

$$\mu = 0: \qquad x^2\frac{d^2y}{dx^2} + x\frac{dy}{dx} + \left(x^2 - \nu^2\right)y = 0, \qquad W(x) = \frac{W_0}{x}. \tag{9.430a–c}$$

Next are obtained some properties of the gamma (digamma) functions [subsection 9.5.13 (9.5.16)] to be used when deriving the regular integrals of the first (second) kind [subsections 9.5.14–9.5.15 (9.5.17–9.5.21)] of the generalized Bessel differential equation (9.428a–f).

9.5.13 Gamma Function (Weierstrass 1856) as a Generalization of the Factorial

The gamma function (note III.1.8) may be defined (III.1.149b) ≡ (9.431b) by the **Euler integral of the first kind (1729)** in the right-hand half-complex plane (III.1.149a) ≡ (9.431a):

$$\operatorname{Re}(\nu) > 0: \qquad \Gamma(\nu) \equiv \int_0^x x^{\nu-1} e^{-x}\, dx. \qquad (9.431\text{a, b})$$

From (9.431b) follows the initial value (III.1.152) ≡ (9.432a) and the recurrence formula (III.1.155b) ≡ (9.432b, c):

$$\Gamma(1) = 1; \quad \operatorname{Re}(\nu + n - 1) > 0: \qquad \Gamma(\nu + n) = (\nu + n - 1)(\nu + n - 2)....(\nu + 1)\, \nu\Gamma(\nu). \qquad (9.432\text{a–c})$$

Setting $\nu = 1$ in (9.432c) and using (9.432a) it follows that the gamma function reduces to the factorial (9.433b) for a positive integer argument (9.433a):

$$n = 1, 2, ...: \qquad \Gamma(n + 1) = n(n - 1)...2.1.\Gamma(1) = n! \qquad (9.433\text{a, b})$$

Thus *the gamma function is (standard CCCII) the generalization of the factorial (9.433b) from positive integer values of the argument (9.433a) to the whole complex* $\nu -$ *plane: (i) starting with (9.431b) in the right-half plane (9.431a); and (ii) using (9.432c) ≡ (9.434b) to perform analytic continuation to (9.432b) ≡ (9.434a):*

$$\operatorname{Re}(\nu) > 1 - n: \qquad \Gamma(\nu) = \frac{\Gamma(\nu + n)}{(\nu + n - 1)(\nu + n - 2)....(\nu + 1)\nu}. \qquad (9.434\text{a, b})$$

From (9.434a, b) also follows that the gamma function (9.431a, b) is analytic in the whole complex plane (9.434a, b) except for simple poles (9.435b) for non-positive integer values (9.435a):

$$m = 0, -1, -2, ...: \qquad \Gamma(\nu) = \frac{\Gamma_{-1}}{\nu + m} + O(1), \qquad \Gamma_{-1} = \frac{(-)^m}{m!}, \qquad (9.435\text{a–c})$$

with residues (9.435c) ≡ (I.1.158c). The residues (9.239b) are calculated by (9.436a):

$$\Gamma_{-1} = \lim_{\nu \to -m} (\nu + m)\Gamma(\nu) = \lim_{\nu \to -m} \frac{\Gamma(\nu + m + 1)}{(\nu + m - 1)...\nu} = \frac{\Gamma(1)}{(-1)...(-m)} = \frac{(-)^m}{m!}, \qquad (9.436\text{a–d})$$

using (9.432b) [(9.432a)] in (9.436b) [(9.436c)] to prove (9.436d) ≡ (9.435c). The pole of the gamma function for non-positive integer values (9.437a) could be understood symbolically as (9.437b):

$$n=0,1,\ldots: \qquad \Gamma(-n)=(-n-1)(-n-2)(-n-3)\ldots.=\infty, \tag{9.437a, b}$$

although the correct interpretation is (9.345a–c).

The inverse of the gamma function is bounded in the complex plane (9.438a) and has simple zeros (9.438c) at the points (9.438b), leading by the extended Mittag-Leffler theorem (subsection II.1.4.3) to (II.1.71) ≡ (9.438e) the **Weierstrass (1856) infinite product** where (9.438d) is the Euler-Mascheroni constant (subsection I.29.5.2):

$$\frac{1}{|\Gamma(\nu)|}<B; \qquad m=0,-1,-2,\ldots:$$

$$\frac{1}{\Gamma(m)}=0;-\gamma\equiv\frac{\Gamma'(1)}{\Gamma(1)}: \qquad \frac{1}{\Gamma(\nu)}=\nu e^{\gamma\nu}\prod_{m=1}^{\infty}\left(1+\frac{\nu}{m}\right)e^{-\nu/m}. \tag{9.438a–e}$$

The product of the gamma functions of $\pm\nu$ simplifies (9.438e) to (9.439a):

$$\frac{1}{\Gamma(\nu)\Gamma(-\nu)}=-\nu^2\prod_{m=1}^{\infty}\left(1-\frac{\nu^2}{m^2}\right): \quad \sin(\pi\nu)=\pi\nu\prod_{m=1}^{\infty}\left(1-\frac{\nu^2}{m^2}\right), \tag{9.439a, b}$$

that may be compared with the infinite product (subsection II.1.5.2) for the circular sine (II.1.75) ≡ (9.439b). From the comparison of (9.439a, b) follows (9.440b):

$$\nu\neq 0,\pm1,\pm2,\ldots: \qquad \frac{\pi}{\sin(\pi\nu)}=-\nu\,\Gamma(-\nu)\,\Gamma(\nu)=\Gamma(1-\nu)\,\Gamma(\nu), \tag{9.440a–c}$$

and also (9.440c) using (9.432b) with $\nu\rightarrow-\nu, n=1$. Thus *the infinite product (9.438d, e) for the gamma function leads to (standard CCCIII) the* ***symmetry formula*** *(9.440b) ≡ (9.440c) excluding (9.440a) positive (9.433a) [non-positive (9.435a)] integer values, when it reduces to the factorial (9.433b) [has a simple pole (9.435b) with residue (9.435c)].* The gamma function appears often in the regular integrals of differential equations, such as (subsection 9.5.14) the generalized Bessel differential equation (9.428a–f).

9.5.14 Generalized Bessel Differential Equation (Campos et al. 2019)

The generalized Bessel differential equation (9.428f) in the form (9.377a) ≡ (9.441c) has coefficients (9.441a, b) that are analytic functions (9.376a, b) in a circle of finite radius with center at the origin that is a regular singularity:

$$p(x)=1-\frac{\mu}{2}x^2, \quad q(x)=x^2-\nu^2: \quad x^2y''+x\,p(x)\,y'+q(x)\,y=0. \tag{9.441a–c}$$

Thus there are two linearly independent regular integrals, and at least one is of the first kind (9.377b), leading on substitution in (9.428f) to (9.442):

$$0=\sum_{k=0}^{\infty} x^{a+k}\, c_k(a)\left[(k+a)^2-\nu^2\right]+\sum_{\ell=0}^{\infty} x^{a+\ell+2}\, c_\ell(a)\left[1-\frac{\mu}{2}(\ell+a)\right]. \qquad (9.442)$$

The change of variable of summation (9.443a) leads to (9.443b):

$$\ell+2=k: \quad 0=\sum_{k=0}^{\infty} x^k\left\{c_k(a)\left[(k+a)^2-\nu^2\right]+c_{k-2}\left[1-\frac{\mu}{2}(k+a-2)\right]\right\}. \qquad (9.443\text{a, b})$$

Setting (9.444a) leads to (9.444b), where $c_0(a)=0$ would lead to all $c_k(a)=0$ in (9.443b) and hence (9.377b) a trivial solution $y(x)=0$; thus a non-trivial solution requires (9.444c), leading to the indicial equation (9.444d) with roots (9.444e):

$$k=0: \quad \left(a^2-\nu^2\right)c_0(a)=0; \quad c_0(a)\neq 0: \quad a^2=\nu^2, \quad a_\pm=\pm\nu. \qquad (9.444\text{a–e})$$

Thus the indices (9.444e) are specified by the order ν as in the original Bessel equation, (9.430b); if $+\nu$ is an index then $-\nu$ must also be an index because the generalized Bessel differential equation (9.428f) is unchanged when the sign of ν is reversed. The recurrence formula (9.443b) for the coefficients (9.445a):

$$c_{2k}(a)=-\frac{1-(\mu/2)(a+2k-2)}{(2k+a)^2-\nu^2}c_{2k-2}(a)=-\frac{1-\mu(k-1+a/2)}{(2k+a-\nu)(2k+a+\nu)}c_{2k-2}(a), \qquad (9.445\text{a, b})$$

shows that they depend (9.445b) also on the degree μ. Appling k times (9.445b) leads to the explicit coefficients (9.446a):

$$\begin{aligned} c_{2k}(\nu)&=(-)^k c_0(\nu)\prod_{j=1}^{k}\frac{1-\mu(j-1+\nu/2)}{4j(j+\nu)} \\ &=c_0(\nu)\frac{(-1/4)^k}{k!}\frac{\Gamma(1+\nu)}{\Gamma(1+k+\nu)}\prod_{j=1}^{k}\left[1-\mu(j-1+\nu/2)\right], \end{aligned} \qquad (9.446\text{a, b})$$

using the recurrence formula (9.432b) for the gamma function in (9.446b). For the original Bessel differential equation (9.447a), the last factor is unity leading to the usual expression (9.447c) using (9.447b) for consistency with common practice:

$$\mu=0: \quad c_0(\nu)=\frac{2^{-\nu}}{\Gamma(1+\nu)}: \quad c_{2k}(\nu)=\frac{2^{-\nu}(-1/4)^k}{k!\,\Gamma(1+k+\nu)}. \qquad (9.447\text{a–c})$$

Thus the generalized Bessel function of the first kind, order ν, and degree μ is given by (9.377b) with index $a=\nu$ in (9.444e) and coefficients (9.446b; 9.447b) leading to (9.448):

$$J_\nu^\mu(x)=\left(\frac{x}{2}\right)^\nu\sum_{k=0}^{\infty}\frac{\left(-x^2/4\right)^k}{k!\Gamma(1+k+\nu)}\prod_{j=0}^{k-1}\left[1-\mu\left(j+\nu/2\right)\right], \qquad (9.448)$$

valid for all μ. It is understood that when $k=0$ the product in (9.448) is replaced by unity.

In the case of the original Bessel function the degree is zero $\mu=0$, and the last factor in (9.448) is omitted, leading to the usual series expansion that is alternating for real variable x and has fixed sign for imaginary variable. The last factor that distinguishes the generalized Bessel function is: (i) positive for $\mu<0$ and does not change the sign of the terms of the series; and (ii) for $\mu>0$ the sign of the terms of the series is fixed for $\mu\left(j+\nu/2\right)>1$, and in particular if $\mu\nu/2>1$ the terms of the series have the same sign. For example if μ,ν are real such that $\mu\nu/2>1$, then the series for the generalized Bessel function (9.448) has fixed sign for real x, and alternating sign for imaginary x; this is the reverse of the series for the original Bessel function when the last factor in (9.448) is omitted. If the degree is not zero (9.449a), the last factor in the coefficients (9.446b) may be written (9.449b) and using (9.432b) leads to (9.449c):

$$\mu\neq 0:\ \prod_{j=0}^{k-1}\left[1-\mu\left(j+\nu/2\right)\right]=(-\mu)^k\prod_{j=0}^{k-1}\left(j+\nu/2-1/\mu\right)=(-\mu)^k\frac{\Gamma(k+\nu/2-1/\mu)}{\Gamma(\nu/2-1/\mu)}; \qquad (9.449a\text{–}c)$$

substitution of (9.449c) in (9.448) leads to (9.450b):

$$\mu\neq 0:\qquad J_\nu^\mu(x)=\frac{(x/2)^\nu}{\Gamma\left(\nu/2-1/\mu\right)}\sum_{k=0}^{\infty}\frac{\left(\mu x^2/4\right)^k}{k!}\frac{\Gamma\left(k+\nu/2-1/\mu\right)}{\Gamma(1+k+\nu)}; \qquad (9.450a, b)$$

this is an alternative expression (9.450b) for the generalized Bessel function (9.448) when the degree is not zero (9.450a) and involves powers of $\mu x^2/4$ rather than of $-x^2/4$, hence omitting the alternating sign and inserting the factor μ. Thus *the general integral of the generalized Bessel equation (9.428a–f) is (standard CCCIV) a linear combination with arbitrary constants $C_\pm$ of the Bessel functions of the first kind (9.451c) for the indices (9.444e):*

$$\nu\neq 0,1,2,\ldots\equiv n\in|N_0:\quad 0\leq|x|<\infty:\quad Q(x)=C_+\,J_\nu^\mu(x)+C_-\,J_{-\nu}^\mu(x), \qquad (9.451a\text{–}c)$$

provided that they be linearly independent; that is, the order is not an integer (9.451a). Since the generalized Bessel differential equation has, besides the origin, only one more singularity at infinity, the solution (9.451c) is valid for finite x; that is, it excludes (9.451b) only the asymptotic limit $x \to \infty$. The general integral (9.451c) fails for integer order (9.451a) because in that case the generalized Bessel functions $J^{\mu}_{\pm n}(x)$ are linearly dependent, as shown next (subsection 9.5.15).

9.5.15 Order and Degree of the Generalized Bessel Function

If the order is zero $\nu = 0$, the generalized Bessel functions in (9.451c) coincide, so there is only one arbitrary constant of integration $C_+ + C_-$, and the general integral fails; in this case, of a double root $a = \pm\nu = 0$ of the indicial equation (9.444d, e), a particular integral linearly independent of J^{μ}_0 is (subsection 9.5.9) a regular integral of the second–kind, first type Y^{μ}_0, designated the Neumann (subsections 9.5.16–9.5.20) function, that has a logarithmic singularity. A logarithmic singularity could also appear in the regular integral of second kind, second type (subsection 9.5.10) when (9.407a) the differences of indices (9.444e) is an integer $s = a_+ - a_- = 2\nu$, leading to two cases, namely: for even $2\nu = 2s$ (odd $2\nu = 2s+1$) the order is an integer $\nu = s$ (integer-plus-one-half $\nu = s + 1/2$) corresponding to the cylindrical (spherical) Bessel functions [subsection(s) 9.5.22 (9.5.23–9.5.26)]:

$$a_+ - a_- = s = \begin{cases} s = 2n \Rightarrow \nu = n: & \text{cylindrical functions} \\ s = 2n+1 \Rightarrow \nu = n + 1/2: & \text{spherical functions} \end{cases}. \tag{9.452a–c}$$

In order to check if the generalized Bessel function orders $\pm\nu$ in the general integral (9.451c) are linearly independent it is sufficient subsection 1.2.3) to determine their Wronskian at one point (subsection 9.5.12); choosing the origin and using the limit as $x \to 0$ of (9.448) leads to (9.453a, b):

$$J^{\mu}_{\pm\nu}(x) = \frac{(x/2)^{\pm\nu}}{\Gamma(1\pm\nu)}\left[1 + O\left(x^2\right)\right], \qquad \frac{d}{dx}\left[J^{\mu}_{\pm\nu}(x)\right] = \pm\frac{\nu}{2}\frac{(x/2)^{\pm\nu-1}}{\Gamma(1\pm\nu)}\left[1 + O\left(x^2\right)\right]. \tag{9.453a, b}$$

The Wronskian (9.425b) is given near the origin by (9.453c):

$$W\left(J^{\mu}_{\nu}(x), J^{\mu}_{-\nu}(x)\right) = -\frac{\nu}{2}\frac{2}{x}\frac{2}{\Gamma(1-\nu)\Gamma(1+\nu)} = -\frac{2/x}{\Gamma(\nu)\Gamma(1-\nu)} = -\frac{2}{\pi x}\sin(\pi\nu), \tag{9.453c–e}$$

using the properties (9.432c) [(9.440c)] of the Gamma function in (9.453d) [(9.453e)].

Comparing the Wronskian (9.453c) near the origin with the general form (9.429c) follows (9.454a):

$$W_0 = -\frac{2}{\pi}\sin(\pi\nu): \quad W\left(J^{\mu}_{\nu}(x), J^{\mu}_{-\nu}(x)\right) = -\frac{2}{\pi x}\sin(\pi\nu)\exp\left(\frac{\mu x^2}{4}\right), \tag{9.454a, b}$$

and hence, substituting (9.454a) in (9.429c) the Wronskian is given for all x by (9.454b). *The Wronskian (9.454b) of the (standard CCCV) generalized Bessel functions (9.448) vanishes (9.454a) both for the original* $\mu = 0$ *(generalized* $\mu \neq 0$*) Bessel functions if (9.454d) the order is an integer (9.454e):*

$$W\left(J_\nu^\mu(x), J_{-\nu}^\mu(x)\right) = 0 \Rightarrow \sin(\pi\nu) = 0 \quad \Rightarrow \quad \nu = 0, \pm 1, \pm 2, \ldots \in | Z, \qquad (9.454\text{c–e})$$

which is the case when the general integral (9.451c) fails (9.451a). Thus cylindrical (9.452b) [spherical (9.452c)] generalized Bessel functions of order equal to an integer (integer plus a half) have zero (9.455a) [non-zero (9.455b)] Wronskian (9.454b):

$$W\left(J_\nu^\mu(x), J_{-\nu}^\mu(x)\right) = 0, \quad W\left(J_{n+1/2}^\mu(x), J_{-n-1/2}^\mu(x)\right) = \frac{(-)^{n+1}2}{\pi x}\exp\left(\frac{\mu x^2}{4}\right), \qquad (9.455\text{a, b})$$

and hence are not (are) linearly independent.

The vanishing of the Wronskian (9.455a) for (9.455c) implies that there is a linear relation between the generalized Bessel functions of orders $\pm n$ that can be obtained, noting that if the order $\nu = n$ is a positive integer in the second solution J_{-n}^μ, the gamma function $\Gamma(1 - n + k) = \infty$ has a pole (9.435a–c) for $k = 1, 2, \ldots, n-1$ by (9.437a, b); this factor in the denominator of (9.450b) suppresses the first n terms, leading to (9.456b):

$$\ell = k - n: \qquad \Gamma\left(-\frac{n}{2} - \frac{1}{\mu}\right) J_{-n}^\mu(x) = \left(\frac{x}{2}\right)^{-n} \sum_{k=n}^{\infty} \left(\frac{\mu x^2}{4}\right)^k \frac{\Gamma(k - n/2 - 1/\mu)}{k!(k-n)!}$$

$$= \left(\frac{x}{2}\right)^{-n} \sum_{\ell=0}^{\infty} \left(\frac{\mu x^2}{4}\right)^{n+\ell} \frac{\Gamma(\ell + n/2 - 1/\mu)}{\ell!(n+\ell)!}$$

$$= \mu^n \left(\frac{x}{2}\right)^n \sum_{\ell=n}^{\infty} \left(\frac{\mu x^2}{4}\right)^\ell \frac{\Gamma(\ell + n/2 - 1/\mu)}{\ell!(n+\ell)!}$$

$$= \mu^n \Gamma\left(\frac{n}{2} - \frac{1}{\mu}\right) J_n^\mu(x), \qquad (9.456\text{a, b})$$

where the substitution (9.456a) was made. The recurrence formula (9.432b) for the gamma function:

$$\Gamma\left(\frac{n}{2} - \frac{1}{\mu}\right) = \Gamma\left(-\frac{n}{2} - \frac{1}{\mu}\right) \prod_{j=1}^{n} \left(\frac{n}{2} - \frac{1}{\mu} - j\right), \qquad (9.457)$$

may be used in (9.456b).

The comparison of (9.457) with (9.449b) suggests the introduction of the **matching coefficient:**

$$\frac{1}{A(\mu,n)} \equiv (-\mu)^n \frac{\Gamma(n/2-1/\mu)}{\Gamma(-n/2-1/\mu)} = \prod_{j=0}^{n-1}\left[1-\mu(j-n/2)\right], \qquad (9.458a, b)$$

that establishes (9.456b) the linear relation between the generalized Bessel functions (9.459b) of arbitrary degree and integer order (9.459a):

$$n = 0,1,2,\ldots \in | N_0: \qquad J^{\mu}_{-n}(z) = \frac{(-)^n}{A(\mu,n)} J^{\mu}_{n}(z). \qquad (9.459a, b)$$

It has been shown that *the generalized Bessel functions of integer order (9.459a) are (standard CCCVI) linearly dependent (9.459b) with a coefficient independent of the variable x and given by (9.458b) [(9.458a)] for arbitrary (non-zero) degree. Thus the general integral (9.451c) of the generalized Bessel differential equation (9.428a–f) of order* ν *and degree* ν *is a linear combination of the orders* $\pm\nu$ *if they are not integers (9.451a).* In the case of integer order, a particular integral independent from the generalized Bessel function $J^{\mu}_{\nu}(x)$ is (subsections 9.5.16–9.5.21) the generalized Neumann function; that is, a regular integral of the second kind (subsections 9.5.9–9.5.10). The coefficients in the series expansions of the regular integrals of the first (second) kinds [subsection(s) 9.5.8 (9.5.9–9.5.10)] often involve the gamma (digamma) function [subsection 9.5.13 (9.5.16)].

9.5.16 The Digamma Function as the Logarithmic Derivative of the Gamma Function

The **digamma function** (9.460a) is defined as the logarithmic derivative of the gamma function:

$$\psi(\nu) \equiv \frac{d}{d\nu}\{\log[\Gamma(\nu)]\} = \frac{\Gamma'(\nu)}{\Gamma(\nu)}:$$

$$\Gamma'(\nu) = \psi(\nu)\Gamma(\nu), \qquad \left[\frac{1}{\Gamma(\nu)}\right]' = -\frac{\Gamma'(\nu)}{[\Gamma(\nu)]^2} = -\frac{\psi(\nu)}{\Gamma(\nu)}, \qquad (9.460a–c)$$

implying that differentiation of the gamma function (its inverse) is equivalent to multiplication by plus (9.460b) [minus (9.460c)] the digamma function. The infinite product (9.438e) for the gamma function is uniformly convergent, and as for uniformly convergent series (section I.21.6), operators like the logarithm (9.461):

$$\log[\Gamma(\nu)] = -\gamma\nu - \log\nu - \sum_{m=1}^{\infty}\left[\log\left(1+\frac{\nu}{m}\right) - \frac{\nu}{m}\right], \qquad (9.461)$$

and differentiation (9.462b) may be applied term by term:

$$\psi(\nu) = \frac{d}{d\nu}\{\log[\Gamma(\nu)]\} = -\gamma - \frac{1}{\nu} + \sum_{m=1}^{\infty}\left(\frac{1}{m} - \frac{1}{m+\nu}\right) = -\gamma - \frac{1}{\nu} + \nu\sum_{m=1}^{\infty}\frac{1}{m(m+\nu)}; \tag{9.462a–c}$$

the series of fractions (9.462c) specifies the digamma function (9.462a). From (9.462c) follows that, like the gamma function (9.435b), the digamma function also has simple poles (9.463b) for non-positive integer values of the variable (9.435a) ≡ (9.463a) with residue minus unity (9.463c) instead of (9.435c):

$$m = 0, -1, -2, \ldots: \qquad \psi(\nu) = \frac{\psi_{-1}}{\nu+m} + O(1), \quad \psi_{-1} = -1; \tag{9.463a–c}$$

the residue (9.239b) is calculated by (9.464a):

$$\psi_{-1} = \lim_{\nu\to -k}(\nu+k)\psi(\nu) = \lim_{\nu\to -k}\frac{\nu(k+\nu)}{k(k+\nu)} = -1, \tag{9.464a–c}$$

where (9.462c) was used in (9.464b) leading to (9.464c) ≡ (9.463c).

Taking the logarithm of the recurrence (9.432b) [symmetry (9.440c)] formula for the gamma function leads to (9.465a) [(9.465b)]:

$$\log[\Gamma(\nu+n)] = \sum_{m=0}^{n-1}\log(\nu+m) + \log[\Gamma(\nu)], \tag{9.465a}$$

$$\log[\Gamma(\nu)] + \log[\Gamma(1-\nu)] = \log\pi - \log[\sin(\pi\nu)], \tag{9.465b}$$

and differentiation proves the recurrence (9.466a) [symmetry (9.466b)] formula for the digamma function:

$$\psi(\nu+n) = \psi(\nu) + \frac{1}{\nu} + \frac{1}{\nu+1} + \ldots + \frac{1}{\nu+n-1}, \quad \psi(\nu) + \pi\cot(\pi\nu) = \psi(1-\nu). \tag{9.466a, b}$$

From (9.466a) with $n = 1$ follows (9.467a), that substituted in (9.466a) [(9.462c)] leads to (9.467b) [(9.467c)]:

$$\psi(1+\nu) = \psi(\nu) + \frac{1}{\nu}: \qquad \psi(\nu+n) = \psi(1+\nu) + \frac{1}{\nu+1} + \frac{1}{\nu+2} + \ldots + \frac{1}{\nu+n-1}, \tag{9.467a, b}$$

$$\psi(1+\nu) = -\gamma + \nu\sum_{m=1}^{\infty}\frac{1}{m(m+\nu)}. \tag{9.467c}$$

The value of the Euler-Mascheroni constant is given by (9.468a, b):

$$-\gamma = \psi(1) = \frac{\Gamma'(1)}{\Gamma(1)}: \qquad \psi(1) = -\gamma - 1 + \lim_{m\to\infty}\left(1 - \frac{1}{m}\right) = -\gamma, \tag{9.468a–c}$$

that follows from (9.462b) for $\nu = 1$ leading to (9.468c). It has been shown that *the digamma function defined as the logarithmic derivative of the gamma function (9.460a–c) is (standard CCCVII) analytic in the whole complex plane except for simple poles (9.463b) with residue (9.463c) for non-positive integers (9.463a). The digamma function is specified by the series of fractions (9.467c) ≡ (9.462c) involving the Euler-Mascheroni constant (9.468a, b) and has recurrence (symmetry) formulas (9.466a) [(9.466b)]*. The digamma function is used next in the derivation of the generalized Neumann function that is a regular integral of the second kind (subsections 9.5.17–9.5.18) that is needed in the general integral of the generalized Bessel differential equation (subsection 9.5.19) when the order is an integer.

9.5.17 Generalized Neumann Function of Integer Order

When the order (9.428d) of the generalized Bessel differential equation (9.428a, b, c, e, f) is a non-negative integer (9.469a), in the general integral (9.451c) the generalized Bessel function $J^{\mu}_{-n}(x)$ of order $-n$ is replaced (9.409d) by a regular integral of the second kind (9.469b):

$$\nu = 0,1,2,,\ldots \equiv n: \qquad Y^{\mu}_{n}(x) = \frac{2}{\pi}\lim_{a\to -n}\frac{\partial}{\partial a}\left[(a+n)y_a(x)\right]; \tag{9.469a, b}$$

the regular integral of the first kind (9.377b) satisfies the recurrence formula (9.445b) for the coefficients, leading to (9.470):

$$y_a(x) = c_0(a)x^a\sum_{k=0}^{\infty}\left(-x^2\right)^k\prod_{\ell=1}^{k}\frac{1-\mu(\ell-1+a/2)}{(2\ell+a+n)(2\ell+a-n)}, \tag{9.470}$$

and thus is linearly independent from the generalized Bessel function. In the **generalized Neumann function** (9.469b; 9.470) with non-negative integer order (9.469a) the constant factor $2/\pi$ was introduced for consistency with the literature on the original Neumann function.

For $k = n$ and $\ell = k = n$ there is a term $2\ell + a - n = a + n$ in the denominator of (9.470) that cancels with $(a+n)$ in (9.469b). This cancellation does not occur for the first n terms $k = 0,\ldots,n-1$ that are separated to form a **preliminary function**:

$$X^{\mu}_{n}(x) = \frac{2}{\pi}\lim_{a\to -n}\frac{\partial}{\partial a}\left\{(a+n)c_0(a)\sum_{k=0}^{n-1}(-)^k\, x^{a+2k}\prod_{\ell=1}^{k}\frac{1-\mu(\ell-1+a/2)}{(2\ell+a+n)(2\ell+a-n)}\right\}. \tag{9.471}$$

If the derivative $\partial/\partial a$ is not applied to $(a+n)$, this term remains and leads to zero when $a \to -n$; thus the only non-zero terms in (9.471) arise differentiating $\partial(n+a)/\partial a = 1$; that is, suppressing the factor $n+a$ and taking the limit $a \to -n$ in the remaining terms, leading to (9.472a, b):

$$X_n^\mu(x) = \frac{2}{\pi} c_0(-n) \sum_{k=0}^{n-1} (-)^k x^{2k-n} \prod_{\ell=1}^{k} \frac{1-\mu(\ell-1-n/2)}{4\ell(\ell-n)}$$
$$= \frac{2}{\pi} c_0(-n) x^{-n} \sum_{k=0}^{n-1} \frac{(x/2)^{2k}}{k!} \frac{1}{(n-1)\ldots(n-k)} \prod_{j=0}^{k-1} \left[1-\mu(j-n/2)\right]. \quad (9.472a, b)$$

Choosing the leading coefficient:

$$c_0(-n) = -(n-1)!2^{n-1} \left\{ \prod_{j=0}^{n-1} \left[1-\mu(j-n/2)\right] \right\}^{-1}, \quad (9.473)$$

and substituting in (9.472b) specifies the preliminary function (9.474a, b):

$$X_n^\mu(x) = -\frac{1}{\pi}\left(\frac{x}{2}\right)^{-n} \sum_{k=0}^{n-1} \frac{(x/2)^k}{k!} \frac{(n-1)!}{(n-1)\ldots(n-k)} \left\{ \prod_{j=k}^{\ell-1} \left[1-\mu(j-n/2)\right] \right\}^{-1}$$
$$= -\frac{1}{\pi}\left(\frac{x}{2}\right)^{-n} \sum_{k=0}^{n-1} \left(\frac{x}{2}\right)^k \frac{(n-k-1)!}{k!} \left\{ \prod_{j=k}^{n-1} \left[1-\mu(j-n/2)\right] \right\}^{-1},$$

(9.474a, b)

that has powers x^{-1} up to x^{-n} corresponding to a pole of order n. The first two factors in (9.473) apply for $\mu = 0$ to the preliminary function for the original Neumann function; the factor in curly brackets is relevant for non-zero degree and affects only the generalized Neumann function. The latter involves, besides the preliminary function (subsection 9.5.18), two other terms; namely, a logarithmic singularity and a complementary function (subsection 9.5.19), as expected for a regular integral of the second kind second type (subsection 9.5.10).

9.5.18 Preliminary and Complementary Functions and Logarithmic Term

Subtracting the preliminary function (9.471) from the generalized Neumann function (9.469b; 9.470) leaves the term of the series starting with $k = n$ in (9.475):

$$\frac{\pi}{2}\left[Y_n^\mu(x) - X_n^\mu(x)\right] = \lim_{a \to -n} \frac{\partial}{\partial a} \left\{ (a+n) c_0(a) x^a \sum_{\alpha=n}^{\infty} \left(-x^2\right)^\alpha \prod_{\beta=1}^{\alpha} \frac{1-\mu(\beta-1+a/2)}{(2\beta+a+n)(2\beta+a-n)} \right\}. \quad (9.475)$$

The leading coefficient is chosen (9.476):

$$c_0(a) = 2^{-2n-a}\frac{(-)^n}{n+a}\prod_{\beta=1}^{n}\frac{(2\beta+a+n)(2\beta+a-n)}{1-\mu(\beta-1+a/2)}, \tag{9.476}$$

to suppress the first n factors in (9.475) leaving in (9.477) only the factors from $\beta = n+1$ to $\beta = \alpha$:

$$\begin{aligned}&\frac{\pi}{2}\left[Y_n^\mu(x) - X_n^\mu(x)\right]\\&= \lim_{a\to -n}\frac{\partial}{\partial a}\left\{(-)^n 2^{-2n}\left(\frac{x}{2}\right)^a\sum_{\alpha=n}^{\infty}\left(-x^2\right)^\alpha\prod_{\beta=n+1}^{\alpha}\frac{1-\mu(\beta-1+a/2)}{(2\beta+a+n)(2\beta+a-n)}\right\}.\end{aligned} \tag{9.477}$$

The changes of summation indices (9.478a, b) lead from (9.477) to (9.478c):

$$\begin{aligned}k = \alpha - n, \ell = \beta - n: \quad &\frac{\pi}{2}\left[Y_n^\mu(x) - X_n^\mu(x)\right]\\&= \lim_{a\to -n}\frac{\partial}{\partial a}\left\{2^{-2n}x^{2n}\left(\frac{x}{2}\right)^a\sum_{k=0}^{\infty}\left(-x^2\right)^k\prod_{\ell=1}^{k}\frac{1-\mu(\ell-1+n+a/2)}{(2\ell+a+3n)(2\ell+a+n)}\right\}.\end{aligned} \tag{9.478a–c}$$

Differentiating the power in (9.478c) leads to a logarithmic term (9.479a):

$$\begin{aligned}&\log\left(\frac{x}{2}\right)\left\{\sum_{k=0}^{\infty}\left(-x^2\right)^k\prod_{\ell=1}^{k}\frac{1-\mu(\ell-1+n/2)}{4\ell(\ell+n)}\right\}\lim_{a\to -n}\left(\frac{x}{2}\right)^{a+2n}\\&= \log\left(\frac{x}{2}\right)\left(\frac{x}{2}\right)^n\sum_{k=0}^{\infty}\frac{\left(-x^2/4\right)^k}{k!(k+n)!}\prod_{j=0}^{k-1}\left[1-\mu(j+n/2)\right]\\&= J_n^\mu(x)\log\left(\frac{x}{2}\right),\end{aligned} \tag{9.479a–c}$$

multiplied by (9.479b) the generalized Bessel function (9.448) in (9.479c).
Substituting (9.479c) in (9.478c) leads to (9.480a):

$$\begin{aligned}&\frac{\pi}{2}\left[Y_n^\mu(x) - X_n^\mu(x)\right] - \log\left(\frac{x}{2}\right)J_n^\mu(x) = \frac{\pi}{2}Z_n^\mu(x)\\&= \lim_{a\to -n}\left(\frac{x}{2}\right)^{a+2n}\sum_{k=0}^{\infty}\left(-x^2\right)^k\frac{\partial}{\partial a}\left\{\prod_{\ell=1}^{k}\frac{1-\mu(\ell-1+n+a/2)}{(2\ell+a+3n)(2\ell+a+n)}\right\},\end{aligned} \tag{9.480a, b}$$

specifying the third term in the generalized Neumann function; that is, the **complementary function**:

$$Z_n^\mu(x) = \frac{2}{\pi}\left(\frac{x}{2}\right)^n \sum_{k=0}^{\infty}\left(-x^2\right)^k \lim_{a\to -n}$$

$$\left\{\prod_{\ell=1}^{k}\frac{1-\mu(\ell-1+n+a/2)}{(2\ell+a+3n)(2\ell+a+n)}\right.$$

$$\left.\times\sum_{m=1}^{k}\left(-\frac{1}{2m+a+3n}-\frac{1}{2m+a+n}+\frac{1}{2m-2+2n+a-2/\mu}\right)\right\}$$

$$= \frac{1}{\pi}\left(\frac{x}{2}\right)^n \sum_{k=0}^{\infty}\frac{\left(-x^2/4\right)^k}{k!(n+k)!}$$

$$\times\left\{\prod_{\ell=1}^{k}\left[1-\mu(\ell-1+n/2)\right]\times\sum_{m=1}^{k}\left(-\frac{1}{m+n}-\frac{1}{m}+\frac{1}{m-1+n/2-1/\mu}\right)\right\}. \tag{9.481a, b}$$

The digamma function (9.466a) may be used in the last factor in (9.481b):

$$\sum_{m=1}^{k}\left(\frac{1}{m}+\frac{1}{m+n}-\frac{1}{m-1+n/2-1/\mu}\right)$$

$$= \psi(1+k)+\psi(1+k+n)-\psi(k+n/2-1/\mu)-\left[\psi(1)+\psi(1+n)-\psi(n/2-1/\mu)\right]. \tag{9.482}$$

The term in square brackets in (9.482) is a constant and multiplies in (9.481b) the generalized Bessel function (9.448); thus it may be incorporated in the arbitrary constant C_+ in the first term of the general integral (9.451c); the term outside the square bracket in (9.482) appears in the generalized Neumann function $Y_n^\mu(x)$ in (9.480b) involving (9.481b; 9.482) the complementary function, that has a zero of order n:

$$Z_n^\mu(x) = -\frac{1}{\pi}\left(\frac{x}{2}\right)^n \sum_{k=0}^{\infty}\frac{\left(-x^2/4\right)^k}{k!(n+k)!}\times\prod_{j=0}^{k-1}\left[1-\mu(j+n/2)\right] \tag{9.483}$$

$$\times\left[\psi(1+k)+\psi(1+k+n)-\psi(k+n/2-1/\mu)\right].$$

This completes the general integral of the generalized Bessel differential equation (9.428a–f) when the order is an integer (subsection 9.5.19).

9.5.19 General Integral in the Case of Integer Order

The generalized Bessel differential equation (9.428a–f), in the case of integer order $\nu = n$, has as particular integral linearly independent from the generalized Bessel function (9.448), the generalized Neumann function:

$$Y_n^\mu(x) = X_n^\mu(x) + \frac{2}{\pi}\log\left(\frac{x}{2}\right)J_n^\mu(x) + Z_n^\mu(x), \tag{9.484}$$

corresponding to (9.474b; 9.483) ≡ (9.485):

$$\begin{aligned} Y_n^\mu(x) = & -\frac{1}{\pi}\left(\frac{x}{2}\right)^{-n}\sum_{k=0}^{n-1}\left(\frac{x}{2}\right)^{2k}\frac{(n-k-1)!}{k!}\times\left\{\prod_{j=k}^{n-1}\left[1-\mu(j+n/2)\right]\right\}^{-1} \\ & -\frac{1}{\pi}\left(\frac{x}{2}\right)^{n}\sum_{k=0}^{\infty}\frac{\left(-x^2/4\right)^k}{k!\,(n+k)!}\times\prod_{j=0}^{k-1}\left[1-\mu(j+n/2)\right] \\ & \times\left[\psi(1+k)+\psi(1+k+n)-\psi(k+n/2-1/\mu)\right]+\frac{2}{\pi}\log\left(\frac{x}{2}\right)J_n^\mu(x). \end{aligned} \tag{9.485}$$

For zero degree $\mu = 0$ the products reduce to unity and the original Neumann (1867) function is regained; for zero order $n = 0$ the first preliminary function on the r.h.s. of (9.485) is omitted. Thus *the general integral of the generalized Bessel differential equation (9.428a–f) valid (standard CCCVIII) for finite variable (9.486b) and non-negative integer order (9.486a):*

$$\nu = 0,1,2,\ldots \equiv n \in |N_0; \quad 0 \le |x| < \infty: \quad y(x) = D_+ J_n^\mu(x) + D_- Y_n^\mu(x), \tag{9.486a–c}$$

is a linear combination (9.486c) with arbitrary constants $D_\pm$ of the Bessel (9.448) ≡ (9.487):

$$J_n^\mu(x) = \left(\frac{x}{2}\right)^n \sum_{k=0}^{\infty}\frac{\left(-x^2/4\right)^k}{k!(n+k)!}\prod_{j=0}^{k-1}\left[1-\mu(j+n/2)\right]. \tag{9.487}$$

and the Neumann (9.485) functions.

If the degree is not zero: (i) using (9.449a, c) the generalized Bessel function of integer order (9.468) becomes (9.450a, b) leading for integer order to (9.488b):

$$\mu \ne 0: \qquad J_n^\mu(x) = \frac{(x/2)^n}{\Gamma(n/2-1/\mu)}\sum_{k=0}^{\infty}\frac{\left(\mu x^2/4\right)^k}{k!(k+n)!}\Gamma(k+n/2-1/\mu); \tag{9.488a, b}$$

(ii) using (9.489a–c):

$$\left\{\prod_{j=k}^{n-1}\left[1-\mu\left(j-n/2\right)\right]\right\}^{-1} = \left(-\mu\right)^{k-n+1}\prod_{j=k}^{n-1}\left(j-n/2-1/\mu\right)^{-1}$$

$$= \left(-\mu\right)^{k-n+1}\left[\left(n/2-1-1/\mu\right)....\left(k-n/2-1/\mu\right)\right]^{-1} = \left(-\mu\right)^{k-n+1}\frac{\Gamma\left(k-n/2-1/\mu\right)}{\Gamma\left(n/2-1/\mu\right)}, \tag{9.489a–c}$$

the preliminary function (9.474b), becomes (9.490a, b):

$$\mu \neq 0: \quad X_n^\mu\left(x\right) = \frac{\mu}{\pi}\frac{\left(-\mu x/2\right)^{-n}}{\Gamma\left(n/2-1/\mu\right)}\sum_{k=0}^{n-1}\left(-\frac{\mu x^2}{4}\right)^k\frac{\left(n-k-1\right)!}{k!}\Gamma\left(k-n/2-1/\mu\right); \tag{9.490a, b}$$

and (iii) using (9.449a, c) the complementary function (9.483) becomes (9.491a, b):

$$\mu \neq 0: \qquad Z_n^\mu\left(x\right) = -\frac{1}{\pi}\frac{\left(x/2\right)^n}{\Gamma\left(n/2-1/\mu\right)}\sum_{k=0}^{n-1}\frac{\left(\mu x^2/4\right)^k}{k!\left(n+k\right)!}\Gamma\left(k-n/2-1/\mu\right) \tag{9.491a, b}$$

$$\left[\psi\left(1+k\right)+\psi\left(1+k+n\right)-\psi\left(k+n/2-1/\mu\right)\right].$$

Thus *there are alternate expressions for (standard CCCIX) arbitrary order (non-zero) order of: (i) the generalized Bessel function (9.448) [(9.450a, b)]; (ii) the preliminary function (9.474b) [(9.490a, b)]; and (iii) the complementary function (9.483) [(9.491a, b)]. The former three (i–iii) appear (iv) in (9.484) in the generalized Neumann function of arbitrary (9.485) [non-zero (9.492a, b)] order:*

$$\mu \neq 0: \; \Gamma\left(n/2-1/\mu\right)Y_n^\mu\left(x\right) = \frac{\mu}{\pi}\left(-\frac{\mu x}{2}\right)^{-n}\sum_{k=0}^{n-1}\left(-\frac{\mu x^2}{4}\right)^k\frac{\left(n-k-1\right)!}{k!}\Gamma\left(k-n/2-1/\mu\right)$$

$$-\frac{1}{\pi}\left(\frac{x}{2}\right)^n\sum_{k=0}^{\infty}\frac{\left(\mu x^2/4\right)^k}{k!\left(k+n\right)!}\Gamma\left(k+n/2-1/\mu\right)$$

$$\left[\psi\left(1+k\right)+\psi\left(1+k+n\right)-\psi\left(k+n/2-1/\mu\right)-2\log\left(x/2\right)\right]. \tag{9.492a, b}$$

The generalized Neumann function is extended next (subsection 9.5.20) from non-negative integer to arbitrary order. The general integrals (9.451c) [(9.486c)] of the generalized Bessel differential equation (9.428a–f) hold for finite variable (9.451b) [≡ (9.486b)] and non-integer (9.451a) [integer (9.486a)] order, and involve only (also) generalized Bessel (Neumann) functions; they can be replaced by a single expression using the generalized Neumann function with order extended from integer to complex (subsection 9.5.21); the extension uses some properties of Wronskians (subsection 9.5.20).

9.5.20 Wronskians of Generalized Bessel and Neumann Functions

The generalized Neumann function involves in the third term of the r.h.s. of (9.484) the product of a logarithm by the generalized Bessel function; thus the generalized Bessel and Neumann functions cannot be constant multiples, that is they must be linearly independent, implying that their Wronskian must be non-zero. In order to confirm that the generalized Bessel and Neumann functions of integer order are linearly independent as assumed in the general integral (9.486a–c) of the generalized Bessel differential equation (9.428a–f) it is sufficient to show that their Wronskian is not zero. The Wronskian for non-zero degree (9.493a) may be calculated near the origin: (i) using (9.453a, b) for the generalized Bessel functions of integer order (9.493b, c):

$$n \neq 0: \quad J_n^\mu(x) = \frac{(x/2)^n}{n!}\left[1+O\left(x^2\right)\right], \quad \frac{d}{dx}\left[J_n^\mu(x)\right] = \frac{1}{2}\frac{(x/2)^{n-1}}{(n-1)!}\left[1+O\left(x^2\right)\right]; \tag{9.493a–c}$$

(ii) using (9.494b) the leading term of the generalized Neumann function (9.485) for non-zero degree (9.494a) where may be substituted (9.458b) leading to (9.494c):

$$\begin{aligned} n \neq 0: \quad Y_n^\mu(x) &= -\frac{(n-1)!}{\pi}\left(\frac{x}{2}\right)^{-n}\left\{\prod_{j=0}^{n-1}\left[1-\mu\left(j-n/2\right)\right]\right\}^{-1}\left[1+O\left(x^2\right)\right] \\ &= -\frac{(n-1)!}{\pi}\left(\frac{x}{2}\right)^{-n} A(\mu,n)\left[1+O\left(x^2\right)\right], \end{aligned} \tag{9.494a–c}$$

and implying (9.495a, b):

$$n \neq 0: \quad \frac{d}{dx}\left[Y_n^\mu(x)\right] = \frac{n!}{2\pi}\left(\frac{x}{2}\right)^{-n-1} A(\mu,n)\left[1+O\left(x^2\right)\right]; \quad \mu = 0: \quad A(0,n) = 1, \tag{9.495a–d}$$

the coefficient (9.458a, b) is unity (9.495d) for the original Neumann function (9.495c) and can be omitted from (9.494c; 9.495b) in that case. Substitution of (9.493b, c) and (9.494c; 9.495b) in (9.425a) leads to the Wronskian (9.496b) of the generalized Bessel and Neumann functions of non-zero integer order (9.496a) near the origin:

$$n \neq 0: \quad W\left(J_n^\mu(x), Y_n^\mu(x)\right) = \frac{2}{\pi x} A(\mu,n)\left[1+O\left(x^2\right)\right], \tag{9.496a, b}$$

the Wronskian (9.496b) agrees with (9.429c) for (9.497a), specifying the exact Wronskian (9.497b):

$$W_0 = \frac{2}{\pi} A(\mu, n): \qquad W\left(J_n^\mu(x), Y_n^\mu(x)\right) = \frac{2}{\pi x} A(\mu, n) \exp\left(\frac{\mu x^2}{4}\right). \tag{9.497a, b}$$

In the case of zero order (9.498a), the leading terms (9.498b) [(9.498c)] of the generalized Bessel (9.448) [Neumann (9.485)] functions and their derivatives (9.498d) [(9.498e)] lead to the Wronskian (9.498f):

$$n = 0: \qquad J_0^\mu(x) \sim 1, \qquad J_0^\mu(x) \sim \frac{2}{\pi} \log\left(\frac{x}{2}\right), \qquad \frac{d}{dx}\left[J_0^\mu(x)\right] \sim -\frac{x}{2},$$
$$\frac{d}{dx}\left[Y_0^\mu(x)\right] \sim \frac{2}{\pi x}, \qquad W\left(J_0^\mu(x),\ Y_0^\mu(x)\right) \sim \frac{2}{\pi x}, \quad A(0, \mu) = 1, \tag{9.498a–g}$$

that coincides with (9.498f) ≡ (9.496b), bearing in mind (9.495d). *The Wronskian (9.497b) holds (standard CCCX) for any order, and does not vanish, proving that the generalized Bessel and Neumann functions of integer order are linearly independent.*

As a preliminary to the extension of the generalized Neumann function from integer to complex order is proved the **lemma of Wronskians**: *if two Wronskians coincide (9.499a) and one of the functions is common (standard CCCXI) the other two functions differ (9.499c) by a constant multiple (9.499b) of the common function:*

$$W(J, Y) = W(J, Z) \quad \Rightarrow \quad C = const: \qquad Z(x) - Y(x) = CJ(x). \tag{9.499a–c}$$

The equality (9.499a) of the Wronskians (9.425b) leads to (9.500a) that implies (9.500b):

$$JY' - J'Y = JZ' - J'Z: \qquad \frac{Z' - Y'}{Z - Y} = \frac{J'}{J}; \ \log[Z - Y] = \log C + \log J, \tag{9.500a–c}$$

integrating (9.500b) leads to (9.500c) ≡ (9.499c). QED. The converse of (9.500a–c) is also true:

$$C = const: \qquad W(J, J) = 0, \ \ W(J, Y + CJ) = W(J, Y) + CW(J, J) = W(J, Y); \tag{9.501a–c}$$

that is, *adding to the second function (standard CCCXII) a constant (9.501a) multiple of the first function (9.501b) does not change the Wronskian (9.501c).* Using the lemma of the Wronskians and the Wronskian for Bessel (9.454b) [Neumann (9.497b)] functions of complex (integer) order the generalized Neumann functions can be extended from integer to complex order (subsection 9.5.21).

9.5.21 Generalized Neumann Function with Complex Order

The ***generalized Neumann function*** *with complex order is defined (standard CCCXIII) by (9.502b) using the* ***extended matching coefficient*** *(9.502a):*

$$A(\mu,\nu)=(-\mu)^{-\nu}\frac{\Gamma(-\nu/2-1/\mu)}{\Gamma(\nu/2-1/\mu)}:\quad Y_\nu^\mu(x)=\frac{J_\nu^\mu(x)\cos(\pi\nu)-A(\mu,\nu)\,J_{-\nu}^\mu(x)}{\sin(\pi\nu)},\tag{9.502a, b}$$

that generalizes (9.458b) from integer n to complex ν.

The definition (9.502a, b) must be consistent with the case of integer order, when the coefficient (9.502a) simplifies (9.503a) to (9.458b):

$$\lim_{\nu\to n}A(\mu,\nu)=A(\mu,n):\qquad \lim_{\nu\to n}Y_\nu^\mu(x)=Y_n^\mu(x),\tag{9.503a, b}$$

and thus (9.502b) leads to (9.503b) that must be satisfied by the Neumann function of arbitrary order and integer degree. The proof of (9.502b) can be made in eight stages: (i) since (9.502b) is a linear combination of solutions $J_{\pm\nu}^\mu(x)$ of the generalized Bessel differential equation it is also a solution; (ii) for ν integer the denominator of (9.502b) is zero and from (9.459b) it follows that the numerator is also zero; (iii) thus the limit (9.502b) is an indetermination of 0:0 type, and it must be shown that it leads to the finite result (9.503b); (iv) the key step is to calculate the Wronskian (9.504b) of the generalized Bessel and Neumann functions of complex order (9.504b):

$$W\left(J_\nu^\mu(x),J_\nu^\mu(x)\right)=0:\quad W\left(J_\nu^\mu(x),Y_\nu^\mu(x)\right)=-\frac{A(\mu,\nu)\,W\left(J_\nu^\mu(x),J_{-\nu}^\mu(x)\right)}{\sin(\pi\nu)},\tag{9.504a, b}$$

bearing in mind that the Wronskian of the same function is zero (9.504a).

Thus (9.454b) leads (v) from (9.504b) to (9.504c):

$$W\left(J_\nu^\mu(x),Y_\nu^\mu(x)\right)=\frac{2}{\pi x}A(\mu,\nu)\exp\left(\frac{\mu x^2}{4}\right),\tag{9.504c}$$

that in limit (9.504d, e):

$$\lim_{\nu\to n}W\left(J_\nu^\mu(x),Y_\nu^\mu(x)\right)=\frac{2}{\pi x}A(\mu,n)\exp\left(\frac{\mu x^2}{4}\right)=W\left(J_n^\mu(x),Y_n^\mu(x)\right),\tag{9.504d, e}$$

coincides with the Wronskian (9.497b) ≡ (9.504e); (vi) in the case of integer order (9.505a) the equal Wronskians (9.504b) ≡ (9.504c) share the same function $J_\nu^\mu(x)$ and the lemma of the Wronskians (9.498a–c) implies (9.505b):

$$\nu=n:\qquad \lim_{\nu\to n}Y_\nu^\mu(x)-Y_n^\mu(x)=CJ_n^\mu(x);\tag{9.505a, b}$$

(vii) inserting the r.h.s. of (9.505b) in (9.502b) the numerator would no longer be zero as in (9.502b) and since the denominator is zero the whole expression would diverge; and (viii) the divergence of the limit can be avoided only by setting $C = 0$ in (9.505b) that then coincides with (9.503b). QED. It has been shown that *the general integral of the generalized Bessel differential equation (9.428a–f) is (standard CCCXIV) a linear combination of generalized Bessel and Neumann functions (9.506b) with arbitrary constants* $D_\pm$:

$$|x| < \infty: \qquad y(x) = D_+ J_\nu^\mu(x) + D_- Y_\nu^\mu(x), \tag{9.506a, b}$$

that holds for: (i) finite variable (9.506a); and (ii) all complex orders and degrees because the Wronskian (9.504b) is not zero and the generalized Bessel and Neumann functions are linearly independent. The preceding results apply both to the original (generalized) Bessel differential equation and Bessel and Neumann functions [subsection(s) 9.5.22 (9.5.14–9.5.21)].

9.5.22 Cylindrical Bessel Differential Equation (Euler 1764, Bessel 1824, Neumann 1867, Hankel 1869)

Most, though not all, of the results for the generalized Bessel differential equation (9.428a–f) simplify for the original Bessel differential equation (9.430b) with zero degree (9.430a) ≡ (9.495c) and the constant (9.495d) in (9.502b). These results may be summarized as follows: *the general integral of the original Bessel differential equation (9.430b) for finite values of the variable (9.507a) is (standard CCCXV) a linear combination with arbitrary constants* $C_\pm$ *of:*

$$|x| < \infty: \qquad y(x) = \begin{cases} C_+ J_\nu(x) + C_- J_{-\nu}(x) & \text{if} \quad \nu \neq 0, \pm 1, \pm 2, \ldots, \\ C_+ J_n(x) + C_- Y_n(x) & \text{if} \quad n = 0, 1, \pm 2, \ldots, \\ C_+ J_\nu(x) + C_- Y_\nu(x) & \text{if} \quad \text{all } \nu \in |C, \end{cases} \tag{9.507a–d}$$

(i) Bessel functions (Euler 1764, Bessel 1824) of orders $\pm\nu$ *that are linearly independent, that is, have non-zero (9.508a) Wronskian (9.454b) for non-integer order (9.507b) and are related by (9.509a) for integer order; (ii) Bessel and Neumann (Neumann 1867, Hankel 1869) functions of integer order (9.507c) that are linearly independent because their Wronskian (9.497b) is not zero (9.508b); (iii) Bessel and Neumann functions of any order (9.507d) that have (9.504a) the same Wronskian:*

$$W\left(J_\nu(x), J_{-\nu}(x)\right) = -\frac{2}{\pi x}\sin(\pi\nu), W\left(J_n(x), Y_n(x)\right) = \frac{2}{\pi x} = W\left(J_\nu(x), Y_\nu(x)\right). \tag{9.508a–c}$$

$$J_{-n}(x) = (-)^n J_n(x); \qquad Y_\nu(x) = \frac{J_\nu(x)\cos(\nu\pi) - J_{-\nu}(x)}{\sin(\nu\pi)}, \tag{9.509a, b}$$

(iv) the Bessel and Neumann function are related (9.501b) by (9.509b); (v) the Bessel functions (9.448) are given by (9.510a) [(9.510b)] for complex (non-negative integer) order:

$$J_\nu(x) = \left(\frac{x}{2}\right)^\nu \sum_{k=0}^{\infty} \frac{(-x^2/4)^k}{k!\Gamma(1+k+\nu)}, \qquad J_n(x) = \left(\frac{x}{2}\right)^n \sum_{k=0}^{\infty} \frac{(-x^2/4)^k}{k!(k+n)!}; \qquad (9.510a, b)$$

and (v) the Neumann functions (9.485) of integer order are given by (9.511):

$$Y_n(x) = \frac{2}{\pi}\log x J_n(x) - \frac{1}{\pi}\left(\frac{x}{2}\right)^{-n} \sum_{k=0}^{n-1} \left(\frac{x}{2}\right)^{2k} \frac{(n-k-1)!}{k!}$$
$$- \frac{1}{\pi}\left(\frac{x}{2}\right)^n \sum_{k=0}^{\infty} \frac{(-x^2/4)^k}{k!(n+k)!}\left[\psi(1+k) + \psi(1+k+n)\right]. \qquad (9.511)$$

In the case (standard CCCXVI) of zero order (9.512a), the original Bessel differential equation (9.430b) simplifies to (9.451b):

$$\nu = 0: \qquad xy'' + y' + xy = 0, \qquad y(x) = C_+ J_0(x) + C_- Y_0(x), \qquad (9.512a–c)$$

whose general integral (9.451c) is a linear combination with arbitrary constants $C_\pm$ of: (i) the Bessel function of zero order (9.451a):

$$J_0(x) = \sum_{k=0}^{\infty} \frac{(-x^2/4)^k}{(k!)^2}; \quad Y_0(x) = \frac{2}{\pi}\log x\, J_0(x) - \frac{2}{\pi}\sum_{k=0}^{\infty} \frac{(-x^2/4)^k}{(k!)^2}\psi(1+k), \qquad (9.513a, b)$$

and (ii) the Neumann function of zero order (9.513b), that does not involve a preliminary function; that is, the second term on the r.h.s. of (9.511) is absent for $n = 0$. The designation cylindrical (spherical) Bessel differential equation and functions [subsection(s) 9.5.22 (9.5.23–26)] relates to their appearance [note 8.4 (8.5)] in the solution of the isotropic equation of mathematical physics (notes 8.1–8.3) in cylindrical (spherical) coordinates and their relation with cylindrical (spherical) waves [notes 7.42–7.43 (7.44–7.45)].

9.5.23 Spherical Bessel Differential Equation

The isotropic equation of mathematical physics (8.340) has harmonic solutions (8.342a) with frequency ω, leading to the Helmholtz equation (8.343b) with wavenumber (8.343a). The Helmholtz equation in cylindrical (8.349) [spherical (8.357)] coordinates has radial $r(R)$ dependence (8.353b) [(8.361a, b)] specified by a cylindrical (9.514c) ≡ (9.430b) [spherical (9.515c)] Bessel differential equation:

$$x = \bar{k}r; \qquad y(x) = X(r): \qquad x^2 y'' + x y' + \left(x^2 - m^2\right) y = 0, \tag{9.514a–c}$$

$$x = kR; \qquad z(x) = X(R): \qquad x^2 z'' + 2xz' + \left[x^2 - n(n+1)\right] z = 0, \tag{9.515a–c}$$

with: (i) variables (9.514a, b) [(9.515a, b)] in agreement with (8.354a, b) [8.362)]; (ii) integer m corresponding (8.355) [(8.363)] to the azimuthal wavenumber. The change of dependent variable (9.516a) where α is an arbitrary constant leads to (9.516b, c):

$$z(x) = x^\alpha y(x): \; z' = x^\alpha \left(y' + \frac{\alpha}{x} y \right), z'' = x^\alpha \left[y'' + \frac{2\alpha}{x} y' + \frac{\alpha(\alpha-1)}{x^2} y \right]. \tag{9.516a–c}$$

Substitution of (9.516a–c) in the spherical Bessel differential equation (9.515c) leads to (9.517):

$$x^2 y'' + 2x(1+\alpha) y' + \left[x^2 + \alpha(\alpha+1) - n^2 - n\right] y = 0; \tag{9.517}$$

the choice (9.518a) for the constant leads from (9.517) to (9.518c):

$$\alpha = -\frac{1}{2}; \qquad m = n + \frac{1}{2}: \qquad x^2 y'' + x y' + \left[x^2 - \left(n + \frac{1}{2} \right)^2 \right] y = 0, \tag{9.518a–c}$$

that is a cylindrical Bessel differential equation (9.514a–c) of order integer plus a half (9.518b).

Thus *two solutions of the* ***spherical Bessel differential equation*** *(9.515c) are (standard CCCXVII) the* ***spherical Bessel (Neumann) function*** *(9.519a) [(9.519b)]:*

$$j_n(x) \equiv \sqrt{\frac{\pi}{2x}} J_{n+1/2}(x), \qquad y_n(x) \equiv \sqrt{\frac{\pi}{2x}} Y_{n+1/2}(x) = (-)^{n+1} \sqrt{\frac{\pi}{2x}} J_{-n-1/2}(x), \tag{9.519a–c}$$

that: (i) relate to the cylindrical Bessel functions of orders $\pm m = \pm(n+1/2)$ *in (9.518b); (ii) involve the factor* $x^{-1/2}$ *from (9.516a; 9.518a); (iii) the constant* $\sqrt{2/\pi}$ *was inserted for consistency with the literature; (iv) the Neumann function (9.519b) of order integer plus one half is related (9.509b) to the Bessel function of order minus integer minus a half by (9.520a) leading from (9.519b) to (9.519c):*

$$\begin{aligned} Y_{n+1/2}(x) &= (-)^{n+1} J_{-n-1/2}(x); W\left(J_{n+1/2}(x), J_{-n-1/2}(x)\right) \\ &= \frac{(-)^{n+1} 2}{\pi x}, W\left(J_{n+1/2}(x), Y_{n+1/2}(x)\right) = \frac{2}{\pi x}, \end{aligned} \tag{9.520a–c}$$

(v) the Bessel functions of order plus or minus integer-and–a–half are linearly independent because their Wronskian (9.508a) is not zero (9.520b); and (vi) the Bessel and Neumann functions of order integer-plus-a–half are (9.509b) related by (9.519c) and also linearly independent (9.520c), in agreement with (9.520a, b) ≡ (9.520c).

The indices of the cylindrical Bessel equation (9.514c) are (9.444e) ≡ (9.521a) and hence (9.519a–c) the factor $x^{-1/2}$ leads to the indices (9.521b, c) for the spherical Bessel equation (9.515c):

$$a_{\pm} = \pm m, \quad \bar{a}_{\pm} = -\frac{1}{2} \pm \left(n + \frac{1}{2} \right) = n, -n-1; \quad a_+ - a_- = 2m, \quad \bar{a}_+ - a_- = 2n+1. \tag{9.521a–e}$$

the indices of the cylindrical (9.521a) [spherical (9.521c)] Bessel differential equation (9.514c) [(9.515c)] differ by an even (9.521d) [odd (9.521e)] integer. In both cases the method of regular integrals [subsection 9.5.9 (9.5.10)] for coincident indices (9.403a) [indices differing by an integer (9.407a)] suggests the possible need in the general integral (9.406c) [(9.415b)] of the second kind type one (9.405a, b) [type two (9.416; 9.414b)] involving a logarithmic singularity. This need not be always the case, as shown by the contrast between: (a) the cylindrical Bessel differential equation (9.514c) leading to Bessel functions of integer orders $\pm n$ that are linearly dependent (9.509a) so that the general integral (9.507c) involves Neumann functions (9.511); (b) *the spherical Bessel differential equation (9.515c) leading (standard CCCXVIII) to spherical Bessel and Neumann functions (9.519a, b) that are equivalent (9.520a) to (9.522b) Bessel functions of opposite orders integer plus one half whose linear combination with arbitrary constants* $E_{\pm}$ *specifies the general integral (9.522c) for finite variable (9.522a):*

$$|x| < \infty: \qquad z(x) = E_+ j_n(x) + E_- y_n(x) = \sqrt{\frac{\pi}{2x}} \left[E_+ J_{n+1/2}(x) + E_- (-)^{n-1} J_{-n-1/2}(x) \right]. \tag{9.522a–c}$$

The linear independence of the spherical Bessel (9.519a) and Neumann (9.519b) ≡ (9.519c) functions with be confirmed next (subsection 9.5.24) from their explicit series expansions.

9.5.24 Spherical Bessel and Neumann Functions

The spherical Bessel (9.519a) [Neumann (9.519b) ≡ (9.519c)] functions have series expansions (9.523a) [(9.523b)] that are of the first kind (9.510a):

$$j_n(x) = \sqrt{\frac{\pi}{2x}} \left(\frac{x}{2} \right)^{n+1/2} \sum_{k=0}^{\infty} \frac{\left(-x^2/4\right)^k}{k!\Gamma(k+n+3/2)}, \tag{9.523a}$$

$$y_n(x) = (-)^{n+1} \sqrt{\frac{\pi}{2x}} \left(\frac{x}{2} \right)^{-n-1/2} \sum_{k=0}^{\infty} \frac{\left(-x^2/4\right)^k}{k!\Gamma(k-n+1/2)}. \tag{9.523b}$$

The gamma functions of variable integer plus one-half in (9.523a) are related (9.524b, c) to the gamma function of one-half (I.1.165b) ≡ (9.524a) by the recurrence formula (9.432b):

$$\Gamma(1/2)=\sqrt{\pi}: \qquad \Gamma(k+n+3/2)=(k+n+1/2)(k+n-1/2)...(1/2)\Gamma(1/2)$$
$$=(2k+2n+1)(2k+2n-1)...3.1.2^{-k-n}\sqrt{\pi}\equiv(2k+2n+1)!!2^{-k-n}\sqrt{\pi}. \tag{9.524a–c}$$

Substitution of (9.524c) in (9.523a) leads to the power series for the spherical Bessel functions (9.525a, b):

$$j_n(x)=x^n\sum_{k=0}^{\infty}\frac{\left(-x^2/2\right)^k}{k!(2n+2k+1)!!}$$
$$=\frac{x^n}{1.3.5...(2n+1)}\left[1-\frac{x^2/2}{1!(2n+3)}+\frac{\left(x^2/2\right)^2}{2!(2n+3)(2n+5)}\cdots\right], \tag{9.525a, b}$$

that have a zero of order n.

In the spherical Neumann function (9.523b) are separated the first (9.526a) [remaining (9.526c)] terms involving the gamma functions (9.526b) [(9.526d)]:

$$k=0: \quad \Gamma\left(\frac{1}{2}-n\right)=\frac{\Gamma(1/2)}{(-1/2)(-3/2)...(1/2-n)}=\frac{2^n(-)^n\sqrt{\pi}}{1.3...(2n-1)}=\frac{(-)^n\sqrt{\pi}}{(2n-1)!!2^{-n}}, \tag{9.526a, b}$$

$$k=1,2,...: \quad \Gamma\left(k-n+\frac{1}{2}\right)=\left(k-n-\frac{1}{2}\right)\left(k-n-\frac{3}{2}\right)\left(\frac{1}{2}-n\right)\Gamma\left(\frac{1}{2}-n\right)$$
$$=(2k-2n-1)(2k-2n-3)...(1-2n)2^{-k}\Gamma\left(\frac{1}{2}-n\right). \tag{9.526c, d}$$

Substitution of (9.526b, d) in (9.523b) leads to the power series for the spherical Neumann function (9.527a, b), that has a pole of order $n+1$:

$$y_n(x)=-x^{-n-1}(2n-1)!!\left\{1+\sum_{k=1}^{\infty}\left[\frac{\left(-x^2/2\right)^k}{k!(1-2n)...(2k-1-2n)}\right]\right\}$$
$$=-\frac{1.3.5...(2n-1)}{x^{n+1}}\left[1-\frac{x^2/2}{1!(1-2n)}+\frac{\left(x^2/2\right)^2}{2!(1-2n)(3-2n)}\cdots\right]. \tag{9.527a, b}$$

The power series expansions for (standard CCCXIX) the spherical Bessel (9.519a) ≡ (9.526a) ≡ (9.526b) [Neumann (9.519b) ≡ (9.527a) ≡ (9.527b)] function show that it is analytic (singular) at the origin where it has a zero (pole) or order $n(n+1)$ and hence they are linearly independent, as assumed in the general integral (9.522a–c) of the spherical Bessel differential equation (9.515c). The cylindrical (9.514c), spherical (9.515c), original (9.430b), and generalized (9.428f) Bessel differential equations all have a regular singularity at the origin, and the cylindrical and spherical Bessel and Neumann functions provide examples of all the six possible cases of regular integrals (subsection 9.5.25).

9.5.25 Classification of Six Cases of Regular Integrals

A singular integral can arise only from a singular linear differential equation, because a linear differential equation with analytic coefficients can have only analytic integrals (subsection 9.4.9). The inverse is not true: *a linear differential equation with a regular singularity can have (standard CCCXX) out of six possible cases two analytic (i–ii) [four singular (iii–vi)] integrals; that is, the integrals can be: (i/ii) an analytic function (9.233a, b) if the regular integral of the first kind (9.377b) has a zero (9.528b) [positive integer n in (9.528a)] exponent corresponding to a finite value (9.253b) [zero of order n (9.253a)], for example the first spherical Bessel function (9.526a, b); (iii) a singular integral with a pole (9.231a, b) if the regular integral of the first kind (9.377b) has an index that is a negative integer (9.528c), for example the second spherical Bessel function (9.527a, b) has a pole of order $n+1$; (iv) a power branch-point if the regular integral of the first kind (9.377b) or second kind first (9.405a, b) [second (9.413)] type has a non-integer index (9.528d), for example the Bessel function (9.510a) of non-integer order; and (v/vi) a logarithmic (9.528e) branch-point (9.248a–c) possibly combined with any of the preceding (i) to (iii) for a regular integral of the second kind first (9.405a, b) or second (9.413) type for example the Neumann function (9.511):*

$$\text{integrals near a regular singularity}\left\{\begin{array}{lll} j_n(x) & \text{with } n \in |N: & \text{zero of order } n \\ j_0(x) & \text{with } n=0: & \text{finite value} \\ j_{1-n}(x) & \text{with } n \in |N: & \text{pole of order } n \\ J_\nu(x) & \text{with } \nu \in |C-|Z & \text{branch-point} \\ Y_\nu(x) & \text{with } a_+ - a_- \in |Z & \text{logarithmic singularity} \end{array}\right. \tag{9.528a–e}$$

An integral of a linear differential equation can have an essential singularity (9.228a–e) only if (9.256a–d) the differential equation has an irregular singularity. An example of essential singularity at the point at infinity is provided by the spherical Bessel functions (subsection 9.5.24) expressed in terms of circular sines and cosines (subsection 9.5.26).

9.5.26 Relation between Spherical Bessel and Elementary Functions

The spherical Bessel differential equation (9.515c) of order zero (9.529a) takes the form (9.529b) ≡ (9.529c) that has solutions (9.529d, e):

$$n=0:\quad 0 = xz'' + 2z' + xz = (xz)'' + xz, \quad xz_{1,2}(x) = \sin x, -\cos x. \tag{9.529a–e}$$

The function in (9.529d) [(9.529e)] is analytic (9.235a–e) [has a simple pole (9.236a–c)] at the origin and thus should coincide with the spherical Bessel (9.530a) [Neumann (9.531a)] function of order zero, to within a multiplying constant. It is shown next that the multiplying constant is unity, and that the spherical Bessel (9.530b) [Neumann (9.531b)] function of order n can be obtained by differentiation in terms of elementary functions (9.530c) [(9.531c)]. It follows that (9.529d) [(9.529e) specify *the spherical Bessel (Neumann) function (9.530a) [(9.531a)] of order zero:*

$$j_0(x) = \frac{\sin x}{x}, \qquad j_n(x) = x^n\left(-\frac{1}{x}\frac{d}{dx}\right)^n j_0(x) = x^n\left(-\frac{1}{x}\frac{d}{dx}\right)^n \frac{\sin x}{x}, \tag{9.530a–c}$$

$$j_0(x) = -\frac{\cos x}{x}, \qquad y_n(x) = -x^n\left(-\frac{1}{x}\frac{d}{dx}\right)^n y_0(x) = -x^n\left(-\frac{1}{x}\frac{d}{dx}\right)^n \frac{\cos x}{x}, \tag{9.531a–c}$$

and that the application of the same differential operator (9.530b) [≡ (9.531b)] leads to the ***Rayleigh formulas*** *(1904) for the spherical Bessel (Neumann) function of order n expressing it (standard CCCXXI) in terms of derivatives of elementary functions (9.530c) [(9.531c)].* The proof of (9.530c) [(9.531c)] can be made substituting the power series for the circular sine (9.235a) [cosine (9.236a)] and showing that the power series for the first (9.526a) [second (9.527a)] spherical Bessel function is regained.

Substituting (9.235a) in (9.530c) leads to (9.532a):

$$\begin{aligned} j_n(x) &= x^n\left(-\frac{1}{x}\frac{d}{dx}\right)^n \sum_{j=0}^{\infty} \frac{(-)^j}{(2j+1)!} x^{2j} \\ &= (-)^n \sum_{j=n}^{\infty} \frac{(-)^j}{(2j+1)!} x^{2j-n} 2j(2j-2)\ldots(2j-2n+2) \\ &= (-)^n x^{-n} \sum_{j=n}^{\infty} \frac{(-)^j x^{2j}}{(2j+1)!} \frac{(2j)!!}{(2j-2n)!!} \\ &= (-)^n x^{-n} \sum_{j=n}^{\infty} \frac{(-)^j}{(2j+1)!!} \frac{x^{2j}}{(j-n)!\, 2^{j-n}}, \end{aligned} \tag{9.532a–d}$$

where: (i) the derivation of even powers in (9.532a) starts at $j = n$ in (9.532b); and (ii) the properties of factorials (9.433b) and double factorials (9.524a–c; 9.526a–d) are used in (9.532c, d). The change of index of summation (9.533a) leads to (9.533b):

$$k = j - n: \qquad j_n(x) = (-)^n x^n \sum_{k=0}^{\infty} \frac{(-)^k}{(2k+2n+1)!!} \frac{x^{2k}}{k!2^k}, \tag{9.533a, b}$$

that coincides with (9.533b) ≡ (9.525a).

Substitution of (9.236a) in (9.531c) leads to (9.534a–d):

$$\begin{aligned} y_n(x) &= -x^n \left(-\frac{1}{x}\frac{d}{dx} \right)^n \sum_{k=0}^{\infty} \frac{(-)^k}{(2k)!} x^{2k-1} \\ &= (-)^{n+1} x^n \sum_{k=0}^{\infty} \frac{(-)^k}{(2k)!} x^{2k-2n-1} (2k-1)....(2k-2n+1); \end{aligned} \tag{9.534a, b}$$

substitution of:

$$\begin{aligned} (2k-1)...(2k-2n+1) &= (-)^n (2n-1-2k)...(1-2k) \\ &= (-)^n (2n-1-2k)...\left[2n-1-2(k+n-1)\right] \\ &= (-)^n \frac{(2n-1).....1...(1-2k)}{(2n-1)...(2n+1-2k)} = (-)^n \frac{(2n-1)!!(2k-1)!!}{(1-2n)...(2k-1-2n)}, \end{aligned} \tag{9.535a–d}$$

leads to:

$$y_n(x) = -x^{-n-1} \sum_{k=0}^{\infty} \frac{\left(-x^2\right)^k}{(2k)!!} \frac{(2n-1)!!}{(1-2n)...(2k-1-2n)}, \tag{9.536}$$

that coincides with (9.536) ≡ (9.527a). *The series expansions (standard CCCXXII) involve unending ascending powers for the: (i/ii) original Bessel (Neumann) functions of integer (9.510b) [(9.511)] or complex (9.510a) [(9.509b)] order; (iii/i) spherical Bessel (9.526a, b) [Neumann (9.527a, b)] functions; (v/vi) generalized Bessel (9.448) [Neumann (9.485)] functions. In all cases (i–vi) the solution has at most a branch-point (always an essential singularity) at the origin (point at infinity), that is thus a regular (irregular) singularity of the (i/ii) original (9.430b), (iii/iv) spherical (9.515c) and (v/vi) generalized (9.428a–f) Bessel differential equation.* It is shown next (section 9.6) that in all cases (i–iv) the irregular integrals in the neighborhood of the irregular singularity at infinity are of the normal type (9.256b, c; 9.257a–d).

9.6 Irregular Singularities and Asymptotic Normal Integrals (Thome 1883, Poincaré 1886, Campos 2001)

If in the neighborhood of an irregular singularity of a linear differential equation of order N there are $0 \le M < N$ linearly independent regular integrals (subsection 9.6.2) then the remaining $M - N$ particular integrals must be irregular (subsection 9.6.1). A particular case of an irregular integral is the normal integral that multiplies the regular integral by an exponential of a polynomial of inverse powers (subsection 9.6.3). Normal integrals appear most often as asymptotic solutions of linear differential equations whose point at infinity is an irregular singularity (subsection 9.6.4). The normal integrals often involve asymptotic expansions (subsection 9.6.5) rather than asymptotic series because the convergence theorem for regular integrals (subsection 9.5.11) does not apply. If the normal integral has in the exponential factor a leading inverse power with exponent k, then the corresponding irregular singularity of the linear differential equation is of degree k. For example, the original, cylindrical, and spherical (generalized) Bessel differential equation has at the point at infinity [subsections 9.6.6–9.6.8 (9.6.9–9.6.12)] an irregular singularity of degree one (two). The asymptotic expansions for the spherical Bessel functions (subsections 9.5.23–9.5.26) can be obtained [subsection 9.6.6 (9.6.7)] most readily to leading order (to all orders) from the Rayleigh formulas (using the method of normal integrals). The asymptotic expansions for the cylindrical and original Bessel functions can be obtained (subsection 9.6.8) alternatively from those of spherical Hankel functions again by the method of normal integral(s). The asymptotic expansions for the first (second) generalized Hankel functions [subsection 9.6.9 (9.6.10)], that are linearly independent asymptotic solutions of the generalized Bessel differential equation (subsections 9.5.11), are also obtained by the method of normal integrals. There is a contrast (subsection 9.6.12) between the original Bessel and Neumann functions (Hankel functions) that can (cannot) be obtained as the limit of zero degree of the generalized Bessel and Neumann (Hankel) functions because there is no (there is) a bifurcation for the degree [subsection 9.6.13 (9.6.14)] at the regular (irregular) singularity at the origin (infinity). The numerical computation of Bessel functions is performed most accurately using the series (asymptotic) expansion for small (large) variable (subsection 9.6.15).

9.6.1 Regular/Irregular Integrals of a Linear Differential Equation

The number of regular integrals of linear differential equation is the degree of the characteristic polynomial; that is, the number of roots of the indicial equation. *For example, consider a linear second-order differential equation (9.537c) where (standard CCCXXIII) the coefficient of the dependent variable (9.537b) [of its derivative (9.537a)] has a pole of order* $\beta(\alpha)$*:*

$$P(x) = \sum_{k=0}^{\infty} P_k x^{k-\alpha} = O\left(x^{-\alpha}\right), Q(x) = \sum_{k=0}^{\infty} Q_k x^{k-\beta} = O\left(x^{-\beta}\right); y'' + P(x)y' + Q(x)y = 0, \tag{9.537a–c}$$

If a solution as a regular integral (9.377b) exists, then apart from the common factor (9.538a) the lowest powers in the three terms of the differential equation (9.537c) are respectively (9.538b–d):

$$c_0 x^a:\ y''(x) \sim a(a-1)x^{-2},\ P(x)y'(x) \sim P_0 a x^{-1-\alpha},\ Q(x)y(x) \sim Q_0 x^{-\beta}, \tag{9.538a–d}$$

and three cases II to IV can arise. Table 9.4 *includes case I of* $\alpha = 0 = \beta$ *of analytic coefficients (9.279a–c) and solutions (9.280c). In case II, when the coefficient of the dependent variable (its derivative) has in (9.537b) [(9.537a)] a double (9.539a) [single (9.539b)] pole:*

$$\beta = 2, \alpha = 1: \qquad 0 = a(a-1) + P_0 a + Q_0 = P_2(a) = (a - a_+)(a - a_-); \tag{9.539a–d}$$

the characteristic polynomial (9.539c) ≡ (9.396e) is of the second degree, and its roots specify (9.539d) two indices, leading to two linearly independent regular integrals (subsections 9.5.8–9.5.10) to obtain the general integral. In case III, when the coefficient of the derivative of the dependent variable (9.537b) has a pole of order at least two (9.540a) and the coefficient of the dependent variable (9.540b) a pole of order unity higher:

$$\beta - 1 = \alpha = 2, \ldots: \qquad 0 = P_0 a + Q_0 = P_1(a), \qquad a = -\frac{Q_0}{P_0}, \tag{9.540a–d}$$

the characteristic polynomial is of the first degree (9.540c) and has only one root (9.540d) or index, so only one regular integral exists, and a second linearly

TABLE 9.4

Second-Order Linear Differential Equation: Linearly Independent Particular Integrals

Case	$P(x)$	$Q(x)$	Particular Integrals
I	$O(1)$	$O(1)$	two analytic integrals
II	$O\left(x^{-1}\right)$	$O\left(x^{-2}\right)$	two regular integrals
III	$O\left(x^{-\alpha}\right)$ with $\alpha = 2, 3, \ldots$	$O\left(x^{\alpha-1}\right)$	One regular integral plus one irregular integral
IV	$O\left(x^{-\alpha}\right)$ with $\alpha = 2, 3, \ldots$	$O\left(x^{-\beta}\right)$ with $\beta \neq \alpha + 1$	two irregular integrals

independent irregular integral is needed to form the general integral. In case IV when the conditions (9.540a, b) are not met the indicial equation is a trivial identity $0 = 0$*; it determines no indices, there are no regular integrals, and two linearly independent irregular integrals are needed to form the general integral.* In the indicial equation (9.539c) [(9.540c)] it is possible to have $P_0 = 0 = Q_0 \, (Q_0 = 0)$ because this would still leave two roots (one root).

9.6.2 Regular Integral near an Irregular Singularity

As an example, consider (9.540a–c) case III with a double (9.541a) [triple (9.541b)] pole of the coefficient of the dependent variable (9.537a) [its derivative (9.537b)] when substitution of the regular integral (9.377b) in the differential equation (9.537c) ≡ (9.376e) leads to (9.541c):

$$\alpha = 2, \beta = 3: \qquad 0 = \sum_{m=0}^{\infty} c_m(a)(m+a)(m+a-1)x^{m+a-2} + \sum_{k,j=0}^{\infty} c_k(a)\left[(k+a)P_j + Q_j\right]x^{a+k+j-3}. \tag{9.541a–c}$$

The changes of variables of summation (9.542a, b) lead from (9.541c) to (9.542c):

$$m+1 = n = k+j: \qquad 0 = \sum_{n=1}^{\infty} x^{n-3}\left[(n+a-1)(n+a-2)c_{n-1}(a) + \sum_{j=0}^{\infty}\left[(n-j+a)P_j + Q_j\right]c_{n-j}(a)\right]. \tag{9.542a, b}$$

The lowest power (9.543a) in (9.541c) has coefficient (9.543b) leading (9.543c) to the indicial equation (9.540c) with a single root (9.543d) ≡ (9.540d):

$$x^{-3}: \qquad (P_0 a + Q_0)c_0(a) = 0; \quad c_0(a) \neq 0: \quad a = -\frac{Q_0}{P_0}. \tag{9.543a–d}$$

Equating the coefficients of powers in (9.542b) to zero leads to the recurrence formula for the coefficients (9.544b):

$$\left[(n+a)P_0 + Q_0\right]c_n(a) = nP_0 c_n(a) = -\left[(n+a-1)(n+a-2) + (n+a)P_1 + Q_1\right]c_{n-1}(a) - \sum_{j=2}^{n}\left[(n-j+a)P_j + Q_j\right]c_{n-j}(a), \tag{9.544a, b}$$

where (9.543f) was used in (9.544a). Thus *the linear second-order differential equation (9.537c) ≡ (9.545c) with (standard CCCXXIV) coefficient of the dependent variable (its derivative) having a triple (9.537b; 9.541b) ≡ (9.545b) [double (9.537a; 9.541a) ≡ (9.545a)] pole:*

$$p(x)=\sum_{k=0}^{\infty} p_k x^{k-2}, \quad Q(x)=\sum_{k=0}^{\infty} Q_k x^{k-3}: \quad y''+P(x)y'+Q(x)y=0, \tag{9.545a–c}$$

has a regular integral (9.377a) ≡ (9.546a) with index (9.543d) and recurrence formula (9.544b) for the coefficients:

$$y(x)=x^{-Q_0/P_0}\sum_{n=0}^{\infty} c_n(-Q_0/P_0)x^n; \qquad c_n/c_{n-1}\sim O(n), \tag{9.546a, b}$$

the theorem of convergence of regular integrals (subsection 9.5.11) does not apply because the singularity of the differential equation is irregular, and indeed the coefficients (9.546b) diverge. Thus the solution (9.546a) can be used only truncating the series and for sufficiently small $|x|$ as an expansion (subsection 9.6.4). Since there is only one regular integral, a second linear independent integral must be irregular; that is, must have an essential singularity. An example of essential singularity at the origin is the exponential (9.238a–c) of an inverse variable. Thus a possible form of an irregular integral, valid in the neighborhood of an irregular singularity at the origin, is the product of an exponential of inverse powers by a regular integral; this particular form of irregular integral is called a normal integral and its existence is considered next (subsection 9.6.3).

9.6.3 Existence of a Normal Integral near an Irregular Singularity

Case III of (subsection 9.4.6) a linear first-order differential equation (9.254b) whose coefficient has a multiple pole (9.260a) leads to: (i) an irregular singularity of the differential equation; and (ii) an irregular singularity in the solution (9.260b) ≡ (9.256d; 9.257d) specified by a **normal integral** (9.547b) consisting of the product of a regular integral (9.377b) by an exponential of a polynomial of inverse powers (9.547a):

$$\Omega\left(\frac{1}{x}\right)\equiv\sum_{m=1}^{M}\frac{\Omega_m}{x^m}: \qquad y(x)=\exp\left[\Omega\left(\frac{1}{x}\right)\right]x^a\sum_{n=0}^{\infty}x^n c_n(a). \tag{9.547a, b}$$

There is no assurance that the preceding result extends to irregular singularities of linear differential equations of order higher than the first, yet the normal integral (9.547a, b) is perhaps the simplest form of irregular integral that could be tried. A linear differential equation has an **irregular singularity**

of degree M if in its neighborhood all integrals are normal (9.547b) and the highest inverse power in any exponential coefficient is M. The conditions for the existence of a normal integral (9.547b) ≡ (9.548a) where (9.377b) ≡ (9.548b) is a regular integral:

$$y(x) = e^{\Omega(1/x)} z(x): \qquad z(x) = x^a \sum_{n=0}^{\infty} x^n c_n(a). \tag{9.548a, b}$$

are investigated next for a second-order differential equation (9.537c) whose coefficients (P, Q) may have singularities at the origin.

From (9.548a) follow (9.549a, b) by two successive differentiations:

$$y' = e^{\Omega}(z' + \Omega' z), \qquad y'' = e^{\Omega}\left[z'' + 2\Omega' z' + \left(\Omega'^2 + \Omega''\right) z\right], \tag{9.549a, b}$$

leading to (9.550) on substitution in (9.537c):

$$z'' + (P + 2\Omega')z' + \left(Q + \Omega' P + \Omega'^2 + \Omega''\right) z = 0; \tag{9.550}$$

the linear differential equation (9.550) ≡ (9.551a) has coefficients (9.551b, c):

$$z'' + P_2(x) z' + Q_2(x) z = 0:$$
$$P_2(x) \equiv P + 2\Omega' = O\left(x^{-\alpha}\right), \quad Q_2(x) \equiv Q + \Omega' P + \Omega'^2 + \Omega'' = O\left(x^{-\beta}\right); \tag{9.551a–c}$$

to which apply the same four cases as in subsection 9.6.1. Thus *a linear second-order differential equation (9.537c) has two linearly independent solutions as normal integrals (9.547a, b) ≡ (9.548a, b) if (standard CCCXXV) a function (9.547a) can be found such that (9.551b) [(9.551c)] has a simple (double) pole (9.552a):*

$$\textit{existence of normal integrals} \begin{cases} 2 & \text{if} \quad \alpha = 1, \beta = 2, & (9.552a) \\ 1 & \text{if} \quad \beta - 1 = \alpha = 2, 3...., & (9.552b) \\ 0 & \textit{otherwise} & (9.552c) \end{cases}$$

If (9.551b) has a pole of order at least two and (9.551c) a pole of order one unit higher then (9.540a–d) there is one normal integral (9.552b). Otherwise (9.552c) there are no normal integrals. In the cases when only one (no) normal integral exists (exist) then one (two) irregular integrals must be sought in another more general form (section 9.7). The linear differential equation with constant coefficients (homogenous derivatives) has exponential (power) solutions [section 1.3 (1.6)], that correspond to an essential singularity (pole) at infinity. Likewise many linear differential equations with analytic coefficients (regular singularities) have power series solutions [section 9.4 (9.5)] with an essential singularity at infinity; an essential singularity of the solution must correspond to an irregular singularity of the differential equation.

Thus the point at infinity of the differential equations in the cases mentioned above must be an irregular singularity. The normal integrals are used most often for differential equations that have an irregular singularity at infinity (subsection 9.6.4).

9.6.4 Singularity of a Differential Equation at the Point at Infinity

The point at infinity (subsection 9.4.7) is obtained by inversion of the origin (9.265a, b) ≡ (9.553a, b):

$$\xi \equiv \frac{1}{x}, \quad y(x) = w(\xi) = w\left(\frac{1}{x}\right):$$

$$\frac{d}{dx} = -\xi^2 \frac{d}{d\xi}, \quad \frac{d^2}{dx^2} = \xi^2 \frac{d^2}{d\xi}\left(\xi^2 \frac{d}{d\xi}\right) = \xi^4 \frac{d^2}{d\xi^2} + 2\xi^3 \frac{d}{d\xi}, \tag{9.553a–e}$$

leading to (9.266) ≡ (9.553c) and (9.553d, e). Substitution of (9.553a, b, c, e) in the linear second-order differential equation (9.537c) leads to (9.554):

$$\xi^4 w'' + \left[2\xi^3 - \xi^2 P\left(\frac{1}{\xi}\right)\right] w' + Q\left(\frac{1}{\xi}\right) w = 0. \tag{9.554}$$

The differential equation (9.554) ≡ (9.555a) is linear with coefficients (9.555b, c):

$$w'' + P_3(\xi) w' + Q_3(\xi) w = 0:$$

$$P_3(\xi) \equiv \frac{2}{\xi} - \frac{1}{\xi^2} P\left(\frac{1}{\xi}\right) = O(\xi^\alpha), Q_3(\xi) \equiv \frac{1}{\xi^4} Q\left(\frac{1}{\xi}\right) = O(\xi^\beta), \tag{9.555a–c}$$

that specify the type of singularity at infinity, namely:

point at infinity:

regular:	$P_3(\xi) = O(1) = Q_3(\xi)$,	(9.556a)
regular singularity:	$P_3(\xi) = O(\xi^{-1}), Q_3(\xi) = O(\xi^{-2})$,	(9.556b)
irregular singularity:	otherwise	(9.556c)

a regular point (9.556a) or a regular (9.556b) [irregular (9.556c)] singularity of the differential equation (9.555a–c) ≡ (9.537c; 9.553a–c).

Thus *the point at infinity (9.553a–c) of a linear second-order differential equation (9.537c) ≡ (9.555a–c) can be classified (9.556a–c) into (standard CCCXXVI) three cases I to III, namely; (case I) a regular point (9.557a, b) in which case there exist analytic integrals specified by a descending asymptotic series (9.557c–e):*

$$2x - x^2 P(x) = O(1) = x^4 Q(x): \qquad w(\xi) = \sum_{n=0}^{\infty} \xi^n c_n = \sum_{n=0}^{\infty} x^{-n} c_n = y(x); \tag{9.557a–e}$$

(case II) a regular singularity (9.558a, b) in which case there exist regular integrals specified by convergent descending series (9.558c–e):

$$2 - xP(x) = O(1) = x^3 Q(x):$$

$$w(\xi) = \xi^a \sum_{n=0}^{\infty} c_n(a)\xi^n = x^{-a} \sum_{n=0}^{\infty} x^{-n} c_n(a) = y(x); \tag{9.558a–e}$$

and (case III) an irregular singularity (9.559a, b) in which case there exists at least one irregular integral involving unending descending powers (9.559c–e):

$$\frac{2}{x} - P(x) = O(1) \text{ and/or } \quad x^2 Q(x) \sim 1:$$

$$w(\xi) = \xi^a \sum_{n=-\infty}^{+\infty} \xi^n c_n(a) = x^{-a} \sum_{n=-\infty}^{+\infty} x^{-n} c_n(a) = y(x), \tag{9.559a–e}$$

Since the convergence theorem for regular integrals (subsection 9.5.11) does not apply near an irregular singularity, the irregular integrals in general (9.559c–e), and the normal integrals in particular (9.547a, b) involve power expansions that may not converge as infinite series, and must be taken as asymptotic expansions (subsection 9.6.5).

9.6.5 Convergent Series versus Asymptotic Expansions

An asymptotic series (9.560a, b) is (section I.21.1) convergent (9.560c) if for any number however small (9.560d) there is an order (9.560e) beyond which (9.560f) the sum of the remaining terms of the series does not exceed that number (9.560g, h):

$$y(x) = \lim_{N\to\infty} y_N(x) = \lim_{N\to\infty} \sum_{k=0}^{N-1} c_k\, x^{-k} = \sum_{k=0}^{\infty} c_k\, x^{-k} \tag{9.560a–c}$$

$$\Leftrightarrow \quad \forall_{\varepsilon>0} \exists_{n\in|N} \forall_{N\geq n}: \qquad \left| y(x) - \sum_{k=0}^{N-1} c_k\, x^{-k} \right| = \left| \sum_{k=N}^{\infty} c_k\, x^{-k} \right| < \varepsilon. \tag{9.560d–h}$$

In contrast, an asymptotic expansion (9.561a): (i) does not converge when all terms are summed (9.561c):

$$u_N(x) = O\left(x^{-N}\right) \sim \sum_{k=0}^{N} c_k x^{-k}; \quad \lim_{N\to\infty} u_N(\infty) = \infty \wedge \lim_{|x|\to\infty} x^N u_N(x) = O(1), \tag{9.561a–d}$$

(ii) if it is truncated at some order N, then it will converge to a finite value (9.561c) as $|x| \to \infty$ when (9.560d) multiplied by x^N. The implication of (9.561c) is that if a function is approximated (9.562a) by an asymptotic expansion truncated at some order N, the difference between them (9.562d) can be made as small as needed (9.562c) by choosing sufficiently large x in (9.562b):

$$u_N(x) \sim \sum_{k=0}^{N} c_k x^{-k}: \quad \forall_{\varepsilon>0} \exists_{R>0}: \qquad |x| > R \Rightarrow \left| u_N(x) - \sum_{k=0}^{N} c_k x^{-k} \right| < \varepsilon. \tag{9.562a–d}$$

Thus asymptotic expansion (9.561a–d) provides any required level of approximation if it is truncated and the variable is sufficiently large (9.562a–d); that is, $\varepsilon \to 0$ as $R \to \infty$. However, if x is kept fixed and $N \to \infty$, the asymptotic expansion diverges, in contrast with an asymptotic series that converges. *An asymptotic series (9.560a–h) provides (standard CCCXXVII) required level of approximation for all non-zero values of the variable provided that a sufficient number of terms of the series is summed. Thus a asymptotic series is a particular case of asymptotic expansion, because: (i) truncating the asymptotic series after N terms leads to an asymptotic expansion of order N, even if the series does not converge; and (ii) an asymptotic expansion of order N leads to an asymptotic series if it converges as* $N \to \infty$.

The asymptotic expansions have similar properties to series in sense (standard CCCXXVIII) that: (i) the sum of two asymptotic expansions (9.561a) and (9.563a) is an asymptotic expansion (9.563b):

$$v_N(x) \sim \sum_{k=0}^{N} d_k x^{-k}: \qquad u_N(x) + v_N(x) \sim \sum_{k=0}^{N} (c_k + d_k) x^{-k}; \tag{9.563a, b}$$

(ii) the product of asymptotic expansions (9.561a; 9.563a) is an asymptotic expansion to which applies the ***Cauchy rule*** *of sum by diagonals (I.21.25a–c) ≡ (9.564):*

$$u_N(x) v_N(x) \sim \sum_{k=0}^{N} x^{-k} \sum_{j=0}^{k} c_j d_{k-j}; \tag{9.564}$$

(iii/iv) the derivative (9.565a) [primitive or indefinite integral (9.565b)] of an asymptotic expansion (9.561a) of order N is an asymptotic expansion of order $N+1(N-1)$:

$$u_N'(x) \sim -\sum_{k=0}^{N} k c_k x^{-k-1}, \quad \int^x u_N(\xi)\, d\xi \sim c_0 x + c_1 \log x - \sum_{k=2}^{N} c_k \frac{x^{1-k}}{k-1}. \tag{9.565a, b}$$

As examples it will be shown [subsections 9.6.6–9.6.9 (9.6.10–9.6.14)] that the original (9.430b), cylindrical (9.514c) and spherical (9.515c) [generalized (9.428a–f)] Bessel differential equation has an irregular singularity of degree 1(2) at the point at infinity (subsection 9.6.4) and thus two linearly independent normal integrals exist (subsection 9.6.3) involving asymptotic expansions (subsection 9.6.5). The normal integrals will be considered in the sequence cylindrical/spherical/generalized first and second Hankel functions (subsections 9.6.6/9.6.7–9.6.8/9.6.9–9.6.11) and then compared to establish a bifurcation property (subsections 9.6.12–9.6.14).

9.6.6 Spherical and Cylindrical Hankel (1869) Functions

The **first (second) spherical Hankel (1860) functions** are related by (9.566a) [(9.567b)] to the first (second) spherical Bessel functions (9.526a, b) [(9.527a, b)] and conversely by (9.566c, d):

$$h_n^{(1,2)}(x) = j_n(x) \pm i y_n(x): \quad 2j_n(x) = h_n^{(1)}(x) + h_n^{(2)}(x), \quad 2iy_n(x) = h_n^{(1)}(x) - h_n^{(2)}(x); \tag{9.566a–d}$$

it follows that in the case of real variable (9.567a) the Hankel functions are complex conjugate (9.567b) and their real (imaginary) part specifies the **spherical Bessel** (9.567c) [**Neumann** (9.567d)] functions:

$$x \in |R: \quad \left[h_n^{(1)}(x)\right]^* = h_n^{(2)}(x), \quad \mathrm{Re}\left[h_n^{(1)}(x)\right] = j_n(x) = \mathrm{Re}\left[h_n^{(2)}(x)\right], \tag{9.567a–c}$$

$$\mathrm{Im}\left[h_n^{(1)}(x)\right] = y_n(x) = -\mathrm{Im}\left[h_n^{(2)}(x)\right]. \tag{9.567d}$$

The spherical Bessel and Neumann functions are linearly independent (9.520c), and thus the *general integral of the spherical Bessel equation (9.515c) is (standard CCCXXXIX) a linear combination (9.568a) of first and second spherical Hankel functions:*

$$y(x) \sim E^+ h_n^{(1)}(x) + E^- h_n^{(2)}(x): \quad 2E^\pm = E_+ \mp iE_-, \quad E_+ = E^+ + E^-, \quad E_- = i\left(E^+ - E^-\right), \tag{9.568a–e}$$

with arbitrary constants related (9.522a) by (9.568b, c) ≡ (9.568d, e).

Substituting (9.530c; 9.531c) in (9.566a, b) specifies the spherical Hankel functions (9.570a) in terms of elementary functions (9.569b, c):

$$h_n^{(1,2)}(x) = x^n \left(-\frac{1}{x}\frac{d}{dx}\right)^n \left(\frac{\sin x \mp i\cos x}{x}\right) = x^n \left(-\frac{1}{x}\frac{d}{dx}\right)^n \left[\mp i \frac{e^{\pm ix}}{x}\right], \tag{9.569a–c}$$

implying that the leading term of the asymptotic expansion is (9.570b) where was used (9.570a):

$$\mp i(-)^n (\pm i)^n = (-)^n (\pm i)^{n-1} = e^{\mp i\pi n}\left(e^{\pm i\pi/2}\right)^{n-1} = e^{\mp i\pi(n+1)/2}: \quad h_n^{(1,2)}(x) \sim x^{-1}\exp\{\pm i[x-(n+1)\pi/2]\}. \tag{9.570a, b}$$

The ***first (second) cylindrical Hankel functions*** *are related (standard CCCXXX) by (9.571a–d) to the corresponding cylindrical Bessel and Neumann functions (9.567a–d):*

$$H_\nu^{(1,2)}(x) = J_\nu(x) \pm iY_\nu(x), \quad H_\nu^{(1)}(x) \pm H_\nu^{(2)}(x) = \{2J_\nu(x), 2iY_\nu(x)\}; \quad W\left(H_\nu^{(1)}(x), H_\nu^{2}(x)\right) = -\frac{4i}{\pi x}; \tag{9.571a–e}$$

the first and second Hankel functions are linearly independent, as follows from their Wronskian (9.571e) calculated (9.508c) by (9.572a) ≡ (9.572b) ≡ (9.571e):

$$W\left(J_\nu(x)+iY_\nu(x), J_\nu(x)-iY_\nu(x)\right) = -iW\left(J_\nu(x), Y_\nu(x)\right) + iW\left(Y_\nu(x), J_\nu(x)\right) = -\frac{4i}{\pi x}. \tag{9.572a, b}$$

Thus *the general integral of the Bessel differential equation (9.430b) is a linear combination of Hankel functions of the first and second kinds (9.573a):*

$$y(x) = C^+ H_\nu^{(1,2)}(x) + C^- H_\nu^{(1,2)}(x), \tag{9.573a}$$

with the arbitrary constants $C^\pm$ related to $C_\pm$ (9.507d) as $\left(E^\pm, E_\pm\right)$ in (9.568b–e). The cylindrical (9.572a, b) [spherical (9.566a, b)] Hankel functions are (standard CCCXXXI) related (9.519a, b) by (9.573c) that involve a change of order (9.573b):

$$\nu = n + 1/2: \qquad H_\nu^{(1,2)}(x) = \sqrt{\frac{2x}{\pi}}\, h_n^{(1,2)}(x) \sim \sqrt{\frac{2}{\pi x}}\exp\left[\pm i(x - \nu\pi/2 - \pi/4)\right], \tag{9.573b–d}$$

that leads (9.570b) to the leading asymptotic term (9.573d). The leading exponential term in the asymptotic expansion (9.573c) can be tentatively explained as follows: (i) for large variable (9.574a, b) the Bessel differential equation (9.430b) simplifies to (9.574c):

$$x^2 >> \nu^2, \qquad xy'' >> y': \qquad y'' + y \sim 0; \qquad y(x) = e^{\pm ix}, \tag{9.574a–d}$$

and (ii) the pair of complex conjugate solutions of (9.574c) is (9.574d) in agreement with the leading exponential term in (9.574c). This result coincides with the leading term of the normal integral of the Bessel differential equation around the irregular singularity at infinity, that supplies the remaining terms of the asymptotic expansions for the cylindrical (spherical) Hankel functions beyond the leading order (9.573c) [(9.570b)] as shown next (subsection 9.6.7).

9.6.7 Asymptotic Integrals of the Cylindrical Bessel Differential Equation (Campos 2001)

Since the asymptotic expansions for spherical (9.566a, b) [cylindrical (9.571a, b)] Hankel functions can be derived from each other (9.570b) [(9.573c)], it is indifferent starting from one or the other. Starting from the cylindrical Bessel differential equation (9.430b) the inversion (9.553a–e) for the point at infinity leads to (9.575a) showing that the origin $\xi = 0$ (point at infinity $x = 1/\xi = \infty$) is an irregular singularity due to the double pole in the coefficient of the dependent variable in (9.575b):

$$0 = \left\{ \frac{d}{d\xi}\left(\xi^2 \frac{d}{d\xi}\right) - \xi\frac{d}{d\xi} + \frac{1}{\xi^2} - \nu^2 \right\} w(\xi) = \xi^2 w'' + \xi w' + \left(\frac{1}{\xi^2} - \nu^2\right) w. \quad (9.575\text{a, b})$$

Seeking a solution in the form of a regular integral (9.576a) would lead in (9.575b) to (9.576b):

$$w(\xi) = \xi^a \sum_{k=0}^{\infty} \xi^k c_n(a): \qquad 0 = \sum_{k=0}^{\infty} c_k(a)\left\{\left[(k+a)^2 - \nu^2\right]\xi^k + \xi^{k-2}\right\}, \quad (9.576\text{a, b})$$

that: (i) cannot be satisfied because the power ξ^{k-2} has non-zero coefficient; and (ii) fails to determine an index, since (i) an indicial equation does not exist. Thus the cylindrical Bessel equation has no regular integrals at infinity and a descending series solution is possibly an asymptotic expansion rather than an asymptotic series.

Seeking a solution of the cylindrical Bessel differential equation (9.430b) in the neighborhood (9.575b) of the point at infinity (9.553a–c) in the form (9.577a) of a normal integral (9.548a) leads (9.550) to the differential equation (9.577b):

$$w(\xi) = e^{\Omega(\xi)} z(\xi): \quad \xi^2 z'' + \xi(1 + 2\Omega'\xi) z' + \left[\frac{1}{\xi^2} - \nu^2 + \Omega'\xi + \left(\Omega'^2 + \Omega''\right)\xi^2\right] z = 0. \quad (9.577\text{a, b})$$

The double pole in the coefficient of the dependent variable can be eliminated by the choice (9.578a) that (9.578b) implies that in the normal integral (9.577a) the leading term is (9.578c) as in the Hankel functions (9.574c):

$$\Omega'(\xi) = \mp\frac{i}{\xi^2}, \quad \Omega(\xi) = \pm\frac{i}{\xi} = \pm ix: \qquad w(\xi) = e^{\pm i/\xi} z(\xi) = e^{\pm ix} z(1/x); \quad (9.578\text{a–c})$$

substituting (9.578a, b) in (9.577b) leads to the differential equation (9.579b) for which a regular integral solution (9.579a) is sought:

$$z(\xi) = \xi^a \sum_{n=0}^{\infty} \xi^n c_n(a): \qquad \xi^2 z'' + \xi\left(1 \mp \frac{2i}{\xi}\right)z' - \left(\nu^2 \mp \frac{i}{\xi}\right)z = 0. \tag{9.579a, b}$$

It was (will be) shown [subsection 9.6.7 (9.6.8)] that the differential equation (9.575b) [(9.579b)] whose terms in curved brackets have double (simple) poles has no (one) regular integral of the form (9.576a) [(9.579a)]. Since $\xi = 0$ is an irregular singularity of the differential equation (9.579b) there could be (subsection 9.6.1) at most one regular integral, and this with the two signs in (9.578a–c) is sufficient to specify two linearly independent normal integrals (subsection 9.6.8).

9.6.8 Asymptotic Expansions for Bessel, Neumann, and Hankel Functions

Substitution of the regular integral (9.579a) in the differential equation (9.579b) leads to (9.580):

$$0 = \sum_{k=0}^{\infty} c_k(a)\left[(k+a)^2 - \nu^2\right]\xi^k \mp i \sum_{n=0}^{\infty} (2n + 2a - 1) c_n(a) \xi^{n-1}. \tag{9.580}$$

The coefficient of the lowest power (9.581a) in (9.580) is (9.581b) and hence (9.581c) the characteristic polynomial (9.581d) is of the first degree and the indicial equation specifies one root (9.581e):

$$\xi^{-1}: \quad (2a-1)c_0(a) = 0; \quad c_0(a) \neq 0: \quad 0 = (2a-1) \equiv P_1(a); \quad a = 1/2; \tag{9.581a–e}$$

from (9.581e) follows that the leading term (9.579a) in the asymptotic solution is (9.582a, b):

$$z(\xi) \sim \xi^{1/2} = x^{-1/2} \sim z\left(\frac{1}{x}\right), \qquad w(\xi) \sim e^{\pm ix} x^{-1/2} \sim y(x), \tag{9.582a–d}$$

implying (9.578b) that the leading term in the asymptotic solution is (9.582c, d) in agreement with the Hankel functions (9.573c). The remaining terms in the asymptotic expansion (9.579a) involve the coefficients in (9.580) that lead to (9.583b) with the change of summation variable (9.583a):

$$k = n-1: \qquad 0 = \sum_{n=0}^{\infty} \xi^{n-1}\left\{(2n+2a-1)c_n(a) \mp i\left[(n+a-1)^2 - \nu^2\right]c_{n-1}(a)\right\};$$

$$\tag{9.583a, b}$$

from (9.583b) follows the recurrence formula for the coefficients (9.584a):

$$c_n^{\pm}(a) = \mp i \frac{\nu^2 - (n+a-1)^2}{2n+2a-1} c_{n-1}^{\pm}(a): \quad c_n^{\pm}\left(\frac{1}{2}\right) = \mp i \frac{4\nu^2 - (2n-1)^2}{8n} c_{n-1}^{\pm}\left(\frac{1}{2}\right), \tag{9.584a, b}$$

that simplifies to (9.584b) for the value (9.581e) of the index. The recurrence formula for the coefficients (9.584b) leads to (9.585a):

$$c_n^{\pm}\left(\frac{1}{2}\right) = c_0^{\pm}\left(\frac{1}{2}\right) \frac{(\mp i)^n}{n!8^n} \prod_{m=1}^{n} \left[4\nu^2 - (2m-1)^2\right]: \quad w_{\pm}(\xi) = e^{\pm i/\xi} \sum_{n=0}^{\infty} \xi^{1/2+n} c_n^{\pm}\left(\frac{1}{2}\right), \tag{9.585a, b}$$

that are substituted in the normal integrals (9.578c; 9.579a; 9.581e).

Choosing the constants (9.586a) the normal integrals (9.586b) coincide with the Hankel functions (9.573c) as concerns the leading term:

$$c_0\left(\pm\frac{1}{2}\right) = \sqrt{\frac{2}{\pi}} \exp\left[\mp i(\nu\pi/2 + \pi/4)\right]: \qquad w_{\pm}(\xi) = H_\nu^{(1,2)}(x) = w_{\pm}\left(\frac{1}{x}\right). \tag{9.586a, b}$$

Using (9.585a, b) specifies all the following terms in the asymptotic expansions (9.587):

$$H_\nu^{(1,2)}(x) = \sqrt{\frac{2}{\pi x}} \exp\left[\pm i(x - \nu\pi/2 - \pi/4)\right]\left[A_\nu(x) \pm i B_\nu(x)\right], \tag{9.587}$$

where are separated the even (9.588a) [odd (9.588b)] powers:

$$\begin{aligned} A_\nu(x) &= 1 + \sum_{n=0}^{M} \frac{(-)^n}{(2n)!(8x)^{2n}} \prod_{m=1}^{2n} \left[4\nu^2 - (2m-1)^2\right] + O\left(x^{-2M-2}\right) \\ &= 1 - \frac{(4\nu^2-1)(4\nu^2-9)}{2!(8x)^2} + \frac{(4\nu^2-1)(4\nu^2-9)(4\nu^2-25)(4\nu^2-49)}{4!(8x)^4} + O\left(x^{-6}\right), \end{aligned} \tag{9.588a}$$

$$\begin{aligned} B_\nu(x) &= \sum_{n=0}^{M} \frac{(-)^n}{(2n+1)!(8x)^{2n+1}} \prod_{m=0}^{2n+1} \left[4\nu^2 - (2m+1)^2\right] + O\left(x^{-2M-3}\right) \\ &= \frac{4\nu^2-1}{8x} - \frac{(4\nu^2-1)(4\nu^2-9)(4\nu^2-25)}{3!(8x)^3} + O\left(x^{-5}\right). \end{aligned} \tag{9.588b}$$

Thus the *cylindrical Hankel functions have (standard CCCXXXII) the asymptotic expansions (9.587; 9.588a, b): (i) leading (9.571a) to the asymptotic expansions with variable (9.589a) for the Bessel (9.589b) [Neumann (9.589c)] functions:*

$$\zeta \equiv x - \nu\pi/2 - \pi/4: \qquad J_\nu(\zeta) = \sqrt{\frac{2}{\pi x}}\left[A_\nu(x)\cos\zeta - B_\nu(x)\sin\zeta\right], \qquad Y_\nu(\zeta) = \sqrt{\frac{2}{\pi x}}\left[A_\nu(x)\sin\zeta + B_\nu(x)\cos\zeta\right]; \tag{9.589a–c}$$

(iii) the asymptotic expansions for the spherical Bessel/Neumann/Hankel functions follow respectively from (9.589a, b)/(9.589a, c)/(9.587) with (9.588a, b) inserting (9.519a)/(9.519b)/(9.573b) a factor $\sqrt{\pi/(2x)}$ *and using an order integer plus one half (9.574a). The asymptotic solution of the generalized Bessel differential equation (9.428a–f) is (standard CCCXXXIII) a linear combination of Hankel functions of two kinds (9.590a):*

$$y(x) = E_1 H_\nu^{(1)}(x) + E_2 H_\nu^{(2)}(x) = (E_1 + E_2)J_\nu(x) + i(E_1 - E_2)J_\nu(x), \tag{9.590a, b}$$

with arbitrary constants $E_{1,2}$ *related by (9.569d, e) to those in the solution (9.507d) in terms of Bessel and Neumann functions.* The original (9.430b) [generalized (9.428a–f)] Bessel differential equation has an irregular singularity of degree one (two) at the point at infinity, and thus the asymptotic normal integrals [subsections 9.6.6–9.6.8 (9.6.9–9.6.11)] are different, corresponding to a bifurcation with regard to the degree (subsections 9.6.12–9.6.14) as shown in the sequel.

9.6.9 Generalized Hankel Function of the First Kind

The preceding general integrals (9.451a–c)/(9.486a–c)/(9.506a, b) of the generalized Bessel differential equation (9.428a–f) involving the generalized Bessel (9.448) and Neumann (9.485; 9.502a, b) functions do not hold asymptotically as $x \to \infty$. To obtain asymptotic solutions of the generalized Bessel differential equation (9.428a–f) the inversion with regard to the origin (9.553a–e) is used leading to the differential equation (9.591a, b):

$$\begin{aligned} 0 &= \left\{\frac{d}{d\xi}\left(\xi^2 \frac{d}{d\xi}\right) - \xi\left(1 - \frac{\mu}{2\xi^2}\right)\frac{d}{d\xi} + \frac{1}{\xi^2} - \nu^2\right\} w(\xi) \\ &= \xi^2 w'' + \xi\left(1 + \frac{\mu}{2\xi^2}\right)w' + \left(\frac{1}{\xi^2} - \nu^2\right)w. \end{aligned} \tag{9.591a, b}$$

The point at infinity $x = \infty$ of the generalized Bessel equation (9.428a–f) would be a regular singularity if the origin $\xi = 0$ was a regular singularity of (9.591b), and that is not the case because the terms in curved brackets have double poles at $\xi = 0$ instead of being analytic at $\xi = 0$. Thus two linearly independent solutions of (9.591b) as ascending power series (9.592a) of ξ or descending power series (9.592b) of x:

$$w(\xi) = \xi^a \sum_{n=0}^{\infty} \xi^n c_n(a) = x^{-a} \sum_{n=0}^{\infty} x^{-n} c_n(a) = y(x), \tag{9.592a, b}$$

cannot exist. Thus either (i) one power solution (9.592b) exists at most or (ii) none at all.

To ascertain which of (i) or (ii) is the present case the series (9.592a) [(9.592b)] is substituted in the differential equation (9.591b) [(9.428f)] leading by both approaches to the same result:

$$0 = \sum_{n=0}^{\infty} c_n(a)\left[(n+a)^2 - \nu^2\right]\xi^{n+a} + \sum_{k=0}^{\infty} c_k(a)\left[\frac{\mu}{2}(k+a)+1\right]\xi^{k+a-2}. \tag{9.593}$$

The change of summation variable (9.594a) leads to (9.594b):

$$k-2=n: \qquad 0 = \sum_{n=0}^{\infty} \xi^n \left\{\left[\frac{\mu}{2}(n+a+2)+1\right]c_{n+2}(a) + \left[(n+a)^2 - \nu^2\right]c_n(a)\right\}. \tag{9.594a, b}$$

Setting (9.595a) leads to (9.595b) implying (9.595c) that the characteristic polynomial is of the first degree (9.595d) and has one root (9.595e):

$$n=-2: \quad 0 = c_0(a)\xi^{-2}(\mu a + 2); \quad c_0(a) \neq 0: \quad 0 = \mu a + 2 = P_1(a); \quad a = -\frac{2}{\mu}; \tag{9.595a–e}$$

thus the generalized Bessel equation (9.428a–f) has one asymptotic solution (9.591b) as a regular asymptotic expansion (9.592a) of descending powers (9.592b) whose coefficients are obtained next.

From (9.594b) follows the recurrence formula for the coefficients (9.596a) that is evaluated (9.596b) for the index (9.595e):

$$c_n(a) = -\frac{(n+a-2)^2 - \nu^2}{\mu(n+a)/2+1} c_{n-2}(a):$$

$$c_{2n}\left(-\frac{2}{\mu}\right) = -4\frac{(n-1-1/\mu)^2 - (\nu/2)^2}{n\mu} c_{2n-2}\left(-\frac{2}{\mu}\right); \tag{9.596a, b}$$

substitution of (9.596b; 9.595e) in (9.592a) leads to the regular integral (9.597b) choosing the leading coefficient to be unity (9.597b):

$$c_0\left(-\frac{2}{\mu}\right)\equiv 1: \qquad w(\xi)=\xi^{-2/\mu}\left\{1+\sum_{n=1}^{M-1}\frac{(-4)^n\,\xi^{2n}}{n!\,\mu^n}\prod_{m=0}^{n-1}\left[\left(m-\frac{1}{\mu}\right)^2-\frac{\nu^2}{4}\right]+O\left(\xi^{2M}\right)\right\}. \tag{9.597a, b}$$

The regular integral (9.592b; 9.597b) ≡ (9.598a, b) specifies:

$$\mu\neq 0: \quad H^{(1)}_{\mu,\nu}(x)=x^{2/\mu}\left\{1+\sum_{n=1}^{M-1}\frac{\left(-\mu x^2/4\right)^{-n}}{n!}\prod_{m=0}^{n-1}\left[\left(m-\frac{1}{\mu}\right)^2-\frac{\nu^2}{4}\right]+O\left(x^{-2M}\right)\right\}. \tag{9.598a, b}$$

the first asymptotic solution of the generalized Bessel differential equation (9.428a–f) near the point-at-infinity.

As in (9.449a, b) the product in (9.598b) can be replaced (9.432b) ratios of gamma functions (9.599a, b):

$$\begin{aligned}\prod_{m=0}^{n-1}\left[\left(m-\frac{1}{\mu}\right)^2-\frac{\nu^2}{4}\right]&=\prod_{m=0}^{n-1}\left(m-\frac{1}{\mu}-\frac{\nu}{2}\right)\left(m-\frac{1}{\mu}+\frac{\nu}{2}\right)\\&=\frac{\Gamma(n-1/\mu-\nu/2)\,\Gamma(n-1/\mu+\nu/2)}{\Gamma(-1/\mu-\nu/2)\,\Gamma(-1/\mu+\nu/2)}.\end{aligned} \tag{9.599a, b}$$

Substitution of (9.599b) in (9.598b) leads to (9.600a):

$$H^{(1)}_{\mu,\nu}(z)\sim\bar{c}_0(\mu,\nu)\,x^{2/\mu}\left\{\sum_{n=0}^{M-1}\frac{\left(-\mu x^2/4\right)^{-n}}{n!}\Gamma(n+\nu/2-1/\mu)\,\Gamma(n-\nu/2-1/\mu)+O\left(x^{-2M}\right)\right\}, \tag{9.600a}$$

with a different choice (9.600b) of leading constant factor:

$$\bar{c}_0(\mu,\nu)\equiv\left[\Gamma(+\nu/2-1/\mu)\,\Gamma(-\nu/2-1/\mu)\right]^{-1}. \tag{9.600b}$$

Thus *the generalized Hankel function of the first kind (9.598a, b) ≡ (9.600a, b) is (standard CCCXXXIV) an asymptotic regular integral of the generalized Bessel differential equation (9.428a–f), and has growing coefficients* $c_n/c_{n-1}\sim O(n)$ *in (9.596a) and thus does not converge as an asymptotic series as* $M\to\infty$*; it is an asymptotic expansion (subsection 9.6.5) valid with a finite number of terms* $M<\infty$ *as* $|x|\to\infty$. Since the convergence theorem for regular integrals (subsection 9.5.11) does not apply near an irregular singularity, the generalized Hankel function of the first kind can be an asymptotic expansion. As $|x| \to \infty$ the generalized Hankel function of the first kind (9.598b) decays for $\operatorname{Re}(\mu) < 0$ and diverges for $\operatorname{Re}(\mu) > 0$. The powers of $\mu x^2/4$ appear in all of the generalized Bessel (9.450b), Neumann (9.492b), and Hankel functions of the first kind (9.598b) $\equiv$ (9.600a, b) and specify when the sign is alternating or not for real or imaginary variable x. Since the generalized Bessel differential equation (9.428a–f) has an irregular singularity (9.591b) at infinity (9.553a–e), an asymptotic integral linearly independent from the generalized Hankel function of the first kind cannot be a regular integral, and turns out to be a normal integral (subsection 9.6.10).

9.6.10 Generalized Hankel Function of the Second Kind

An asymptotic solution of the generalized Bessel differential equation (9.428a–f) in the neighborhood of the irregular singularity at infinity (9.591b) is sought in the form of a normal integral (9.577a) leading (9.549a, b; 9.550) to (9.601):

$$\xi^2 z'' + \xi\left(1 + \frac{\mu}{2\xi^2} + 2\Omega'\xi\right)z' + \left[\frac{1}{\xi^2} - \nu^2 + \xi\left(1 + \frac{\mu}{2\xi^2}\right)\Omega' + \xi^2\Omega'^2 + \xi^2\Omega''\right]z = 0. \tag{9.601}$$

The choice of the polynomial Ω' in (9.601) should be made so as to lead to the existence of a regular integral for z of the form (9.579a). The simplest choice is an inverse power $\Omega' \sim \xi^{-n}$. For $n = 1$ then $\Omega \sim \xi^{-1}$ leads to $\Omega \sim a \log \xi$ or $e^{\Omega} \sim \xi^{a}$; that is, the regular integral (9.579a). For $n = 2$ the $\Omega' \sim \xi^{-2}$ leads to $\Omega \sim \xi^{-1}$ and $e^{\Omega} \sim \exp(1/\xi) \sim \exp x$ that is the asymptotic scaling of the original Hankel (9.587) function of degree zero $\mu = 0$; it is a solution of the original Bessel equation that has at infinity an irregular singularity of degree one. The generalized Bessel equation of non-zero degree has a stronger irregular singularity at infinity, so the lowest degree would be two, that is $\Omega \sim \xi^{-2}$ or $\Omega' \sim \xi^{-3}$. In order to check if the irregular singularity at infinity of the generalized Bessel equation is of degree two, (9.602a) is substituted in (9.601) leading to the differential equation (9.602b):

$$\Omega'\left(\frac{1}{\zeta}\right) = \frac{b}{\xi^3}: \quad \xi^2 z'' + \xi\left(1 + \frac{2b + \mu/2}{\xi^2}\right)z' + \left(\frac{b(b + \mu/2)}{\xi^4} + \frac{1 - 2b}{\xi^2} - \nu^2\right)z = 0. \tag{9.602a, b}$$

The fourth-order pole in the term in square brackets in (9.602b) may be suppressed, choosing (9.603a) that simplifies the differential equation (9.602b) to (9.603b):

$$b = -\frac{\mu}{2}: \qquad \xi^2 z'' + \xi\left(1 - \frac{\mu}{2\xi^2}\right)z' + \left(\frac{1 + \mu}{\xi^2} - \nu^2\right)z = 0. \tag{9.603a, b}$$

The choices (9.602a; 9.603a) ≡ (9.604a) imply (9.604b):

$$\Omega'(\xi) = -\frac{\mu}{2\xi^3}, \quad \Omega(\xi) = \frac{\mu}{4\xi^2}, \qquad \exp\left[\Omega(\xi)\right] = \exp\left(\frac{\mu}{4\xi^2}\right) = \exp\left(\frac{\mu x^2}{4}\right), \tag{9.604a–c}$$

that the normal integral (9.577a) has a factor (9.604c) that appears in the Wronskian (9.429c) of the generalized Bessel differential equation (9.428a–f) and also shows that it has an irregular singularity of degree two at infinity.

The point at infinity is still an irregular singularity of (9.603b), so there cannot exist two linearly independent regular integrals of the form (9.579a). However, one asymptotic solution (9.597b) of the generalized Bessel equation (9.428a–f) has already been found and thus only one more is needed. Substituting the regular integral (9.579a) in the differential equation (9.603b) leads to (9.605):

$$0 = \sum_{n=0}^{\infty} c_n(a)\left[(n+a)^2 - \nu^2\right]\xi^{n+a} + \sum_{k=0}^{\infty} c_k(a)\left[1 + \mu - \frac{\mu}{2}(k+a)\right]\xi^{n+a-2}. \tag{9.605}$$

Setting to zero the coefficient of (9.606a) leads to (9.606b), implying (9.606c) that the indicial equation (9.606d) has a single root (9.606e):

$$\xi^{a-2}: \quad 0 = c_0(a)\left(1 + \mu - \frac{\mu a}{2}\right); \; c_0(a) \neq 0: \; 0 = (2 + 2\mu - \mu a) = P_1(a), \; a = 2 + 2/\mu. \tag{9.606a–e}$$

The change of summation variable (9.607a) in (9.605) leads to (9.607b):

$$k - 2 = n: \quad 0 = \sum_{n=0}^{\infty} \xi^n \left\{\left[(n+a)^2 - \nu^2\right] c_n(a) + \left[1 - \mu\frac{n+a}{2}\right] c_{n+2}(a)\right\}. \tag{9.607a, b}$$

From (9.607b) follows the recurrence formula for the coefficients (9.608a) that simplifies to (9.608b) for the index (9.606e):

$$c_n(a) = -\frac{(n+a-2)^2 - \nu^2}{1 + \mu - \mu n/2 - \mu a/2} c_{n-2}(a), \quad c_{2n}\left(2 + \frac{2}{\mu}\right) = 4\frac{(n + 1/\mu)^2 - \nu^2/4}{\mu n} c_{2n}\left(2 + \frac{2}{\mu}\right). \tag{9.608a, b}$$

and leads to (9.609b):

$$c_0\left(2 + \frac{2}{\mu}\right) = 1: \qquad c_{2n}\left(2 + \frac{2}{\mu}\right) = \frac{(\mu/4)^{-n}}{n!} \prod_{m=1}^{n} \left[\left(m + \frac{1}{\mu}\right)^2 - \frac{\nu^2}{4}\right], \tag{9.609a, b}$$

with the starting value (9.609a).

Substituting (9.609b; 9.579a; 9.604c) in (9.577a) specifies the second asymptotic solution of the generalized Bessel equation:

$\mu \neq 0$:

$$H^{(2)}_{\mu,\nu}(x) = \exp\left(\frac{\mu x^2}{4}\right) x^{-2-2/\mu} \left\{1 + \sum_{n=1}^{M-1} \frac{\left(\mu x^2/4\right)^{-n}}{n!} \prod_{m=1}^{n} \left[\left(m + \frac{1}{\mu}\right)^2 - \frac{\nu^2}{4}\right] + O\left(x^{-2M}\right)\right\}, \tag{9.610a, b}$$

that may be designated the **generalized Hankel function of the second kind**. Using in the last term on the r.h.s. of (9.610b) a relation similar to (9.599b) with $-1/\mu$ replaced by $1/\mu$ leads to an alternate expression for the generalized Hankel function of the second kind:

$$H^{(2)}_{\mu,\nu}(x) \sim \overline{e}_0(\mu,\nu) \exp\left(\frac{\mu x^2}{4}\right) x^{-2-2/\mu}$$

$$\left\{\sum_{n=0}^{M-1} \frac{\left(\mu x^2/4\right)^{-n}}{n!} \Gamma(1+n+\nu/2+1/\mu)\Gamma(1+n-\nu/2+1/\mu) + O\left(z^{-2M}\right)\right\}, \tag{9.611a}$$

with leading constant (9.609a) replaced by (9.611b):

$$\overline{e}_0(\mu,\nu) = \left[\Gamma(1+\nu/2+1/\mu)\Gamma(1-\nu/2+1/\mu)\right]^{-1}. \tag{9.611b}$$

The generalized Hankel functions of the first and second kind are linearly independent and specify the general asymptotic integral of the generalized Bessel differential equation (subsection 9.6.11).

9.6.11 Wronskians and Alternative General Integrals

It has been shown that *the generalized Bessel differential equation (9.428a–f) in the neighborhood (9.601) of the point at infinity (9.553a–c): (i) has (standard CCCXXXIV) only one asymptotic solution without an essential singularity, namely the generalized Hankel function of the first kind (9.598b) ≡ (9.600a, b) that is a regular asymptotic expansion; (ii) any other solution must involve (standard CCCXXXV) the generalized Hankel function of the second kind (9.610b) ≡ (9.611a, b) that is an asymptotic normal integral with an essential singularity of degree two; and (iii) the linear combination of (i) and (ii) with arbitrary constants* $E_{1,2}$ *specifies (standard CCCXXXVI) for non-zero degree (9.612a) the general asymptotic integral (9.612b):*

$$\mu \neq 0: \qquad y(x) \sim E_1 H^{(1)}_{\mu,\nu}(x) + E_2 H^{(1)}_{\mu,\nu}(x), \tag{9.612a, b}$$

and thus has an essential of degree two (9.604c) at infinity. In contrast, all general integrals (9.507a–d; 9.590a, b) of the original Bessel differential equation (9.430b) have an essential singularity of degree one at infinity (9.587; 9.588a, b; 9.589a–c) that is oscillatory for real variable. Instead, the asymptotic solution (9.612b) of the generalized Bessel equation (9.428a–f) with non-zero degree (9.612a) involves (9.612b) a singularity of degree two (9.604c), that is monotonic for real μ and x. The asymptotic expansions for the solutions of the original (9.587; 9.588a, b) and generalized (9.598b; 9.610b) Bessel equation are different because the irregular singularity at infinity is of different degree, respectively one and two for the original and generalized Bessel differential equation. This example illustrates that the solution of an ordinary differential equation near a singularity may be discontinuous with regard to a parameter (subsection 9.6.12), in this case the degree in the generalized Bessel equation (subsection 9.6.13) that has a bifurcation at the point at infinity (subsection 9.6.14). The bifurcation is considered after obtaining the set of Wronskians of the generalized Bessel, Neumann, and Hankel functions used to prove the linear independence of the generalized Hankel functions of the first and second kinds, that is assumed in the general integral (9.612a, b).

The generalized Hankel functions of the first (9.598b) [second (9.610b)] kind have leading terms (9.613a) [(9.613b)]:

$$H^{(1)}_{\mu,\nu}(x) \sim x^{2/\mu}, \qquad H^{(2)}_{\mu,\nu}(x) \sim x^{-2-2/\mu}\exp\left(\frac{\mu x^2}{4}\right); \tag{9.613a, b}$$

their Wronskian is also calculated to leading order:

$$W\left(H^{(1)}_{\mu,\nu}(x), H^{(1)}_{\mu,\nu}(x)\right) \sim \exp\left(\frac{\mu x^2}{4}\right)\begin{vmatrix} x^{2/\mu} & x^{-2-2/\mu} \\ \frac{2}{\mu}x^{2/\mu-1} & \frac{\mu}{2}x^{-1-2/\mu} \end{vmatrix}$$

$$= \exp\left(\frac{\mu x^2}{4}\right)\frac{\mu}{2x}\left[1 + O\left(x^{-1}\right)\right], \tag{9.614a, b}$$

where: (i) in the lower right corner in (9.614a) only the exponential is differentiated; and (ii) only the product of the main diagonal is used to calculate the determinant to lowest order in (9.614b). Thus *the Wronskian of the generalized Hankel functions of two kinds is given (standard CCCXXXVII) by (9.614b) ≡ (9.615a):*

$$W\left(H^{(1)}_{\mu,\nu}(x), H^{(1)}_{\mu,\nu}(x)\right) = \frac{\mu}{2x}\exp\left(\frac{\mu x^2}{4}\right), \qquad W_0 = \frac{\mu}{2}, \tag{9.615a, b}$$

that: (i) coincides with (9.429c) with the constant given (9.615b); and (ii) does not vanish for non-zero degree (9.612a), proving the linear independence of the two particular integrals in the general integral (9.612b).

The remaining Wronskian to be calculated concerns the generalized Neumann functions of orders $+\nu$ in (9.502b) and $-\nu$ in (9.616):

$$Y_{-\nu}^{\mu}(x) = \frac{A(\mu,-\nu)\, J_{\nu}^{\mu}(x) - J_{-\nu}^{\mu}(x)\cos(\pi\nu)}{\sin(\pi\nu)}, \tag{9.616}$$

bearing in mind that the Wronskian of a function with itself is zero (9.500b), from (9.502b; 9.616) follows (9.617a):

$$\begin{aligned} W\left(Y_{\nu}^{\mu}(x), Y_{-\nu}^{\mu}(x)\right) &= -\frac{A(\mu,\nu)A(\mu,-\nu) + \cos^2(\nu\pi)}{\sin^2(\nu\pi)} W\left(J_{\nu}^{\mu}(x), J_{-\nu}^{\mu}(x)\right) \\ &= \frac{2}{\pi x}\frac{1+\cos^2(\nu\pi)}{\sin(\nu\pi)}\exp\left(\frac{\mu x^2}{4}\right), \end{aligned} \tag{9.617a, b}$$

and substitution of (9.453e) leads to (9.617b) bearing in mind that (9.501a) implies:

$$A(\mu,\nu) \quad A(\mu,-\nu) = 1. \tag{9.618}$$

The numerator in (9.617b) is generally not zero for any degree and the denominator vanishes for integer order, leading to a singular Wronskian. Thus *the generalized Neumann functions $Y_{\pm\nu}^{\mu}(x)$ are (standard CCCXXXVIII) linearly independent for non-integer order (9.619a) and their linear combination with arbitrary constants $F_{\pm}$ specify the general integral (9.561b) of the generalized Bessel differential equation (9.428a–f):*

$$\nu \neq 0, \pm 1, \pm 2, \ldots: \qquad y(x) = F_{+} Y_{\nu}^{\mu}(x) + F_{-} Y_{-\nu}^{\mu}(x). \tag{9.619a, b}$$

Table 9.5 summarizes (standard CCCXXXIX) the four equivalent forms of the general integrals (9.451c)/(9.486c)/(9.506b)/(9.619b), and the related Wronskians (9.454b)/(9.497b)/(9.504c)/(9.615a) and conditions of validity (9.451a)/(9.486a)/(none)/(9.619a) for the generalized Bessel differential equation (9.328a–f). It also applies (standard CCCXL) with zero degree (9.430a) to the original Bessel equation (9.430b) in which case and their integrals are indicated in Table 9.6. The generalized (original) Bessel differential equations, and their solutions in terms of generalized Bessel, Neumann, and Hankel functions are compared next (subsection 9.6.12).

9.6.12 Generalized versus Original Bessel Differential Equations

The generalized Bessel differential equation (9.428a–f) has a regular singularity at the origin (9.441a–c) for all values of the degree μ, that does not appear in the indices (9.444e) since the latter are determined only by the

TABLE 9.5

Alternative General Integrals of the Generalized Bessel Differential Equation

I	II	III	IV	V
Subsection	**Validity**	**Restrictions**	**General Integral**	**Wronskiam**
9.5.12–9.5.16	$\lvert x\rvert<\infty$	$v\neq 0,\pm1,\pm2,\ldots$	$y(x)=C_+J_v^\mu(x)+C_-J_{-v}^\mu(x)$	$-\frac{2}{\pi x}\sin(\pi v)\exp\left(\frac{\mu x^2}{4}\right)$
9.5.17–9.5.21	$\lvert x\rvert<\infty$	–	$y(x)=D_+J_v^\mu(x)+D_-Y_v^\mu(x)$	$\frac{2A(\mu,v)}{\pi x}\exp\left(\frac{\mu x^2}{4}\right)$
9.6.9–9.6.11	$\lvert x\rvert>0$	–	$y(x)=E_1H_{\mu,v}^{(1)}(x)+E_2H_{\mu,v}^{(2)}(x)$	$\frac{\mu}{2x}\exp\left(\frac{\mu x^2}{4}\right)$
9.6.11	$\lvert x\rvert<\infty$	$v\neq 0,\pm1,\pm2$	$y(x)=F_+Y_v^\mu(x)+F_-Y_{-v}^\mu(x)$	$\frac{2}{\pi x}\frac{1+\cos^2(\pi v)}{\sin(\pi v)}\exp\left(\frac{\mu x^2}{4}\right)$

Also apply to the original Bessel differential equation (9.430b) with $\mu=0, A=1$.
$A(\mu,v)$ in (9.502a)

order ν. It follows that in the limit of zero degree, the generalized Bessel (9.448) [Neumann (9.485)] functions tend (9.620a) [(9.620b)] to the original Bessel (9.510a) [Neumann (9.509b)] functions:

$$\lim_{\mu\to0}J_\nu^\mu(z)=J_\nu(z),\qquad \lim_{\mu\to0}Y_\nu^\mu(z)=Y_\nu(z). \tag{9.620a, b}$$

The situation is different (Table 9.6) concerning the asymptotic solutions around the irregular singularity at infinity: (i) both the generalized Hankel

TABLE 9.6

Bessel Differential Equation: Original and Generalized

Case	Original	Generalized
Parameter(s)	Order: v	Degree: μ
Equation	(9.430a, b)	(9.428a–f)
Origin	regular singularity	regular singularity
Series solution	(9.507d; 9.510a; 9.509b)	(9.506a, b; 9.448; 9.502a, b)
Name of functions	Bessel: $J_v(x)$ Neumann: $Y_v(x)$	generalized Bessel: $J_v^\mu(x)$ generalized Neumann: $Y_v^\mu(x)$
Continuity	Yes: uniform as $\mu\to0$	
Point-at-infinity	Irregular singularity of the first degree	Irregular singularity of the second degree
Asymptotic expansion	(9.590a; 9.587; 9.588a, b)	(9.612a, b; 9.598a, b; 9.610a, b)
Name of functions	Hankel: $H_v^{(1,2)}(x)$	Generalized Hankel $H_{\mu,v}^{(1,2)}(x)$
Continuity	no: bifurcation as $\mu\to0$	

function of the first (9.598a, b) and second (9.610a, b) kind do not hold for zero degree; and (ii) the generalized Hankel function of the first kind (9.600a, b) has no essential singularity, the generalized Hankel function of the second kind (9.611a, b) has an essential singularity of degree two, whereas the original Hankel functions of two kinds (9.587; 9.588a, b) have an essential singularity of degree one. Thus continuity as the degree tends to zero is impossible (9.621a, b):

$$\lim_{\mu\to 0} H^{(1,2)}_{\mu,\nu}(z) \neq H^{(1,2)}_{\nu}(z). \tag{9.621a, b}$$

This situation might be expected from the generalized Bessel equation (9.428f) where the degree μ appears only in term $(\mu/2)x^3y'$: (i) as $x \to 0$ this term vanishes, and does not affect the continuity of the generalized and original Bessel (9.620a) and Neumann (9.620b) functions that are expansions in ascending powers of x; and (ii) as $x \to \infty$ the term $(\mu/2)x^3y' = 0$ for $\mu = 0$ whereas for $\mu \neq 0$ it diverges $(\mu/2)x^3y' \to \infty$, and thus the original and generalized Hankel functions are discontinuous (9.621a, b) since they correspond to expansions in descending powers of x. Thus *the generalized Bessel and Neumann functions (Hankel functions of two kinds) tend (9.620a, b) [do not tend (9.621a, b)] to (standard CCCXLI) the cylindrical Bessel and Neumann (Hankel) functions for zero degree because the singularity at the origin remains regular (at infinity changes from irregular of degree two to irregular of degree one).* The question might be raised whether a pair of other asymptotic solutions of the generalized Bessel equation exists that would lead to the original Hankel functions in the limit of zero degree. It will be proved next in two independent ways that this is impossible.

Starting with the generalized Bessel equation (9.428a–f) and seeking an asymptotic (9.553a–c) solution (9.591b) as a first normal integral (9.577a) with leading term (9.604a–c) leads to the differential equation (9.603b). In the case of zero order $\mu = 0$ the leading term (9.604c) is unity, and it could be hoped that the normal integral for the differential equation (9.603b) would lead to the original Hankel functions (9.587; 9.588a, b). In order to ascertain if this is possible, the solution of the differential equation (9.603b) is sought as a second normal integral (9.622a) so that combined with the first (9.577a) the asymptotic solution of the generalized Bessel equation would be (9.622b):

$$z(\xi) = e^{\Theta(1/\xi)} h(\xi): \qquad w(\xi) = e^{\Omega(1/\xi)} e^{\Theta(1/\xi)} h(\xi); \tag{9.622a, b}$$

the function $h(\xi)$ satisfies the differential equation (9.623) obtained (9.548a; 9.549a, b) substituting (9.622a) in (9.603b):

$$\xi^2 h'' + \xi\left(1 - \frac{\mu}{2\xi^2} + 2\Theta'\xi\right)h' + \left[\xi^2\left(\Theta'^2 + \Theta''\right) + \left(\xi - \frac{\mu}{2\xi}\right)\Theta' + \frac{1+\mu}{\xi^2} - \nu^2\right]h = 0. \tag{9.623}$$

The first normal integral was sought (9.602a) with a triple pole for Ω'; a simple pole for Θ' would lead to an asymptotic expansion without an essential singularity. Thus Θ' is chosen with a double pole (9.624a), leading by substitution in (9.623) to the differential equation (9.624b):

$$\Theta' = \frac{g}{\xi^2}: \quad \xi^2 h'' + \xi\left(1 - \frac{\mu}{2\xi^2} + \frac{2g}{\xi}\right)h' + \left[-\frac{\mu g}{2\xi^3} + \frac{1+\mu+g^2}{\xi^2} - \frac{g}{\xi} - \nu^2\right]h = 0. \tag{9.624a, b}$$

The coefficient of v has a triple pole that could be eliminated only by the choice $g = 0$ leading to a trivial solution $\Theta' = 0$ in (9.624a). This is an indicator that the normal integral being sought does not exist as shown next (subsection 9.6.13), implying a parametric discontinuity in the asymptotic integrals.

9.6.13 Parametric Discontinuity in the Asymptotic Integrals

The arbitrary g in (9.624b) can be chosen to cancel (9.625a) the double pole in square brackets in the coefficient of v in (9.624b):

$$g^2 + 1 + \mu = 0: \qquad g = \mp i\sqrt{1+\mu}, \qquad \Theta = -\frac{g}{\xi} = \pm i\frac{\sqrt{1+\mu}}{\xi}. \tag{9.625a–c}$$

The roots (9.625b) lead (9.624a) to (9.625c); using (9.625c) and (9.604b) in (9.622b) leads to (9.626):

$$w(\xi) = \exp\left(\frac{\mu}{4\xi^2} \pm i\frac{\sqrt{1+\mu}}{\xi}\right)h(\xi) = \exp\left(\frac{1}{4}\mu x^2\right)\exp\left(\pm ix\sqrt{1+\mu}\right)h\left(\frac{1}{x}\right), \tag{9.626}$$

consisting of: (i) the dominant term (9.604c) for the generalized Hankel function (9.610b) of the second kind for non-zero degree; (ii) for zero degree $\mu = 0$ this factor is unity and the next leading term $\exp(\pm ix)$ indeed coincides with the asymptotic scaling of the original Hankel functions (9.587); however, (iii) for (9.626) to be a pair of asymptotic solutions of the generalized Bessel equation $h(\xi)$ must be an asymptotic regular integral of the form (9.627a, b):

$$h(\xi) \sim \sum_{n=0}^{\infty} \xi^{a+n} c_n(a) = \sum_{n=0}^{\infty} x^{-a-n} c_n(a), \tag{9.627a, b}$$

that is, one index a must exist; there cannot be two because $\xi = 0$ is an irregular singularity of the differential equation (9.624b). If there is no index the asymptotic solution (9.626) fails, as is shown next.

Substituting (9.625b) the differential equation (9.624b) leads to (9.628):

$$\xi^2 h'' + \xi\left(1 - \frac{\mu}{2\xi^2} \mp \frac{2i\sqrt{1+\mu}}{\xi}\right)h' - \left[\nu^2 \mp \frac{i}{\xi}\left(1 + \frac{\mu}{2\xi^2}\right)\sqrt{1+\mu}\right]h = 0. \quad (9.628)$$

Substitution of (9.627a) in (9.628) leads to (9.629):

$$\begin{aligned} 0 = {} & \sum_{n=0}^{\infty} \xi^n c_n(a)\left[(n+a)^2 - \nu^2\right] \mp i\sqrt{1+\mu}\sum_{k=0}^{\infty} \xi^{k-1} c_k(a)(2k+2a-1) \\ & - \frac{\mu}{2}\sum_{\ell=0}^{\infty} \xi^{\ell-2} c_\ell(a)(\ell+a) \mp \frac{i\mu}{2}\sqrt{1+\mu}\sum_{j=0}^{\infty} \xi^{j-3} c_j(a). \end{aligned} \quad (9.629)$$

The changes of summation indices (9.630a–c) lead to (9.630d):

$$\begin{aligned} n = k-1 = \ell-2 = j-3:\ 0 = \sum_{n=0}^{\infty} \xi^n \Big\{ & c_n(a)\left[(n+a)^2 - \nu^2\right] \mp i\sqrt{1+\mu}(2n+2a+1)c_{n+1}(a) \\ & - \frac{\mu}{2}(n+a+2)c_{n+2}(a) \mp \frac{i\mu}{2}\sqrt{1+\mu}\, c_{n+3}(a)\Big\}. \end{aligned} \quad (9.630a–d)$$

Setting (9.631a) leads to (9.631b), implying that there is no index (9.631c) so all coefficients in (9.627b) vanish (9.631d) leading in (9.627a) to a trivial solution (9.631e):

$$n = -3: \quad 0 = \mp i\mu\sqrt{1+\mu}\; c_0(a), \quad c_0(a) = 0, \quad c_n(a) = 0, \quad h(\xi) = 0. \qquad (9.631a–e)$$

The failure of the indicial equation is due to the tripe pole in the coefficient in square brackets in the differential equation (9.624b). Thus *there is no asymptotic solution of the generalized Bessel equation (9.428a–f) for non-zero degree* μ *that (standard CCCXLII) in the limit* $\mu \to 0$ *tends to the original Hankel functions.* The existence of a bifurcation for the value zero of the degree in the asymptotic solution of the generalized Bessel differential equation can be confirmed by an independent method (subsection 9.6.14).

9.6.14 Bifurcation for the Degree at the Point at Infinity

It can be proved in an independent and simple way by reduction to absurd that *a solution of the generalized Bessel differential equation (9.428a–f) in (standard CCCXLIII) the form (9.626) cannot exist.* Suppose that a solution of the form (9.626) does exist with h a descending asymptotic expansion (9.627b). The solution (9.626) ≡ (9.632) would have to be a linear combination with arbitrary constants $G_{1,2}$ of generalized Hankel functions of the first (9.598b) and second (9.610b) kinds:

$$\exp\left(\frac{1}{4}\mu x^2 \pm ix\sqrt{1+\mu}\right)h\left(\frac{1}{x}\right) = G_1 H^{(1)}_{\mu,\nu}(x) + G_2 H^{(2)}_{\mu,\nu}(x). \qquad (9.632)$$

The r.h.s. of (9.632) contains only even powers of x coming from (9.598b; 9.610b); the l.h.s. of (9.632) has even and odd powers of x coming from the exponential factor. Thus the equality is impossible. It would be possible if the exponential on the l.h.s. did not have the second term, since in that case both sides contain only even powers of x. *In conclusion (standard CCXLIV): (i) the simplest asymptotic solution of the generalized Bessel equation (9.428a–f) is the generalized Hankel function of the first kind (9.598b), because it is the only solution without an essential singularity; (ii) any other solution has the exponential factor (9.604c) corresponding to an essential singularity, for example the generalized Hankel function of the second kind (9.610b). Any other solution would have to be a linear combination of the preceding and thus could not (9.633a) take the form (9.632):*

$$y\left(\frac{1}{x}\right) \neq \exp\left(\frac{1}{4}\mu x^2\right)\exp\left[\pm ix f(\mu)\right]h\left(\frac{1}{x}\right), \qquad f(0)=1, \qquad (9.633\text{a, b})$$

that would ensure continuity (9.633b) with the original Hankel functions; (iv) the discontinuity between the generalized and original Hankel functions (9.621a, b) is a discontinuity of the asymptotic solution of the generalized Bessel equation (9.428a–f) with regard to the parameter μ*; and (v) the reason for the discontinuity is that the irregular singularity at infinity is of different degree, namely two (one) for the generalized* $\mu \neq 0$ *(original* $\mu = 0$*) Hankel functions. This discontinuity is analogous to a Hopf-type bifurcation because in the case of real variable x and order* ν*, the asymptotic solution is: (i) oscillatory for zero degree* $\mu = 0$ *corresponding to the original Hankel functions (9.587; 9.588a, b) for zero degree; and (ii/iii) unstable (stable) for positive (negative) real part of the degree since both the generalized Hankel functions of the first (9.598b) and second (9.610b) kinds diverge (decay) as* $x \to \infty$.

The original Hopf bifurcation (section 4.8.5) concerns an autonomous differential system corresponding to a non-linear second-order differential equation with constant coefficients. The present case (9.428a–f) concerns a linear second-order differential equation with variable coefficients. A simple example for a linear second-order differential equation with constant coefficients is $y'' + \mu y = 0$, which has oscillatory solutions for $\mu > 0$, decaying or unstable solutions for $\mu < 0$, and a linear or monotonic solution for $\mu = 0$. The power series (asymptotic expansions) specify [section 9.5 (9.6)] the special functions that are the solutions of singular linear differential equations, such as the generalized or original Bessel, Neumann, and Hankel functions, and allow their accurate computation for small (large) values of the variable (subsection 9.6.15).

9.6.15 Numerical Computation for Small and Large Variable

As an example of numerical computation the simplest Bessel function of order zero is: (i) a power series (9.513a) ≡ (9.634a) for small variable (9.634b):

$$J_0(x)=\sum_{n=0}^{\infty}(-)^n\left(\frac{x^n}{n!2^n}\right)^2=1-\frac{x^2}{4}+\frac{x^4}{64}-\frac{x^6}{2304}+\frac{x^8}{147456}+O\left(x^{10}\right); \qquad (9.634\text{a, b})$$

and (ii) the asymptotic expansion (9.589a, b; 9.588a, b) for large variable (9.635):

$$J_0(x)\sim\sqrt{\frac{2}{\pi x}}\left\{\left[1-\frac{9}{128x^2}+O\left(\frac{1}{x^4}\right)\right]\cos\left(x-\frac{\pi}{4}\right)\right.$$
$$\left.+\frac{1}{8x}\left[1-\frac{225}{384x^2}+O\left(\frac{1}{x^4}\right)\right]\sin\left(x-\frac{\pi}{4}\right)\right\}, \qquad (9.635)$$

For example, for small variable (9.636a) the first three terms of the power series (9.634b) given seven accurate digits in (9.636b):

$$x=0.1: \qquad J_0(0.1)=1-\frac{0.01}{4}+\frac{0.0001}{64}+O\left(10^{-8}\right)=0.9975016. \qquad (9.636\text{a, b})$$

The convergence of the Bessel series (9.634a) is assured by the convergence theorem on regular integrals (subsection 9.5.11); since the only singularity of the original Bessel differential equation (9.430b) besides the origin is the point at infinity, the series is valid for all finite values of x; that is, it has an infinite radius of convergence. This can be confirmed by writing the Bessel series in the form (9.634a) ≡ (9.637a) with general term (9.637b):

$$J_0(x)=\sum_{n=0}^{\infty}u_n x^{2n}, \qquad u_n\equiv\frac{(-)^n}{(n!)^2}2^{-2n}; \qquad (9.637\text{a, b})$$

the D'Alembert ratio test (subsection I.29.3.2) specifies (subsection I.29.8.1) the radius of convergence (I.29.71a) ≡ (9.586a) showing that it is infinite (9.686b, c):

$$R=\lim_{n\to\infty}\left|\frac{u_n}{u_{n+1}}\right|=\lim_{n\to\infty}\left[\frac{(n+1)!}{n!}\right]^2\frac{2^{-2n}}{2^{-2n-2}}=\lim_{n\to\infty}4(n+1)^2=\infty. \qquad (9.638\text{a–c})$$

The convergence of a series gives no assurance that it is an efficient means of computing the function it represents, as shown by the example of the Bessel function of order zero for values of the variable that are moderate but not small.

As an example, consider the series (9.634a, b) ≡ (9.637a, b) for the Bessel function of order zero (9.639b) and variable (9.639a):

$$x = 10: \quad J_0(x) = \sum_{n=0}^{\infty} (-)^n 10^{2n} |u_n|, |u_{0-4}| = \left\{1, \frac{1}{4}, \frac{1}{64}, \frac{1}{2304}, \frac{1}{147456}\right\}, \tag{9.639a–c}$$

with coefficients (9.639c) as in (9.634b): (i) the terms of the series increase rapidly and only start to decay beyond the order $n \sim 20$; (ii) since the series has an alternating sign the errors of the difference of successive terms will not be small unless many digits are used; (iii) the sum of the series is (9.587) of the order $\sqrt{\pi/2x} \sim 0.4$ and thus small; (iv) thus the accumulated errors may easily exceed the sum of the series, making the result unreliable; and (v) an accurate sum, say with five digits, would require using many more digits in the larger terms of the series. This is why the asymptotic approximation (9.635), although it does not converge as $n \to \infty$ because the coefficients in (9.588a, b) are $O(n^n)$, is a much better approximation with a few terms, even for moderate values of x; for example (9.639a) when substituted in (9.635) gives (9.640) that has four accurate digits:

$$J_0(10) = \frac{1}{\sqrt{5\pi}} \left[\left(1 - \frac{9}{12800}\right) \cos\left(10 - \frac{\pi}{4}\right) + \frac{1}{80}\left(1 - \frac{225}{38400}\right) \sin\left(10 - \frac{\pi}{4}\right) \right] = -0.2459. \tag{9.640}$$

The preceding examples suggest that *the cylindrical, spherical, and generalized Bessel, Neumann, and Hankel functions of two kinds for small (large) variable are (standard CCCXLV) calculated more accurately by a few terms of the series (asymptotic) expansion.* The normal integral (section 9.6) is a particular case of the general irregular integral (section 9.7) in the neighborhood of an irregular singularity of a linear differential equation. The general irregular integral combines a branch-point with an essential singularity in a Laurent series (9.228a–e) with a power factor (9.253a–e) in the case of a single index, with additional logarithmic branch-points for a multiple index (9.263b). The replacement of ascending series by ascending and descending series transforms: (i) the recurrence formulas for the coefficients into an infinite homogenous system of equations; and (ii) the indices instead of being the roots of a characteristic polynomial become the roots of an infinite determinant.

9.7 Essential Singularities and Infinite Determinants

As was expected (subsections 9.4.5–9.4.6), a singular linear differential equation has in general in the neighborhood of an isolated irregular singularity (subsection 9.7.1) an irregular integral of the first kind combining a power type branch-point with an essential singularity (subsection 9.7.2); in the case of a repeated index (subsection 9.7.3) there is also a logarithmic branch-point leading to an irregular integral of the second kind (subsection 9.7.4). The regular integral can be also be of the first kind or second kind first/second types (subsection 9.7.5) leading to a classification of analytic, regular, and irregular integrals (subsection 9.7.6). The most direct method of obtaining the irregular integral in the neighborhood of an irregular singular is to substitute a Laurent series with a power type branch-point leading to: (i) an infinite system of linear algebraic equations to determine all coefficients in terms of one (subsection 9.7.7); and (ii) the indices as the roots of an infinite determinant that acts as the indicial equation (subsection 9.7.8). The infinite determinants raise convergence issues (subsections 9.7.9–9.7.10) like the series, infinite products, and continued fractions (chapters I.21, I.23, I.25, I.27, I.29; sections II.1.2–II.1.9, II.9.2–II.9.6). In the case of the Hill differential equation (subsections 9.7.11–9.7.14) that generalizes the Mathieu differential equation (subsection 4.3.2 and 4.3.7–4.3.11), leads to: (i) an infinite linear algebraic system for the coefficients (subsection 9.7.14); and (ii) a full infinite determinant, that is, a determinant with no zero elements, that can be evaluated analytically (subsections 9.7.15–9.7.16).

9.7.1 Existence of Eigenvalues and of Eigenintegrals

Consider two linearly independent particular integrals $y_\pm(x)$, a linear second-order differential equation (9.641c) whose coefficients have an isolated singularity at the point x_0 and are analytic (9.641b) in a ring with inner (outer) radius $\varepsilon(R)$ around it (9.641a):

$$0<\delta<R; \quad P,Q \in A\left(\varepsilon<|x-x_0|<R\right): \qquad y''_\pm + P(x)y'_\pm + Q(x)y_\pm = 0. \quad \text{(9.641a–c)}$$

In the complex x-plane (Figure 9.12), if the (9.642b) point x describes a closed curve or loop C, say a circle (9.642c) of radius δ within (9.642a) the ring (9.641a, b), the coefficients of the differential equation (9.641c) return to the same value, and the corresponding solutions at the start $y_\pm(x)$ and end $y_\pm(\overline{x})$ of the loop must be related linearly (9.642e, f):

$$\varepsilon<\delta<R; \quad x = x_0+\varepsilon; \quad \overline{x} = x_0+\varepsilon e^{i2\pi}; \quad 0 \neq A = \operatorname{Det}(a_{\pm\pm}) \equiv a_{++}a_{--} - a_{+-}a_{-+}: \quad \text{(9.642a–d)}$$

$$y_+(\overline{x}) = a_{++}y_+(x) + a_{+-}y_-(x), \qquad y_-(\overline{x}) = a_{-+}y_+(x) + a_{--}y_-(x), \quad \text{(9.642e, f)}$$

where (9.642d) ensures that $\overline{y}_{1,2}$ remain linearly independent if $y_{1,2}$ are linearly independent. An **eigenintegral** or **multiplied solution or principal integral** is transformed by multiplication by an **eigenvalue** (9.643a, b):

$$y_\pm(\overline{x}) = \lambda y_\pm(x); \qquad y(x) = C_+y_+(x) + C_-y_-(x), \quad \text{(9.643a–c)}$$

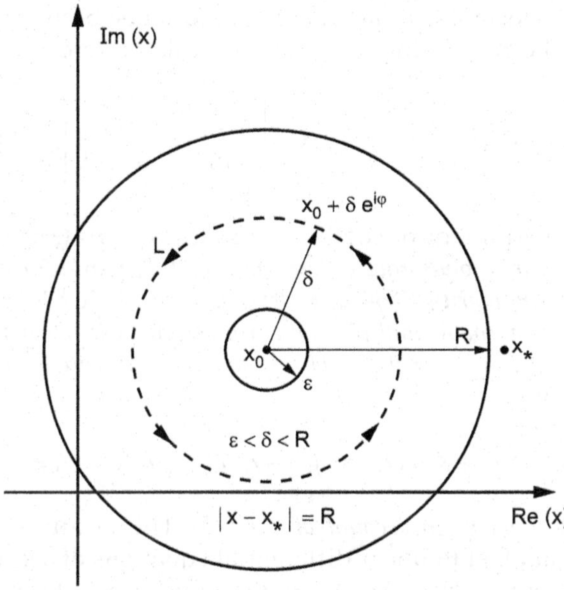

FIGURE 9.12
If x_0 is an isolated singularity (Figure 9.10a) describing a closed regular path around it like a circle of radius $|\delta|$ in the region of analicity $\varepsilon < |\delta| < R$ returns $0 \le \phi \le 2\pi$ to the same point $x_0 + \delta$ in the domain and: (i) also in the range for a single-valued function (Figure 9.8a); (ii) not in the range for a multi-valued function (Figure 9.8b) due to the crossing of the branch-cut in the domain (Figure 9.9b) and passage to another sheet of the Riemann surface (Figure 9.9a).

and the general integral (9.643c) is a linear combination of particular integrals (9.641c) where $C_\pm$ are arbitrary constants.

The general integral (9.643c) ≡ (9.644a) is transformed (9.642e, f) to (9.644b):

$$\begin{aligned} y(\bar{x}) &= C_+ y_+(\bar{x}) + C_- y_-(\bar{x}) \\ &= (C_+ a_{++} + C_- a_{-+}) y_+(x) + (C_+ a_{+-} + C_{--} a_-)_- \, y_-(x) \\ &= \lambda\left[C_+ y_+(x) + C_- y_-(x)\right], \end{aligned} \qquad (9.644\text{a–c})$$

and coincides with (9.644c) if the eigenintegrals (9.643a, b) exist. Since the particular integrals $y_\pm(x)$ are linearly independent, their coefficients in (9.644b) ≡ (9.644c) must coincide, implying (9.645a) ≡ (9.645b):

$$\begin{bmatrix} a_{++} & a_{-+} \\ a_{+-} & a_{--} \end{bmatrix} \begin{bmatrix} C_+ \\ C_- \end{bmatrix} = \lambda \begin{bmatrix} C_+ \\ C_- \end{bmatrix} \Leftrightarrow \begin{bmatrix} a_{++} - \lambda & a_{-+} \\ a_{+-} & a_{--} - \lambda \end{bmatrix} \begin{bmatrix} C_+ \\ C_- \end{bmatrix} = 0. \qquad (9.645\text{a, b})$$

The arbitrary constants of integration $C_\pm$ cannot be both zero (9.646b) otherwise (9.646a) the general integral (9.643c) would be zero:

$$y(x) \neq 0 \Rightarrow (C_+, C_-) \neq (0, 0): \qquad 0 = \begin{vmatrix} a_{++} - \lambda & a_{-+} \\ a_{+-} & a_{--} - \lambda \end{vmatrix}, \tag{9.646a–c}$$

and thus the determinant of coefficients must be zero (9.646c). It has been shown that *a linear second-order differential equation (9.641c) whose coefficients have an isolated singularity (9.641a, b) has (standard CCCXLVI) eigensolutions (9.643a, b) that transform by multiplication by an eigenvalue, when describing a loop around the singularity (Figure 9.12), where the eigenvalues are the roots (9.647b) of (9.646c) ≡ (9.647a):*

$$0 = \lambda^2 - (a_{++} + a_{--})\lambda + A = (\lambda - \lambda_+)(\lambda - \lambda_-), \qquad \lambda_+\lambda_- \equiv A \neq 0, \tag{9.647a–c}$$

and are not zero (9.647c) on account of (9.642d). This result is similar to the Floquet theory applied to linear differential equations of second-order with periodic coefficients (subsection 4.3.3) and is used next to demonstrate the existence of irregular integrals of the first and second kinds (subsection 9.7.2).

9.7.2 Irregular Integrals of the First Kind

If there are two distinct eigenvalues (9.648a), the (standard CCCXLVII) corresponding eigenintegrals are linearly independent (9.648b):

$$\lambda_+ \neq \lambda_- \quad \Leftrightarrow \quad \frac{y_+(\bar{x})}{y_-(\bar{x})} \neq const \equiv C: \quad C = \frac{y_+(\bar{x})}{y_-(\bar{x})} = \frac{\lambda_+}{\lambda_-}\frac{y_+(x)}{y_-(x)} = \frac{\lambda_+}{\lambda_-}C \Rightarrow \lambda_+ = \lambda_-, \tag{9.648a–d}$$

otherwise a contradiction arises, namely *linearly dependent eigenintegrals must (standard CCCXLVIII) correspond to the same eigenvalue (9.648c, d).* A loop around the singularity is equivalent to multiplication (9.649c) of the eigenintegral (9.643a) ≡ (9.649b) by the eigenvalue that is related to the **index** by (9.649a):

$$\lambda_\pm \equiv \exp(i2\pi a_\pm): \qquad y_\pm(\bar{x}) = \lambda_\pm y_\pm(x) = e^{i2\pi a_\pm} y_\pm(x); \tag{9.649a–c}$$

$$(\bar{x} - x_0)^{a_\pm} = \left(\varepsilon e^{i2\pi}\right)^{a_\pm} = (x - x_0)^{a_\pm} e^{i2\pi a_\pm}, \tag{9.650a–c}$$

the power (9.650a) with the same exponent is also multiplied (9.650b) by the same eigenvalue (9.650c) when describing a loop (9.649a) around the singularity (Figure 9.12). Thus *the eigenintegral (9.643a) with the eigenvalue (9.649a) and the power (9.650a) with exponent (9.650b, c) have (standard CCCXLIX) the* *same branch-point at $x = x_0$, and thus their ratio (9.651a) is a single-valued function, that is expressed as a Laurent series (9.228a–e):*

$$\frac{y_\pm(x)}{(x-x_0)^{a_\pm}} = \sum_{n=-\infty}^{+\infty} (x-x_0)^n c_n(a_\pm) \begin{cases} A.C.: & \delta < |x-x_0| < R, \\ T.C.: & \delta < \bar{\delta} \le x - x_0 \le \underline{R} < R; \end{cases} \qquad (9.651a\text{–}c)$$

the series (9.651a) is absolutely (and uniformly) convergent in the open ring (9.651b) [closed sub-ring (9.651c)] or punctured (9.641a) disk (Figure 9.12) of analyticity of the coefficients (9.641a, c) of the second-order linear differential equation (9.641c) with an isolated singularity at $x = x_0$.

Two eigenintegrals are (standard CCCL) linearly independent (9.648b) ≡ (9.652a) if: (i) the eigenvalues are distinct (9.648a) ≡ (9.652b); and (ii) the indices (9.652c) do not coincide or differ by an integer (9.652d, e):

$$y_+(x) \ne C y_-(x) \Leftrightarrow \lambda_+ \ne \lambda_- \Leftrightarrow e^{i2\pi a_+} \ne e^{i2\pi a_-} \Leftrightarrow \operatorname{Re}(a_+) \ge \operatorname{Re}(a_-): \quad a_+ - a_- \ne 0, 1, 2, \ldots \qquad (9.652a\text{–}e)$$

In this case, (9.652a–e), the general integral of the linear second-order differential equation (9.641c) in the neighborhood of an isolated irregular singularity (9.641a, b), is a linear combination (9.643c) ≡ (9.653a) with arbitrary constants $C_\pm$ of two ***irregular integrals of the first kind*** *(9.651a–c) one for each index (9.653b, c):*

$$y(x) = C_+ y_+(x) + C_- y_-(x): \quad y_\pm(x) = (x-x_0)^{a_\pm} \sum_{n=-\infty}^{\infty} (x-x_0)^n c_n(a_\pm). \qquad (9.653a\text{–}c)$$

If the indices coincide or differ by an integer (subsection 9.7.3) there is only one irregular integral of the first kind, and a second linearly independent integral is an irregular integral of the second kind (subsection 9.7.4).

9.7.3 Case of Indices Differing by an Integer

If the eigenvalues coincide there is only one eigenvalue equation (9.643a) ≡ (9.654a) and the second transformed integral is a linear combination of the first two (9.654b):

$$y_+(\bar{x}) = \lambda_+ y_+(x), \qquad y_-(\bar{x}) = a_{-+} y_+(x) + a_{--} y_-(x). \qquad (9.654a, b)$$

The general integral (9.643c) ≡ (9.655a) is given by (9.655b):

$$y(\bar{x}) = C_+ y_+(\bar{x}) + C_- y_-(\bar{x}) = (\lambda_+ C_+ + a_{-+} C_-) y_+(x) + a_{--} C_- y_-(x), \qquad (9.655a, b)$$

instead of (9.644a–c). From the comparison of (9.655a, b) ≡ (9.644a–c) or (9.642e, f) ≡ (9.654a, b) follows (9.656a, b):

$$a_{++} = \lambda_+, a_{+-} = 0; \quad 0 = \begin{vmatrix} \lambda_+ - \lambda & a_{-+} \\ 0 & a_{--} - \lambda \end{vmatrix} = (\lambda_+ - \lambda)^2 \Rightarrow a_{--} = \lambda_+, \tag{9.656a–e}$$

the determinant (9.646c) with (9.656a, b) simplifies to (9.656c) and since its has a double root (9.656d) follows (9.656e). The first eigenintegral (9.654a) leads in all cases to an irregular integral of the first kind (9.651a–c).

The second eigenintegral (9.654b; 9.656e) ≡ (9.657a):

$$y_-(\bar{x}) = a_{-+} y_+(x) + \lambda_+ y_-(x): \qquad \frac{y_-(\bar{x})}{y_+(\bar{x})} = \frac{y_-(x)}{y_+(x)} + \frac{a_{-+}}{\lambda_+}, \tag{9.657a, b}$$

divided by the first (9.654a) leads to (9.657b) showing that their ratio increases by a_{-+}/λ_+ when describing a loop around the singularity (Figure 9.12). The logarithm changes by $2\pi i$ in a loop around the singularity (9.658a, b) and thus (9.658c):

$$\begin{aligned} \frac{a_{-+}}{2\pi i \lambda_+} \log(\bar{x} - x_0) &= \frac{a_{-+}}{2\pi i \lambda_+} \log\left[(\bar{x} - x_0) e^{i2\pi}\right] \\ &= \frac{a_{-+}}{2\pi i \lambda_+} (\log \varepsilon + i2\pi) \\ &= \frac{a_{-+}}{2\pi i \lambda_+} \log(x - x_0) + \frac{a_{-+}}{\lambda_+}, \end{aligned} \tag{9.658a–c}$$

changes by the same value (9.658c)~(9.657b). Thus the difference of (9.657b) and (9.658c) is a single-valued function (9.659):

$$\frac{y_-(\bar{x})}{y_+(\bar{x})} - \frac{a_{-+}}{i2\pi\lambda_+} \log(\bar{x} - x_0) = \sum_{m=-\infty}^{+\infty} (\bar{x} - x_0)^m e_m(a_-), \tag{9.659}$$

that can be expanded in a Laurent series (9.228a–e).

The equation (9.659) may be re-written (9.660a–c):

$$b \equiv \frac{a_{-+}}{i2\pi\lambda_+}: \qquad y_-(x) = b \log(x - x_0) y_+(x) + y_+(x) \sum_{m=-\infty}^{+\infty} (x - x_0)^m e_m(a_-); \tag{9.660a–c}$$

the Cauchy rule of multiplication of series by diagonals applied to the last term on the r.h.s. of (9.660c) leads (9.651a) to (9.661c–e):

$$d_n(a_-) = \sum_{m=-\infty}^{+\infty} e_m(a_-) c_{n-m}(a_-); \qquad m+k=n: \tag{9.661a, b}$$

$$y_+(x) \sum_{m=-\infty}^{+\infty} (x-x_0)^m e_m(a_-) = \sum_{m,k=-\infty}^{\infty} (x-x_0)^{m+k} e_m(a_-) c_k(a_-) = \sum_{n=0}^{\infty} (x-x_0)^n d_n(a_-), \tag{9.661c–e}$$

with coefficients (9.661a) via the change of summation index (9.661b). Substitution (9.661e) in (9.660c) leads to:

$$a_+ - a_- \equiv s = 0,1....: \quad \bar{y}_-(x) = b\log(x-x_0) y_+(x) + (x-x_0)^{a_+} \sum_{n=-\infty}^{+\infty} (x-x_0)^n d_n(a_-), \tag{9.662a, b}$$

as the **irregular integral of the second kind** with a combined essential singularity and power-type branch-point. It has been shown that *if the linear second-order differential equation (9.641c) with coefficients having an isolated singularity (9.641a, b) has (standard CCCLI) equal eigenvalues (9.663a), or equivalently (9.649a) indices (9.663b) differing by an integer (9.652d, e) ≡ (9.662a), then the general integral (9.663b):*

$$\lambda_+ = \lambda_- \Leftrightarrow |a_+ - a_-| \in |N: \qquad y(x) = C_+ y_+(x) + C_- \bar{y}_-(x), \tag{9.663a, b}$$

is a linear combination with arbitrary constants $C_\pm$ of: (i) an irregular integral of the first kind (9.653c) specified by a Laurent series with a power-type branch-point; and (ii) an irregular integral of the second kind (9.662b) consisting of the sum of: (ii-1) the irregular integral of the first kind with a logarithmic branch-point multiplied by a constant b; (ii-2) a complementary function specified by another Laurent series with a power type branch-point. A particular case without essential singularity is the regular integral of the second kind (9.416) that can be obtained by a method (subsection 9.7.4) distinct from the preceding (subsections 9.5.10–9.5.11).

9.7.4 Irregular Integral of Second Kind

From (5.221b) ≡ (9.641c) one particular integral of a linear second-order differential equation can be obtained another particular integral (5.226a–c) given by (9.664a) where (9.664b) ≡ (9.425d) is the Wronskian of the two particular integrals:

$$\bar{y}_-(x) = y_+(x)\int^x \frac{W(\xi)}{[y_+(\xi)]^2}\,d\xi, \qquad W(\xi) = \exp\left\{-\int^\xi P(\eta)\,d\eta\right\}; \tag{9.664a, b}$$

in the case of the linear second-order differential equation with an isolated singularity of the coefficients (9.641a–c) one particular integral is always an irregular integral of the first kind (9.651a), and a second linearly independent particular integral is (9.664a, b) that is obtained as shown next. The single-valued coefficient has a Laurent series (9.665a–c):

$$c \equiv P_{-1}: \qquad P(x) = \sum_{n=-\infty}^{+\infty} P_n (x-x_0)^n = \frac{c}{x-x_0} + \sum_{\substack{m=-\infty \\ m\neq -1}}^{+\infty} P_m (x-x_0)^m, \tag{9.665a–c}$$

where the term with the residue (9.665a) is singled–out in (9.664b) the integration (9.664b) for the Wronskian (9.666a, b):

$$\begin{aligned} W(\xi) &= \exp\left\{-\int^\xi \left[\frac{c}{\eta-x_0} + \sum_{\substack{m=-\infty \\ m\neq -1}}^{+\infty} P_m(\eta-x_0)^m\right] d\eta\right\} \\ &= \exp\left\{-c\log(\xi-x_0) - \sum_{\substack{m=-\infty \\ m\neq -1}}^{+\infty} P_m \frac{(\xi-x_0)^{m+1}}{m+1}\right\} = (\xi-x_0)^{-c} \sum_{k=-\infty}^{+\infty} Q_k (x-x_0)^k, \end{aligned} \tag{9.666a–c}$$

that corresponds to the leading term in (9.666c).

Substitution in (9.664a) of the irregular integral of the first kind (9.653b) together with the Wronskian (9.666c) leads to the irregular integral of the second kind (9.667):

$$\bar{y}_-(x) = y_+(x)\int^x (\xi-x_0)^{-c-2a_+} \sum_{n=-\infty}^{+\infty} (\xi-x_0)^n g_n(a_+)\,d\xi, \tag{9.667}$$

where appears the Laurent series satisfying (9.668):

$$\left\{\sum_{\substack{k=-\infty \\ k\neq 1}}^{+\infty} Q_k(\xi-x_0)^k\right\} = \left\{\sum_{j=-\infty}^{+\infty} (x-x_0)^j c_j(a_+)\right\}^2 \times \sum_{n=-\infty}^{+\infty} (x-x_0)^n g_n(a_+). \tag{9.668}$$

TABLE 9.7

Linear Second-Order Differential Equation: Integrals of the First and Second Kind

Case	A	B
Integral	**First Kind**	**Second Kind**
Eigenvalues	$\lambda_+ \neq \lambda_-$	$\lambda_+ = \lambda_-$
Indices	$a_+ - a_- \notin Z$	$a_+ - a_- \in Z$
Linearly independent particular integrals	$y_\pm(x) = \sum_{n=-\infty}^{+\infty} (x - x_o)^{n+a_\pm}\ c_n\ (a_\pm)$	$\bar{y}_-\ (x) = b\ y_+\ (x)\log(x - x_o) + \sum_{n=-\infty}^{+\infty} (x - x_o)^{n+a_-}\ d_n\ (a_-)$
To be determined	$a_\pm,\ c_k(a_\pm)$	$a_\pm,\ c_k(a_\pm),\ d_n\ (a_\pm)$
General integral	$y(x) = C_+\ y_+\ (x) + C_-\ y_-(x)$	$y(x) = C_+\ y_+(x) + C_-\ \bar{y}_-(x)$

Thus, *the irregular integral of the second kind (9.667; 9.668) of the linear second-order differential equation (9.641c) with an isolated singularity (9.641a, b) may be obtained (standard CCCLII) from the irregular integral of the first kind (9.651a–c) ≡ (9.653a–c) using (9.664a) the Wronskian (9.664b; 9.665a–c; 9.666a–c). The irregular integrals of the first (9.653a–c) [second (9.663a, b; 9.675)] kind are compared in the Table 9.7.* This method of derivation of the second from the first irregular integral (subsection 9.7.4): (i) is an alternative to the preceding method (subsection 9.7.3); and (ii) also applies to regular integrals as shown next (as an alternative to subsection 9.5.10). In the case of a regular singularity the coefficient of the first derivative has a simple pole (9.669a, b):

$$P(x) = \frac{c}{x - x_0} + \sum_{n=0}^{\infty} P_n (x - x_0)^n = \frac{p(x)}{x - x_0}, \qquad p(x) = \sum_{m=0}^{\infty} P_{m-1} (x - x_0)^m, \tag{9.669a–c}$$

and the residue at the pole corresponds (9.669c) to (9.670a, b) and must coincide with (9.670c) in agreement with the roots of the indicial equation (9.396d, e):

$$c \equiv P_{-1} = p_0 = 1 - a_+ - a_-; \qquad -c - 2a_+ = a_- - a_+ - 1 = -s - 1, \tag{9.670a–f}$$

the exponent in (9.667) is given by (9.670d) ≡ (9.670e) and in the case when the indices differ by an integer (9.662a) the exponent is a negative integer (9.670f). In the case of a regular singularity, the series in (9.667) is unilateral from $n = 0$ to $n = \infty$, and its evaluation leads (subsection 9.7.5) to the two types of regular integrals of the second kind (subsections 9.5.10–9.5.11).

9.7.5 Regular Integrals of the Second Kind First/Second Type

Substituting (9.670f) in (9.667) with only the ascending sum, leads to (9.671a, b):

$$\bar{y}_-(x) = y_+(x) \sum_{n=0}^{\infty} \int^x (\xi - x_0)^{n-s-1} g_n(a_+) d\xi$$

$$= y_+(x) \left[g_s(a_+) \log(x - x_0) + \sum_{\substack{n=0 \\ n \neq s}}^{\infty} (x - x_0)^{n-s} \frac{g_n(a_+)}{n-s} \right]. \quad (9.671a, b)$$

If the indices coincide (9.672a, b), then (9.671b) is a regular integral of the second kind first type (9.672b) ≡ (9.405b):

$$a_+ - a_- = 0 = s: \qquad \bar{y}_+(x) = b \log(x - x_0) y_+(x) + (x - x_0)^{a_+} \sum_{n=1}^{\infty} (x - x_0)^n d_n(a_+), \quad (9.672a, b)$$

with coefficients (9.673a, b):

$$b \equiv g_s(a_+), \quad d_n(a_+) = \sum_{\substack{k=0 \\ k \neq s}}^{\infty} \frac{g_k(a_+)}{k-s} c_{n-k}(a_+), \quad (9.673a, b)$$

resulting from the product of the series (9.653b) by that in the last term of (9.671b). If the indices differ by a non-zero integer (9.674a, b) then (9.671b) leads to (9.674c):

$$a_+ - a_- \equiv s \neq 0; \qquad \bar{y}_-(x) = y_+(x) [b \log(x - x_0) + \sum_{n=0}^{s-1} (x - x_0)^{n-s} \frac{g_n(a_-)}{n+1} + \sum_{n=s+1}^{\infty} \frac{(x - x_0)^{n-s}}{n-s} g_n(a_-)], \quad (9.674a–c)$$

that is a regular integral of the second–kind second type (9.674d) ≡ (9.675) ≡ (9.416):

$$\bar{y}_-(x) = b \log(x - x_0) y_+(x) + (x - x_0)^{a_-} \sum_{m=0}^{\infty} (x - x_0)^m e_m(a_-) + (x - x_0)^{a_-} \sum_{n=0}^{a_+ - a_- - 1} (x - x_0)^n d_n(a_-), \quad (9.675)$$

with coefficients (9.673a) and (9.676):

$$e_m(a_-) = \sum_{\substack{k=0 \\ k\neq s}}^{m} g_k(a_-) \quad c_{m-k}(a_-). \tag{9.676}$$

Thus *the regular integrals of the second kind first (9.672a, b; 9.673a, b) [second (9.675; 9.676; 9.673a, b)] type can be obtained (standard CCCLIII) from the irregular integral of the second kind (9.667; 9.668) omitting the descending powers and retaining all other powers;* this is an alternative to the method of subsections 6.5.9 (9.5.10). This completes the list of possible integrals of a linear second-order differential equation that is summarized next (subsection 9.7.6 and tables 9.7–9.8).

9.7.6 Irregular, Regular, and Analytic Integrals

The linear second-order differential equations may be classified (Table 9.8) according to the three related aspects of: (i) properties of the coefficients: analytic, with poles or essential singularities; (ii) types of points: regular points or regular or irregular singularities; (iii) form of the solutions: ascending and/or descending power series with power and/or logarithmic branch points. Consider (standard CCCLIV) a linear second-order differential equation (9.641c) with coefficients that are single-valued analytic functions (9.641a, b) in a ring (Figure 9.12) around an isolated singularity $x = x_0$. If the coefficient of the derivative (the function) has a pole of order higher than one (two) or an essential singularity, then the point is an irregular singularity of the differential equation, and in its neighborhood exists at least one irregular integral of the first kind (9.653b) that has at most an essential singularity (9.228a–e) and a power type branch point (9.253a–e). A second linearly independent integral is obtained as an irregular integral of the first (9.653c) [second (9.662b)] kind if the indices do not differ (9.652e) [do differ (9.662a)] by an integer. A particular case of irregular integral is the normal integral (9.547a, b); two, one, or none may exist in the neighborhood of an irregular singularity if the function Ω can be chosen so that the differential equation (9.550) has a regular singularity.

At a regular singularity of the differential equation the coefficient of the derivative (function) can have at most a simple (9.376c) [double (9.376d)] pole so that the second-order differential equation is of the form (9.376e) where (9.376a, b) are analytic functions. In the neighborhood of a regular singularity of a linear second-order differential, there are two regular integrals that are linearly independent and involve convergent series. In the neighborhood of an irregular singularity there is at most one regular integral; for example, if the coefficient of the function has a pole of order one unit higher than that of the derivative (9.540a–d), but there is no assurance of convergence. In the neighborhood of a regular singularity there is always one regular integral of the first kind (9.377b) consisting of an analytic series multiplied by a power that can have a branch-point, for the index whose real part is not smaller than that of the other index. The other index leads to a linearly independent integral

TABLE 9.8

Second Linear Differential Equation: Classification of Points and Integrals

	Case	I	II	III
Differential Equation	Point	Regular	Regular singular	Irregular singularity
	Coefficients	$P,Q \in \mathcal{A}$	$P(x)=\frac{p(x)}{x-x_0}, Q(x)=\frac{Q(x)}{(x-x_0)^2}$ $P,Q \in \mathcal{A}$	$p \notin \mathcal{A}$ and/or $q \notin \mathcal{A}$
	Type	Analytic	Poles: single for P double for Q	Higher order poles* or essential singularities
Solutions Or integrals	Series	$y(x)=\sum_{k=0}^{+\infty}\frac{(x-x_0)^k}{k}y^{(k)}(x_0)$	$y(x)=(x-x_0)^a\sum_{k=0}^{+\infty}(x-x_0)^k c_k(a)$	$y(x)=(x-x_0)^a\sum_{k-\infty}^{+\infty}(x-x_0)^k c_k(a)$
	Type	Taylor series	Complex power × Taylor series	Complex power × Laurent series
	Point	Regular	Branch-point	Branch – point + essential singularity
	Coefficients	$c_k=\frac{1}{k}y^{(k)}(x_0)$	$c_0(a), c_1(a), c_2(a),\ldots$	$c_0(a), c_{\pm 1}(a), c_{\pm 2}(a),\ldots$
	Index	–	a	a
	Exponents	Ascending	Ascending	Ascending and descending

Higher order poles: $P(x)=\frac{p(x)}{(x-x_0)^\alpha}$, $p \in \mathcal{A}, \alpha \geq 2$: $Q(x)=\frac{q(x)}{(x-x_0)^\beta}$, $q \in \mathcal{A}, \beta \geq 3$; Essential singularity: $\alpha=\infty$ or $\beta=\infty$

that is: (i) another regular integral of the first kind (9.397c) if the indices do not differ by an integer, leading to two exceptions; (ii) if the indices coincide the second linearly independent integral is a regular integral of the second kind first type (9.405a, b) ≡ (9.672a, b; 9.673a, b) that generally includes an additional term with a logarithm multiplying the regular integral of the fist kind; and (iii) if the indices differ by a non-zero integer the second linearly independent integral is a regular integral of the second kind second type (9.416; 9.414a, b) ≡ (9.675; 9.673a, b; 9.676) adding a third term that is a power multiplied by a polynomial.

In the neighborhood of a regular point of the linear second-order differential equation the coefficients are analytic (9.279a–c) and two linearly independent particulars exist as Taylor series (9.280c). Any point x_0 in the finite plane can be moved to the origin by a translation , changing the power series from $(x-x_0)^n$ to x^n. The exception is the point at infinity that is mapped to the origin by inversion (9.553a–e) leading to the differential equation (9.554). The preceding results can be extended to differential equations of (9.279c) order N, that have: (i) analytic integrals (9.280c) if the coefficients are analytic (9.279a, b); (ii) all integrals regular (9.377b) if the coefficients of the n-th derivative has at most a pole (9.380a–d) of order $N-n$; otherwise (iii) at least some integrals will be irregular, possibly of normal type. The regular (irregular) integrals involve: (i) ascending (ascending and descending) power series; (ii) a power factor for each index that does not differ from any other by an integer; and (iii) in the case of indices differing by an integer logarithmic factors can appear. In all cases have to be calculated the coefficients of the series, and indices or other constants, as in the following general case of irregular integrals (subsections 9.7.7–9.7.12) leading to infinite linear systems and determinants.

9.7.7 Infinite Linear System for the Coefficients

Consider a linear differential equation of the second-order with an irregular singularity at the origin so that the coefficients may have a pole of arbitrary order or an essential singularity (9.677a, b) and the solution is an irregular integral (9.677c):

$$\{P(x),Q(x)\}=\sum_{\ell=-\infty}^{+\infty}\{P_\ell,Q_\ell\}x^\ell: \qquad y(x)=\sum_{n=-\infty}^{\infty}x^{n+a}c_n(a). \tag{9.677a–c}$$

Substituting (9.677a–c) in the differential equation (9.678) leads to (9.678b):

$$0=y''+P(x)y'+Q(x)y=\sum_{n=-\infty}^{+\infty}c_n(a)x^{n+a-2}(n+a)(n+a-1)$$
$$+\sum_{k,\ell=-\infty}^{+\infty}c_k(a)x^{k+a+\ell-1}(k+a)P_\ell+\sum_{j,\ell=-\infty}^{+\infty}x^{j+a+\ell}c_j(a)Q_\ell. \tag{9.678a, b}$$

The changes of variable of summation (9.679a, b) lead to (9.625c):

$$n-2=k+\ell-1=j+\ell: \qquad 0=\sum_{n=-\infty}^{+\infty} x^{n-2}\left\{(n+a)(n+a-1)c_n(a) + \sum_{\ell=-\infty}^{+\infty}\left[(n+a-\ell-1)c_{n-\ell-1}(a)P_\ell + c_{n-\ell-2}(a)Q_\ell\right]\right\}, \tag{9.679a–e}$$

where the coefficients of all powers must vanish. This leads to a linear homogenous infinite system of equations (9.680a):

$$\begin{aligned} 0 &= \left[(n+a)(n+a-1)+P_{-1}(n+a)+Q_{-2}\right]c_n(a) \\ &+ \sum_{\substack{\ell=-\infty \\ \ell\neq-1}}^{+\infty}\left[(n+a-\ell+1)c_{n-\ell-1}(a)P_\ell + \sum_{\substack{\ell=-\infty \\ \ell\neq-2}}^{+\infty} c_{n-\ell-2}(a)Q_\ell\right] \\ &\equiv \sum_{\ell=-\infty}^{+\infty} A_{n\ell}(a)c_\ell(a); \end{aligned} \tag{9.680a, b}$$

the coefficients cannot be all zero (9.681a), otherwise a trivial solution would result, so the determinant of the matrix in (9.680b) must vanish (9.681b):

$$\left\{c_0(a), c_{\pm1}(a),\ldots\right\}\neq\{0,0,\ldots\}: \qquad 0=B(a)=\operatorname{Det}\left[A_{n\ell}(a)\right]=C\prod_{s=1}^{n}(a-a_s), \tag{9.681a–c}$$

and its roots specify the indices in (9.681c) where C is a constant. Substituting an index in the infinite linear system (9.680b) all coefficients (9.682a) can be expressed as linear functions (9.682b) of $c_0(a_s)$, leading to the particular integrals (9.682c):

$$m=\pm1,\pm2,\ldots: \quad c_m(a_s)=c_0(a_s)d_m(a_s), \quad y_s(x)=x^{a_s}c_0(a_s)\left[1+\sum_{m=-\infty}^{+\infty}x^m d_m(a_s)\right]. \tag{9.682a–c}$$

There can be at most two linearly independent particular integrals, since the differential equation is of the second-order. The method of irregular integrals is summarized next (subsection 9.7.8) and then applied to the Hill differential equations (subsections 9.7.11–9.7.16) after some considerations on infinite determinants (subsections 9.7.9–9.7.10).

9.7.8 Indices as Roots of an Infinite Determinant

It has been shown (subsection 9.7.7) *that the linear second-order differential equation (9.678a) with an irregular singularity at the origin, corresponding to the Laurent series for the coefficients (9.677a, b) has (standard CCCLV) irregular integrals (9.682c) where: (i) the indices are the roots of the infinite determinant (9.681c) of the matrix (9.680a, b); (ii) the coefficients (9.682a, b) are expressed in terms of one them solving the infinite linear system (9.680a, b) with a specified by that root; (iii) not more than two linearly independent irregular integrals of the first kind (9.682c) can exist; and (iv) if the indices differ by an integer there may exist an irregular integral of the second kind (9.263b).* The 3×3 central part of the infinite linear system (9.680a, b) is written explicitly in (9.629):

$$\begin{bmatrix} \ddots & \vdots & \vdots & \vdots & \iddots \\ \dots (a-2)(a-1)+(a-1)P_{-1}+Q_{-2} & a P_{-2}+Q_{-3} & (a+1)P_{-3}+Q_{-4} & \dots \\ \dots & (a-1)P_0+Q_{-1} & (a-1)a+a P_{-1}+Q_{-2} & (a+1)P_{-2}+Q_{-3} & \dots \\ \dots & (a-1)P_1+Q_0 & a P_0+Q_{-1} & a(a+1)+(a+1)P_{-1}+Q_{-2} & \dots \\ \iddots & \vdots & \vdots & \vdots & \ddots \end{bmatrix} \begin{bmatrix} \vdots \\ c_{-1}(a) \\ c_0(a) \\ c_1(a) \\ \vdots \end{bmatrix} = 0. \tag{9.683}$$

The matrix (9.680b) ≡ (9.683) has the (9.684a) diagonal (9.684b) [non-diagonal (9.630c)] elements:

$$m \neq n: \quad A_{n,n} = (a+n)(a+n-1)+(n+a)P_{-1}+Q_{-2}, A_{n,m} = (a+m)P_{n-m-1}+Q_{n-m-2}; \tag{9.684a–c}$$

these follow from the relations (9.685a–d):

$$P_m = P_{n-\ell-1} \Rightarrow \quad \ell = n-m-1; \qquad Q_m = Q_{n-\ell-2}: \qquad \ell = n-m-2. \tag{9.685a–d}$$

The consideration of infinite determinants raises convergence issues addressed next (subsections 9.6.9–9.6.10).

9.7.9 Five Types of Convergence of Infinite Determinants (Poincare 1886)

The issue of convergence arise for **infinite processes** such as: (i) series (chapters I.21, I.29; sections II.9.4–II.9.6), including power series (chapters I.23, I.25, I.27) and series of fractions (sections II.1.2–II.1.3); (ii) infinite products (sections II.1.4–II.1.5;II.9.2); (iii) continued fractions (sections II.1.6–II.1.9; II.9.3); and (iv) infinite determinants considered here (subsection IV.9.7.10) starting with the definition. The definition of

infinite determinant of an infinite matrix proceeds in three steps: (i) the matrix is truncated (9.686a) to form a square with $2M+1$ elements per side around the central element $(0,0)$; (ii) the determinant of the finite truncated matrix is taken (9.686b):

$$m,n = 0,\pm 1,\dots,\pm M: \quad D_M \equiv Det\left(A_{m,n}\right), \lim_{M\to\infty} D_M = \begin{cases} D<\infty: & \text{convergent} \quad C, \\ \text{other:} & \text{oscillatory} \quad O, \\ \infty: & \text{divergent} \quad D, \end{cases}$$

(9.686a–e)

and (iii) the limit as the number of rows tends to infinity is taken, leading to three possible cases: (a) convergent if the limit is unique and finite (9.686c); (b) divergent if the limit includes infinity (9.686e); and (c) oscillatory if the limit is finite but not unique (9.686d).

The **absolute convergence** (9.687a) requires convergence of the determinant of the moduli of the elements of the matrix (9.687b):

$$D \equiv \lim_{M\to\infty} Det\left(A_{m,n}\right) A.C. \qquad \Leftrightarrow \qquad \bar{D} = \lim_{M<\infty} Det\left(\left|A_{m,n}\right|\right) \geq D, \qquad \text{(9.687a–c)}$$

and is a more stringent condition (9.687c). If the elements of the matrix depend on a variable (9.688a) there is **uniform convergence** if a matrix exists with elements in modulus not smaller (9.988b) whose determinant is convergent (9.688c):

$$D(x) = \lim_{M\to\infty} Det\left(A_{m,n}(x)\right): \qquad \left|A_{m,n}(x)\right| \leq B_{m,n} \wedge \lim_{M\to\infty} Det\left(B_{m,n}\right) = B \geq \left|D(x)\right|.$$

(9.688a–c)

An infinite determinant is **conditionally convergent** (9.689a) if it converges but not absolutely (9.589b):

$$\text{conditionally convergent} - \text{C.C.:} \qquad \text{C. and not A.C.,} \qquad \text{(9.689a, b)}$$

$$\text{totally convergent} - \text{T.C.:} \qquad \text{A.C. and U.C.,} \qquad \text{(9.690a, b)}$$

and is **totally convergent** (9.690a) if it is both absolutely and uniformly convergent (9.690b). Thus *an infinite determinant (9.686a, b) may be (standard CCLVI): (i) divergent (9.686e); (ii) oscillatory (9.686d); or (iii) convergent (9.686c). The convergence may be absolute (9.687a–c) [conditional (9.689a, b)]. The uniform convergence (9.688a–c) combined with absolute convergence leads to total convergence (9.690a, b),* as shown in Diagram I.21.1. The following theorem indicates conditions under which the convergence of an infinite determinant is assured (subsection 9.7.11).

9.7.10 Convergence Theorem for Infinite Determinants (Von Koch 1892)

A sufficient condition for the convergence of the infinite determinant of an infinite matrix (9.691c) is (standard CCCLVII) that both the infinite product of the diagonal element minus one (9.691a) [the double series of the sum of off-diagonal elements (9.691b)] be absolutely convergent:

$$\prod_{m=-\infty}^{+\infty}\left(A_{m,m}-1\right)A.C. \wedge \sum_{\substack{n,m=-\infty \\ n\neq m}}^{+\infty} A_{m,n}\,A.C. \quad \Rightarrow \quad Det\left(A_{m,n}\right)C. \tag{9.691a–c}$$

The proof is based on the infinite product (9.692b), including the diagonal elements (9.692a), that contains all terms of the determinant (9.691a):

$$A_{m,m}=1+a_{m,m}: \qquad E=\prod_{n,m=-\infty}^{+\infty}\left(1+a_{m,n}\right)A.C. \quad \Leftrightarrow \quad G=\sum_{n,m=-\infty}^{+\infty} a_{m,n}\,A.C.. \tag{9.692a–c}$$

The convergence of the infinite product (9.692b) is equivalent (II.9.18b, d) to the convergence of the series (9.692c), and thus (subsection II.9.2.2) the conditions of absolute convergence of (9.691a, b) imply the absolute convergence of (9.692b). The absolute convergence of (9.692b) implies the convergence of the infinite product of moduli (9.693a):

$$F_M=\prod_{n,m=-M}^{M}\left(1+\left|a_{m,n}\right|\right)C: \qquad \lim_{M\to\infty}\left(F_{M+N}-F_M\right)=0, \tag{9.693a, b}$$

and thus the Cauchy convergence principle (subsection I.29.2.2) implies (I.29.18) that the limit (9.693b) is zero. The elements (9.693a) in (9.693b) are the moduli of the elements in (9.687b) and thus not smaller (9.694a):

$$\left|D_{M+N}-D_M\right|\leq\left|F_{M+N}-F_M\right|: \qquad \lim_{M\to\infty}\left|D_{M+N}-D_M\right|=0. \tag{9.694a, b}$$

The limit (9.694b) follows from (9.694a; 9.693b) and proves the convergence of the infinite determinant (9.691c). QED. The convergence theorem will be used in the exact evaluation of the infinite determinant (subsections 9.7.14–9.7.16) that arise from the Hill differential equation (subsections 9.7.12–9.7.13). The Hill (1892) differential equation was introduced in lunar theory, and as a generalization of the Mathieu equation (subsections 4.3.7–4.3.11) it applies to parametric resonance (section 4.3) extended to forcing by a fundamental excitation frequency plus all its harmonics (subsection 9.7.11).

9.7.11 Parametric Resonance Forced by a Fundamental and Harmonics

Consider a linear oscillator (4.84d) with constant mass (9.695a) and spring resilience a function of time, so that the displacement satisfies (9.695b):

$$m = \text{const}: \qquad m\frac{d^2x}{dt^2} + k(t)\,x(t) = 0; \quad k(-t) = k(t) = k(t+\tau_e), \qquad \text{(9.695a–d)}$$

it is assumed that the resilience of the spring is: (i) an even function of time (9.695c); and (ii) has an excitation period τ_e in (9.695d). If the resilience of the spring is (subsection I.27.9.5) also (iii) a function of bounded oscillation (fluctuation/variation) in a period (9.696a) it has (subsection II.5.7.9) a Fourier cosine series (II.5.159a, b) ≡ (9.696b):

$$k \in \mathcal{F}(0,\tau_e): \qquad k(t) = k_0 + 2\sum_{\ell=1}^{\infty} k_\ell \cos\left(\frac{2\pi\ell t}{\tau_e}\right). \qquad \text{(9.696a, b)}$$

Substituting (9.696b) in (9.695b) leads to (9.697b):

$$\omega_e \equiv \frac{2\pi}{\tau_e}: \qquad m\frac{d^2x}{dt^2} + x(t)\left| k_0 + 2\sum_{\ell=0}^{\infty} k_\ell \cos(\ell\omega_e t)\right| = 0, \qquad \text{(9.697a, b)}$$

where (9.697a) is the applied frequency.

Thus *the displacement with small amplitude of an oscillator with constant mass (9.695a) satisfies (standard CCCLVIII) the linear second-order differential equation (9.697b) assuming that the resilience of the spring is an even function of time (9.695c) with applied period (9.695d) [frequency (9.697a)] that is of bounded fluctuation over a period (9.696a) and has Fourier cosine series (9.696b). There are three cases: (I) if the only non-zero coefficient is (9.698a) then (9.697b) leads to the harmonic oscillator (2.54c) with natural frequency (2.54a) ≡ (9.698a):*

$$k_0 \equiv m\omega_0^2; \qquad k_1 = 2mh\omega_0^2; \qquad k_\ell: \qquad \omega_\ell = \omega_e\,\ell, \qquad \text{(9.698a–d)}$$

(II) if there is one more non-zero coefficient (9.698b), then (9.697b) applies (4.149) to the parametric resonance of an oscillator with applied fundamental frequency (9.697a); and (III) the coefficients of higher orders (9.698c) are the amplitudes of forcing at harmonics multiple frequencies (9.698d). Introducing the phase (9.699a) in the displacement (9.699b) leads from (9.697b) to (note 9.33) the **generalized Hill differential equation** (9.699d) with coefficients (9.699c):

$$\theta \equiv \omega_e t,\ u(\theta) \equiv x(t),\ b_\ell = \frac{\omega_e^2}{m}k_\ell: \ \frac{d^2u}{d\theta^2} + \left[b_0 + \sum_{\ell=1}^{\infty} b_\ell \cos(\ell\theta)\right]u(\theta) = 0. \qquad \text{(9.699a–d)}$$

The Hill equation (subsection 9.7.13) is similar to (9.699d) replacing $\ell\theta$ by $2\ell\theta$ to change the period from 2π to π.

9.7.12 Hill (1892) Differential Equation with Trigonometric Coefficients

A linear second-order differential equation (9.281a) can, through the change of dependent variable (9.281b), be written without first order derivative (9.282a) ≡ (9.700a) involving a single coefficient; namely, the invariant (9.282b):

$$\frac{d^2u}{d\theta^2} + I(\theta)u(\theta) = 0: \qquad I(\theta+\pi) = I(\theta) = I(-\theta); \tag{9.700a–c}$$

the Floquet theory (section 9.3) applies if the invariant is a periodic function, in this case (9.700b) with period π. It is also assumed that the invariant is an even function (9.700c) with bounded oscillation (9.701a) so that (subsection II.5.7.6) it has a Fourier series (II.5.169a, b) ≡ (9.701b):

$$I \in \mathcal{F}(0,\pi): \; I(\theta) = b_0 + 2\sum_{\ell=1}^{\infty} b_\ell \cos(2\ell\theta), \; b_\ell = \frac{1}{\pi}\int_0^\pi I(\theta)\cos(2\ell\theta)\,d\theta. \tag{9.701a–c}$$

with coefficients (II.5.171a) ≡ (9.701c).

Assuming that the cosine series (9.701b) is uniformly convergent (section I.21.4) it can be integrated term by term to prove (9.701c). The zero-order coefficient (9.702c) is (9.702b) the mean value of the function in the interval (9.654a):

$$\langle I(\theta)\rangle \equiv \frac{1}{\pi}\int_0^\pi I(\theta)\,d\theta = b_0 + \sum_{m=1}^{\infty} b_m \left[\frac{\sin(2m\theta)}{2m}\right]_0^\pi = b_0. \tag{9.702a–c}$$

The remaining coefficients are calculated from:

$$\begin{aligned}\int_0^\pi I(\theta)\cos(2m\theta)\,d\theta &= 2\sum_{k=1}^{\infty} b_k \int_0^\pi \cos(2m\theta)\cos(2k\theta)\,d\theta \\ &= \sum_{m=0}^{\infty} b_m \int_0^\pi \{\cos[2(m+k)\theta] + \cos[2(m-k)\theta]\}\,d\theta = \pi b_k,\end{aligned} \tag{9.703a–c}$$

where: (i) all integrals are zero (9.704b) for (9.704a):

$$p = m \pm k \neq 0: \qquad \int_0^\pi \cos(2p\theta)\,d\theta = \left[\frac{\sin(2p\theta)}{2p}\right]_0^\pi = 0; \tag{9.704a, b}$$

and (ii) the only remaining integral is the second term with $k = m$ leading to (9.703c) ≡ (9.701c). It has been shown that *any linear second-order differential equation (9.274a) can be transformed (9.281b) to (9.282a, b) the invariant form*

(9.700a) if the invariant is (i) an even function (9.700c), with (ii) (9.700b) period π, and (iii) is of bounded oscillation (subsections I.27.9.5 and II.5.7.5) in a period, leading (standard CCCLIX) to the ***Hill (1896) differential equation*** *in trigonometric form (9.705a):*

$$O = \frac{d^2u}{d\theta^2} + \left[b_0 + 2\sum_{m=1}^{\infty} b_m \cos(2m\theta) \right] u(\theta)$$
$$= \frac{d^2u}{d\theta^2} + \left[b_0 + 2b_1\cos(2\theta) + 2b_2\cos(4\theta) + \ldots \right] u(\theta), \qquad (9.705a, b)$$

that: (i) involves a Fourier cosine series with coefficients (9.701c); and (ii) includes the Mathieu (1873) differential equation (4.89) as the particular case when the r.h.s. of (9.705b) consists only of the first two terms. The Hill differential equation is rewritten with power coefficients (subsection 9.7.13) to identify its singularities and hence the form of the Hill functions that are its solutions (subsection 9.7.14).

9.7.13 Hill Differential Equation with Power Coefficients

The change of variable (9.706a, b) implies (9.706c, d):

$$x = e^{i\theta}; \quad u(\theta) = y(x): \qquad \frac{d}{d\theta} = \frac{dx}{d\theta}\frac{d}{dx} = ie^{i\theta}\frac{d}{dx} = ix\frac{d}{dx}, \qquad (9.706a\text{–}c)$$

$$\frac{d^2}{d\theta^2} = i^2 x\frac{d}{dx} x\frac{d}{dx} = -x^2\frac{d^2}{dx^2} - x\frac{d}{dx}. \qquad (9.706d)$$

and is used together with (II.5.3a) ≡ (9.707a, b):

$$2\cos(2n\theta) = e^{i2n\theta} + e^{-i2n\theta} = x^{2n} + x^{-2n}, \qquad (9.707a, b)$$

to transform the Hill differential equation from trigonometric (9.699d) to polynomial (9.708) coefficients:

$$0 = x^2\frac{d^2y}{dx^2} + x\frac{dy}{dx} - \left[b_0 + \sum_{n=1}^{\infty} b_n\left(x^{2n} + x^{-2n}\right) \right] y = 0. \qquad (9.708)$$

An alternative form is (9.708) ≡ (9.709b):

$$b_{-m} = b_m: \qquad 0 = x^2\frac{d^2y}{dx^2} + x\frac{dy}{dx} - \left(\sum_{m=-\infty}^{+\infty} b_m x^m \right) y = 0, \qquad (9.709a, b)$$

with the identification of coefficients (9.709a).

The Hill differential equation (9.709b) has irregular singularities at the origin and infinity because one coefficient has an essential singularity; also the essential singularity in (9.709b) excludes the existence of solutions in the form of normal integrals (section 9.6). The solution near the origin in the x-plane is the irregular integral (9.710a):

$$y(x) = x^a \sum_{n=-\infty}^{+\infty} x^{2n} c_n(a) = e^{ia\theta} \sum_{n=-\infty}^{+\infty} e^{i2n\theta} c_n(a) = u(\theta), \qquad (9.710\text{a, b})$$

corresponding to the trigonometric series (9.710b). The symmetry of the coefficients (9.709a) implies (9.711a) so that the solution is a series of cosines (9.711b):

$$c_{-n}(a) = c_n(a): \qquad u(\theta) = e^{ia\theta}\left[c_0(a) + \sum_{k=1}^{\infty} c_n(a)\cos(2n\theta)\right]. \qquad (9.711\text{a, b})$$

The irregular integral (9.711b) is similar to the invariant (9.701b) in the Hill differential equation (9.705a) with the index factor $\exp(ia\theta)$ and coefficients c_n to be determined from the b_m in (9.701c). The irregular integral (9.710a, b) is valid in a circle of finite radius in the complex x-plane (9.712a) that maps (9.712b–d):

$$\infty > R > |x| = \left|e^{i\theta}\right| = \left|\exp\left[i\operatorname{Re}(\theta)\right]\exp\left[-\operatorname{Im}(\theta)\right]\right| = \exp\left[-\operatorname{Im}(\theta)\right] \Leftrightarrow \operatorname{Im}(\theta) > -\log R, \qquad (9.712\text{a–e})$$

the complex θ-plane (9.712e) to the upper region containing the real axis (Figure 9.13). Thus *the Hill differential equation with trigonometric (9.705a, b) [power (9.708) ≡ (9.709a, b)] coefficients has (standard CCCLX) the irregular integral solution (9.710b) ≡ (9.711a, b) [(9.710a)] valid (Figure 9.13) in the x-plane (θ-plane) in a circle with center at the origin (9.712a, b) [an upper half plane including the real axis (9.712e)].* The coefficients c_n (index a) are determined from (9.653c) by the solution (roots) of [subsection 9.7.15 (9.7.16)] of an infinite linear system (infinite determinant).

9.7.14 Infinite Linear System for the Coefficients

Using (9.707a; 9.709a) the Hill differential equation (9.705a) becomes (9.713):

$$\frac{d^2u}{d\theta^2} + u(\theta)\sum_{k=-\infty}^{+\infty} b_k e^{i2k\theta} = 0; \qquad (9.713)$$

the substitution in (9.713) of the irregular integral (9.710b) leads to (9.714):

$$0 = -\sum_{n=-\infty}^{+\infty} (2n+a)^2 e^{i(2n+a)\theta} c_n(a) + \sum_{k,m=-\infty}^{+\infty} b_k c_m(a) e^{i(a+2m+2k)\theta}. \qquad (9.714)$$

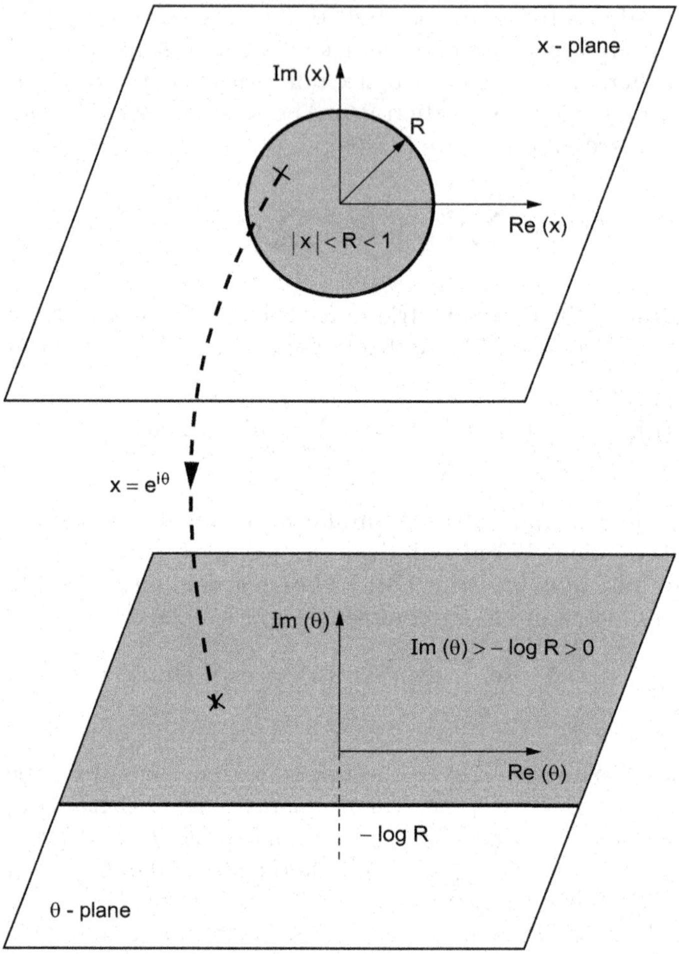

FIGURE 9.13
A Laurent power series in the punctured disk of radius R in the complex x-plane is mapped by $x = e^{i\theta}$ to a Fourier series in the upward half plane $\operatorname{Im}(\theta) > -\log R$ in the complex θ-plane, including the real axis $\operatorname{Im}(\theta) \geq 0$ for $R < 1$.

The change of index of summation (9.715a) transforms (9.714) to (9.715b):

$$n = m + k: \qquad 0 = \sum_{n=-\infty}^{+\infty} e^{i2n\theta} \left[(2n+a)^2 c_n(a) - \sum_{m=-\infty}^{+\infty} b_{n-m} c_m(a) \right]. \qquad (9.715a, b)$$

The vanishing of the factor in square brackets in (9.715b) leads to the infinite linear homogenous system of equation (9.716a):

$$\sum_{m=-\infty}^{+\infty} B_{n,m}(a) c_m(a) = 0: \; n \neq m: \; B_{n,n} = (2n+a)^2 - b_0, \; B_{n,m} = -b_{n-m}, \qquad (9.716a\text{–}d)$$

with matrix (9.716b) having diagonal (non-diagonal) elements (9.716c) [(9.716d)].

The matrix (9.716b–d) has elements $O(n^2)$ along the diagonal leading to a diverging determinant (9.686e). For a converging determinant the diagonal elements (9.692a) should be close to unity. The infinite linear homogenous system of equations in square brackets in (9.715a) ≡ (9.717):

$$\left[(2n+a)^2 - b_0\right] c_n(a) - \sum_{\substack{m=-\infty \\ m\neq 0}}^{+\infty} b_{n-m}\, c_m(a) = 0, \tag{9.717}$$

has the same solution if each equation is multiplied by a factor, for example (9.718a) leads to (9.718b):

$$\frac{1}{4n^2 - b_0} \times: \quad 0 = \frac{(2n+a)^2 - b_0}{4n^2 - b_0} c_n(a) - \sum_{\substack{m=-\infty \\ m\neq 0}}^{+\infty} \frac{b_{n-m}\, c_m(a)}{4n^2 - b_0} = \sum_{m=-\infty}^{+\infty} A_{n,m}(a)\, c_m(a). \tag{9.718a–c}$$

The corresponding matrix (9.718c) has $O(1)$ diagonal elements (9.719b) and non-diagonal elements (9.719c) of $O(n^{-2})$:

$$n \neq m: \; A_{n,n} = \frac{(2n+a)^2 - b_0}{4n^2 - b_0}, \quad A_{n,m} = -\frac{b_{n-m}}{4n^2 - b_0}; \; A = Det(A_{n,m}) = 0, \tag{9.719a–d}$$

the determinant (9.719d) of the matrix (9.719a–c) appears in the linear system:

$$\begin{bmatrix} \ddots & \vdots & \vdots & \vdots & \vdots & \vdots & \iddots \\ \cdots & \frac{(a-4)^2 - b_0}{16 - b_0} & \frac{b_1}{16-b_0} & -\frac{b_2}{16-b_0} & -\frac{b_3}{16-b_0} & -\frac{b_4}{16-b_0} & \cdots \\ \cdots & -\frac{b_1}{4-b_0} & \frac{(a-2)^2 - b_0}{4-b_0} & -\frac{b_1}{4-b_0} & -\frac{b_2}{4-b_0} & -\frac{b_3}{4-b_0} & \cdots \\ \cdots & \frac{b_2}{b_0} & \frac{b_1}{b_0} & 1-\frac{a^2}{b_0} & \frac{b_1}{b_0} & \frac{b_2}{b_0} & \cdots \\ \cdots & -\frac{b_3}{4-b_0} & -\frac{b_2}{4-b_0} & -\frac{b_1}{4-b_0} & \frac{(a+2)^2 - b_0}{4-b_0} & -\frac{b_1}{4-b_0} & \cdots \\ \cdots & -\frac{b_4}{16-b_0} & -\frac{b_3}{16-b_0} & -\frac{b_2}{16-b_0} & -\frac{b_1}{16-b_0} & \frac{(a+4)^2 - b_0}{16-b_0} & \cdots \\ \iddots & \vdots & \vdots & \vdots & \vdots & \vdots & \ddots \end{bmatrix} \begin{bmatrix} c_{-2}(a) \\ c_{-1}(a) \\ c_0(a) \\ c_1(a) \\ c_2(a) \\ \vdots \end{bmatrix} = 0, \tag{9.720}$$

It has been shown that the *Hill differential equation with trigonometric (9.705a) ≡ (9.705b) [power (9.708) ≡ (9.709a, b)] coefficients has (standard CCCLXI) solutions in the form of irregular integrals (9.710b) [(9.710a)] with: (i) the index a being a root of the* ***Hill infinite determinant*** *in (9.719a–d); and (ii) for each value of the index substituted in the infinite linear homogenous system (9.718b) ≡ (9.718c; 9.719a–c) ≡ (9.720) specifies all coefficients (9.682b) in terms of* $c_0(a)$ *leading to the irregular integral (9.682c).* It remains to evaluate the Hill determinant (subsection 9.7.15) whose vanishing acts as indicial equation, so that the indices are specified by its roots.

9.7.15 Exact Analytic Evaluation of the Hill Determinant

The diagonal terms (9.719b) of the Hill determinant differ from unity (9.721a) by a term $O(1/n)$ leading (9.721b) to (9.689a, b) conditional convergence (9.721c) as (section I.21.3) the series with general term $O(1/n)$:

$$A_{n,n}(a)=\left(1-\frac{b_0}{4n^2}\right)^{-1}\left[\left(1+\frac{a}{2n}\right)^2-\frac{b_0^2}{4n^2}\right]\sim 1+\frac{a}{n}+O\left(\frac{1}{n^2}\right): \qquad Det\left\{A_{m,n}(a)\right\}C.C. \tag{9.721a–c}$$

If instead of multiplying by (9.718a) the multiplication is by (9.722a) the recurrence relation (9.717) becomes (9.722b):

$$\times\frac{1}{(2n+a)^2-b_0}: \qquad 0=c_n(a)-\sum_{\substack{m=-\infty\\ m\neq 0}}^{+\infty}\frac{b_{n-m}\,c_m(a)}{(2n+a)^2-b_0} =\sum_{m=-\infty}^{+\infty}D_{n,m}(a)\,c_m(a); \tag{9.722a–c}$$

the infinite linear homogenous system (9.722c) has a matrix (9.723a) with unity diagonal elements (9.723b) and off-diagonal elements (9.723c) of $O(1/n^2)$, so the vanishing (9.723d) determinant is absolutely convergent (9.723e):

$$m\neq n:\quad D_{n,m}(a)=1, \quad D_{n,m}(a)=\frac{b_{n-m}}{b_0-(2n+a)^2}, \qquad 0=D(a)\equiv Det\left[D_{n,m}(a)\right]A.C. \tag{9.723a–e}$$

The linear system (9.722b) ≡ (9.722c; 9.723a–c) ≡ (9.724):

$$\begin{bmatrix} \ddots & \vdots & \vdots & \vdots & \vdots & \vdots & \iddots \\ \cdots & 1 & \frac{b_1}{b_0-(a-4)^2} & \frac{b_2}{b_0-(a-4)^2} & \frac{b_3}{b_0-(a-4)^2} & -\frac{b_4}{b_0-(a-4)^2} & \cdots \\ \cdots & \frac{b_1}{b_0-(a-2)^2} & 1 & \frac{b_1}{b_0-(a-2)^2} & \frac{b_2}{b_0-(a-2)^2} & \frac{b_3}{b_0-(a-2)^2} & \cdots \\ \cdots & \frac{b_2}{b_0-a^2} & \frac{b_1}{b_0-a^2} & 1 & \frac{b_1}{b_0-a^2} & \frac{b_2}{b_0-a^2} & \cdots \\ \cdots & \frac{b_3}{b_0-(a+2)^2} & \frac{b_2}{b_0-(a+2)^2} & \frac{b_1}{b_0-(a+2)^2} & 1 & \frac{b_1}{b_0-(a+2)^2} & \cdots \\ \cdots & \frac{b_4}{b_0-(a+4)^2} & \frac{b_3}{b_0-(a+4)^2} & \frac{b_2}{b_0-(a+4)^2} & \frac{b_1}{b_0-(a+4)^2} & 1 & \cdots \\ \iddots & \vdots & \vdots & \vdots & \vdots & \vdots & \ddots \end{bmatrix} \begin{bmatrix} \vdots \\ c_{-2}(a) \\ c_{-1}(a) \\ c_0(a) \\ c_1(a) \\ c_2(a) \\ \vdots \end{bmatrix} = 0, \tag{9.724}$$

involves the **modified Hill determinant** (9.724) distinct from the original Hill determinant in (9.720).

The original (9.718b, c; 9.719a–d; 9.720) [modified (9.722b, c; 9.723a–d; 9.724)] Hill determinant arise from the same linear homogenous infinite system (9.717) multiplying by different factors (9.718a) [(9.722a)] and thus their ratio is specified by the infinite product (9.725a):

$$\frac{A(a)}{D(a)} = \prod_{n=-\infty}^{+\infty} \frac{(2n+a)^2 - b_0}{4n^2 - b_0} = \prod_{n=-\infty}^{+\infty} \frac{\left(2n+a-\sqrt{b_0}\right)\left(2n+a+\sqrt{b_0}\right)}{\left(2n-\sqrt{b_0}\right)\left(2n+\sqrt{b_0}\right)}. \tag{9.725a, b}$$

Introducing the variables (9.726a, b) the infinite product (9.725b) is evaluated (9.726c) in terms of circular sines (9.726d) using (9.439b) ≡ (9.726c, d):

$$\alpha \equiv \frac{\pi a}{2}, \quad \beta = \frac{\pi\sqrt{b_0}}{2}: \quad \sin\phi = \phi \prod_{m=1}^{\infty}\left(1 - \frac{\phi^2}{m^2\pi^2}\right) = \prod_{m=-\infty}^{+\infty}\left(1 + \frac{\phi}{m\pi}\right). \tag{9.726a–d}$$

Substitution of (9.726a, b, d) in (9.725b) leads to (9.727):

$$A(a) = -D(a)\sin(\alpha-\beta)\sin(\alpha+\beta)\csc^2\beta. \tag{9.727}$$

The evaluation of the determinant (9.723e) specifies the roots (9.723d) of the determinant (9.719d) from (9.727) leading to the indicial equation (subsection 9.7.16).

9.7.16 Indices as Roots of a Transcendental Equation

The determinant (9.723e) in (9.724): (i) is an even function (9.728a); (ii) has period two (9.728b); (iii) as $\mathrm{Im}(a) \to \pm\infty$ all terms vanish except the diagonal so it tends to unity (9.728c); and (iv) it has poles for $(2n+a)^2 - b_0 = 0$, that is (9.728d):

$$D(-a) = D(a) = D(a+2); \lim_{\mathrm{Im}(a)\to\pm\infty} D(a) = 1; \lim_{a\to 2n\mp\sqrt{b_0}} \left(a+2n\pm\sqrt{b_0}\right) D(a) = O(1); \tag{9.728a–d}$$

the same properties apply to the function in square brackets in (9.729a) and thus a constant K exists such that the function defined by (9.681a):

$$E(a) = D(a) - K\left[\cot(\alpha+\beta) - \cot(\alpha-\beta)\right] = const, \tag{9.729a, b}$$

has no poles, is periodic, hence bounded in the whole complex plane, and hence by the Liouville's theorem (section I.27.6) is a constant (9.729b). The limit (9.730a) determines (9.728c) the constant (9.730b):

$$\lim_{\mathrm{Im}(a)\to\pm\infty} E(a) = \lim_{\mathrm{Im}(a)\to\pm\infty} D(a) = 1: \qquad D(a) = 1 + K\left[\cot(\alpha+\beta) - \cot(\alpha-\beta)\right], \tag{9.730a–c}$$

implying (9.730c). Substitution of (9.730c) in (9.727) specifies the Hill determinant:

$$\begin{aligned} &A(a) + \sin(\alpha+\beta)\sin(\alpha-\beta)\csc^2\beta \\ &= -K\left[\cot(\alpha+\beta) - \cot(\alpha-\beta)\right]\sin(\alpha+\beta)\sin(\alpha-\beta)\csc^2\beta \\ &= -K\left[\cos(\alpha+\beta)\sin(\alpha-\beta) - \cos(\alpha-\beta)\sin(\alpha+\beta)\right]\csc^2\beta \\ &= K\sin(2\beta)\csc^2\beta = 2K\cos\beta\csc\beta = 2K\cot\beta, \end{aligned} \tag{9.731a–e}$$

for arbitrary index.

The constant K is determined from the value of the Hill determinant (9.731e) at the origin (9.732a):

$$A(0) - 1 = 2K\cot\beta, \qquad A(a) = A(0) - 1 - \frac{\sin(\alpha+\beta)\sin(\alpha-\beta)}{\sin^2\beta}. \tag{9.732a, b}$$

and substituting (9.732a) in (9.731e) leads to (9.732b). Using (9.685a) leads to (9.733b, c):

$$\sin(\alpha\pm\beta) = \sin\alpha\cos\beta \mp \sin\beta\cos\alpha: \tag{9.733a, b}$$

$$\begin{aligned} \sin(\alpha+\beta)\sin(\alpha-\beta) + \sin^2\beta &= \sin^2\alpha\cos^2\beta + \sin^2\beta\left(1-\cos^2\alpha\right) \\ &= \sin^2\alpha\left(\cos^2\beta + \sin^2\beta\right) = \sin^2\alpha. \end{aligned} \tag{9.733c}$$

Substitution of (9.733c) in (9.732b) leads to:

$$A(a) = A(0) - \frac{\sin^2 \alpha}{\sin^2 \beta}; \quad A(a) = 0: \quad \sin^2\left(\frac{\pi a}{2}\right) = A(0)\sin^2\left(\frac{\pi\sqrt{b_0}}{2}\right), \tag{9.734a–c}$$

and (9.734b) implies (9.734c) using (9.726a, b). Thus *the Hill infinite determinant (9.719a–c) appearing (standard CCCLXII) in the infinite linear homogenous system (9.720) satisfies (9.734a) with (9.726a, b); its vanishing (9.719d) ≡ (9.734b) specifies the indicial equation (9.734c), whose roots appear in the irregular integrals (9.710b) ≡ (9.711a, b) together with the recurrence formula (9.717) for the coefficients.* The solution of linear differential equations in the neighborhood of regular points (regular/irregular) singularities leads [section 9.4 (sections 9.5/9.6–9.7)] to analytic (regular/irregular) power series. A different method of solution of linear differential equations is the use of integral transforms (section 9.8).

9.8 Kernel and Path of Integral Transforms (Laplace 1812; Bateman 1909)

An alternative to the solution of linear differential equations by power series (sections 9.4–9.7) is to use (section 9.8) integral transforms or integral representations that involve: (i) the transform that is a function of an auxiliary variable; (ii) the product by a kernel, that is a function of both the original and auxiliary variables; and (iii) an integration along a path in the complex plane of the auxiliary variable. The simplest integral representations are the Fourier (Laplace) transform [notes 1.11–1.14 (1.15–1.28)] that apply the linear differential equations with constant coefficients (chapter 1), and use: (i) an imaginary (real) exponential as kernel; and (ii) use the whole (positive) real axis as path of integration. In order to solve linear differential equations with variable coefficients it is necessary to relax one or both conditions, leading to a variety of integral transforms (subsection 9.8.5), of which two are considered in more detail: (a) the generalized Laplace transform along a path in the complex plane can be used to solve linear differential equations whose coefficients are linear functions (subsections 9.8.6–9.8.11); and (b) for other types of coefficients a Bateman transform may be needed, using both a path of integration in the complex plane and a kernel that is not an exponential (subsections 9.8.12–9.8.16).

The generalized Laplace transform (subsection 9.8.6) is used to solve the generalized (original) Bessel differential equation [subsections 9.8.7–9.8.8 (9.8.10)]; this leads to parametric integral representations for the generalized (original) Bessel functions [subsections 9.8.9 (9.8.11)] that are equivalent alternatives to the power series representations [subsections 9.5.15–9.5.16 and 9.5.18–9.5.21 (9.5.22)]. The Bateman transform (subsection 9.8.5) may be chosen with a kernel satisfying a partial differential equation (subsection 9.8.12), and a kernel distinct from that in the generalized Laplace transform leads through the adjoint operator and bilinear concomitant (chapter III.7 and subsection 9.8.13) to parametric integral representations for the original Hankel (Neumann) function [subsection 9.8.14 (9.8.15)] and to a second alternative integral representation for the Bessel function (subsection 9.8.16). The series representations for generalized Bessel (Neumann) functions [subsections 9.5.15–9.5.16 (9.5.18–9.5.21)] use the Euler gamma (digamma) function [subsection 9.5.14 (9.5.17)]. The relations between the series expansions (subsections 9.5.15–9.5.16 and 9.5.18–9.5.22) and integral representations (subsections 9.8.5–9.8.11 and 9.8.12–9.8.16) of the generalized and original Bessel, Neumann, and Hankel functions are established using the beta function (subsection 9.8.4), that is another function introduced by Euler. The gamma (beta) function is defined by the Eulerian integral of the first (second) kind [subsection 9.5.14 (9.8.1)] and is a generalization of the factorial (permutation) from integer to complex variables (subsection 9.8.2); this implies the existence of a relation between the beta and gamma functions (subsection 9.8.3).

9.8.1 Eulerian Integral of the Second Kind (Euler 1772)

The Gamma function or Eulerian integral of the first kind (Euler's digamma function) was introduced [subsection 9.5.13 (9.5.16)] in connection with the regular integrals of the first (second) kind [subsection(s) 9.5.9 (9.5.10–9.5.11)] of singular linear differential equations, with the generalized Bessel (Neumann) function [subsections 9.5.14–9.5.15 (9.5.17–9.5.20)] as an example in the case of the generalized Bessel differential equation (subsections 9.5.12 and 9.5.21). In connection with the solution of linear differential equations with variable coefficients and the associated integral representations of special functions (subsections 9.8.3–9.8.14) is introduced next a third Eulerian function (or second Eulerian integral); namely, [subsection 9.8.1.(9.8.2)] the beta function (that is related to the gamma function). The **beta function or Eulerian integral of the second kind** is defined by the definite integral (9.735c) where (9.735a) [(9.735b)] ensure convergence at the lower (upper) boundary point of the unit interval of integration:

$$\operatorname{Re}(\alpha) > 0 < \operatorname{Re}(\beta): \qquad B(\alpha,\beta) \equiv \int_0^1 t^{\alpha-1}(1-t)^{\beta-1}\,dt. \tag{9.735a–c}$$

The changes of variable (9.735a–c) imply (9.736a–c):

$$t = \sin^2\phi, \qquad t = \frac{1}{s}, \qquad t = \tanh^2\psi, \tag{9.736a–c}$$

$$dt = 2\sin\phi\cos\phi, \qquad dt = -\frac{ds}{s^2}, \qquad dt = 2\tanh\psi\,\operatorname{sech}^2\psi, \tag{9.737a–c}$$

and transform the integral (9.735a–c) respectively to (9.738a–e):

$$\text{Re}(\alpha) > 0 < \text{Re}(\beta): \qquad B(\alpha,\beta) = 2\int_0^{\pi/2} \sin^{2\alpha-1}\phi \cos^{2\beta-1}\phi \; d\phi, \tag{9.738a–c}$$

$$= \int_1^{\infty} s^{-\alpha-\beta}(s-1)^{\beta-1}\, ds, \tag{9.738d}$$

$$= 2\int_0^{\infty} \sinh^{2\alpha-1}\psi \cosh^{1-2\alpha-2\beta}\psi \, d\psi. \tag{9.738e}$$

The beta function of variables (9.735a, b) is defined by the integral (9.735c) and (standard CCCLXIII) evaluates the integrals (9.738c–e).

The change of variable (9.739a) shows (9.739b):

$$u = 1 - t: \qquad B(\alpha,\beta) = \int_0^1 (1-u)^{\alpha-1} u^{\beta-1}\, du = B(\beta,\alpha), \tag{9.739a–c}$$

that the beta function is symmetric in the two variables (9.739c) ≡ (9.740a):

$$B(\alpha,\beta) = B(\alpha,\beta); \qquad B(\alpha,1) = \frac{1}{\alpha}, \qquad B(1,\beta) = \frac{1}{\beta}, \tag{9.740a–c}$$

also (9.740b, c) follow immediately from the definition (9.735c) and are consistent with (9.740a). The integration by parts of (9.735c) leads to (9.741a):

$$B(\alpha,\beta) = \frac{1}{\alpha}\int_0^1 (1-t)^{\beta-1}\, d\left(t^{\alpha}\right) \tag{9.741a}$$

$$= \frac{1}{\alpha}\left[(1-t)^{\beta-1} t^{\alpha}\right]_0^1 - \frac{1}{\alpha}\int_0^1 t^{\alpha}\, d\left[(1-t)^{\beta-1}\right] \tag{9.741b}$$

$$= \frac{\beta-1}{\alpha}\int_0^1 t^{\alpha}(1-t)^{\beta-2}\, dt, \tag{9.741c}$$

where: (i) the first term in (9.741b) vanishes for (9.742a, b); and (ii) the remaining second term in (9.741b) leads (9.741c) to (9.742c) that is the **recurrence formula** for the beta function:

$$\text{Re}(\alpha) > 0,\ \text{Re}(\beta) > 1: \qquad B(\alpha,\beta) = \frac{\beta-1}{\alpha} B(\alpha+1,\beta-1). \tag{9.742a–c}$$

Applying (9.742a–c) iteratively n-times (9.743a–c):

$$n \in |N;\ \operatorname{Re}(\alpha) > 1 - n,\ \operatorname{Re}(\beta) > n:\ B(\alpha,\beta) = \frac{(\beta-1)(\beta-2)\ldots(\beta-n)}{\alpha(\alpha+1)\ldots.(\alpha+n-1)} B(\alpha+n,\beta-n). \tag{9.743a–d}$$

leads to the **iterated recurrence formula** (9.743d).

9.8.2 Permutations and Properties of the Beta Function

The gamma function (9.431a, b) of a positive integer coincides with the factorial (9.433a, b) and generalizes it to complex values of the variable. Setting (9.744a–c) in the iterated recurrence formula (9.743a–d) leads to (9.744d):

$$\begin{aligned} n \in |N,\quad \beta = n+1,\quad \operatorname{Re}(\alpha) > n:\quad B(\alpha, n+1) &= \frac{n(n-1)\ldots 1}{\alpha(\alpha+1)\ldots.(\alpha+n-1)} B(\alpha+n,1) \\ &= \frac{n!}{\alpha(\alpha+1)\ldots.(\alpha+n)} = n! \frac{\Gamma(\alpha)}{\Gamma(\alpha+n+1)}, \end{aligned} \tag{9.744a–f}$$

where: (i) the initial value (9.740b) was used in (9.744e); and (ii) the recurrence formula (9.432b) for the gamma function (9.432a, b) was used in (9.744f). Setting (9.745a–c) in (9.744e) leads to (9.745d):

$$m, n \in |N,\ \alpha = m - n \geq 1:\qquad B(m-n, n+1) = \frac{n!\,(m-n-1)!}{m!}. \tag{9.745a–d}$$

Comparing (9.745d) with the permutation (9.746a) expresses the relation (9.746b) with the beta function (9.681c) with integer variables (9.681a–c):

$$\binom{m}{n} \equiv \frac{m!}{n!\,(m-n)!} = \frac{m!}{n!\,(m-n-1)!}\frac{1}{m-n} = \frac{1}{(m-n)\,B(m-n,n+1)}. \tag{9.746a–c}$$

The **generalized permutation** can be defined by (9.746c) for complex (m, n).

The *beta function (9.735c) is (standard CCCLXIV) a generalization of the permutation (9.746a–c) from positive integer (9.745a–d) to complex variables (9.735a, b), and has the following properties: (i) symmetry (9.740a); (ii) initial values (9.740b, c); (iii) simple (9.742a–c) [iterated (9.743a–d)] recurrence relation; and (iv) the symmetric (9.740a) of (9.742a–c) [(9.743a–d)] is (9.747a–c) [(9.748a–d)]:*

$$\operatorname{Re}(\alpha) > 1,\ \operatorname{Re}(\beta) > 0:\qquad B(\alpha,\beta) = \frac{\alpha-1}{\beta} B(\alpha-1,\beta+1), \tag{9.747a–c}$$

$$n \in |N,\ \operatorname{Re}(\alpha) > n,\ \operatorname{Re}(\beta) > 1-n:\ B(\alpha,\beta) = \frac{(\alpha-1)\cdots(\alpha-n)}{\beta(\beta+1)\cdots(\beta+n-1)} B(\alpha-n,\beta+n), \tag{9.748a–d}$$

and performs the analytic continuation of the whole complex $\alpha(\beta)$-planes except for poles at (9.749a, b) [(9.750a, b)] with residues (9.749c, d) [(9.751c, d)]:

$$m \in |N_0: B(\alpha,\beta) = \frac{A_{-1}(\beta)}{\alpha+m} + O(1), A_{-1}(\beta) = \frac{(-)^m}{m!}(\beta-1)\dots(\beta-m) = \frac{(-)^m}{m!}\frac{\Gamma(\beta)}{\Gamma(\beta-m)}, \tag{9.749a–d}$$

$$m \in |N_0: B(\alpha,\beta) = \frac{B_{-1}(\beta)}{\beta+m} + O(1), B_{-1}(\beta) = \frac{(-)^m}{m!}(\alpha-1)\dots(\alpha-m) = \frac{(-)^m}{m!}\frac{\Gamma(\alpha)}{\Gamma(\alpha-m)}. \tag{9.750a–d}$$

The residue (9.749c) is calculated from (9.743a–d) using (9.751a), leading to (9.751b):

$$\begin{aligned} m = n-1: \quad A_{-1}(\beta) &= \lim_{\alpha \to -m} (\alpha+m)\, B(\alpha,\beta) \\ &= \lim_{\alpha \to -m} (\alpha+m) \frac{(\beta-1)(\beta-m-1)}{\alpha(\alpha+1)\dots\dots(\alpha+m)} B(\alpha+m+1, \beta-m-1) \\ &= \frac{(\beta-1)(\beta-2)\dots\dots(\beta-m-1)}{(-m)(-m+1)\dots\dots(-1)} B(1,\beta-m-1) \\ &= \frac{(-)^m}{m!}(\beta-1)(\beta-2)\dots\dots(\beta-m), \end{aligned} \tag{9.751a–e}$$

that simplifies to (9.751c–e) using (9.740b) and coincides with (9.751e) ≡ (9.749d). The residue (9.750d) can be calculated in a similar way to (9.751a–e), or can be obtained from (9.749d) by symmetry (9.740a). The analogies between the properties of the gamma (beta) functions [subsection(s) 9.5.14 (9.8.1–9.8.4)], also known as the Eulerian integrals of the first (1729) [second (1772)] kind, suggests that they are related (subsection 9.8.3).

9.8.3 Relation between the Gamma and Beta Functions

Substituting (9.744b) in (9.744e) leads to *the relation (standard CCCLXV) between the gamma and beta function (9.752a) that holds for all complex values of the variables (9.752a, b) including poles:*

$$\alpha, \beta \in |C: \quad \Gamma(\alpha)\Gamma(\beta) = \Gamma(\alpha+\beta)\, B(\alpha,\beta). \tag{9.752a–c}$$

The relation (9.752c): (i) has been proved (9.744f) for (9.744a–c); (ii) a different proof given next extends it to complex variables satisfying (9.735a, b); (iii) analytic continuation (9.743a–d; 9.748a–d) extends to the whole complex-α and complex-β-planes, except possibly for poles; (iv) it is shown that the

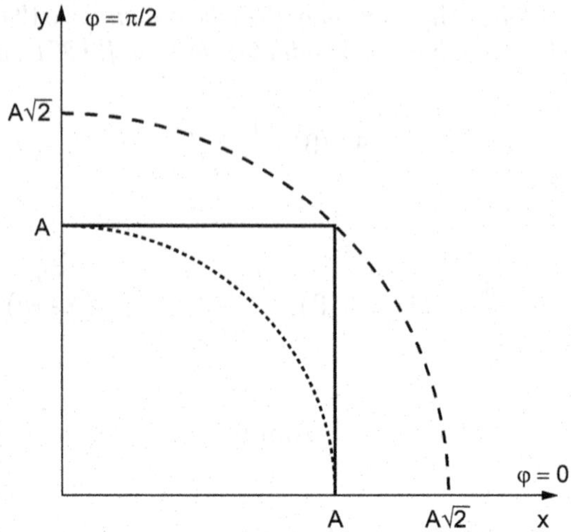

FIGURE 9.14
The proof of the relation between the gamma and beta functions, that is the Eulerian integrals of the first and second kinds, uses a construction similar to the evaluation of the Gaussian integral (Figure III.1.2) namely: (i) for a integrand positive in the first quadrant $x > 0 < y$ the integral over the square of side R has for lower (upper) bound the integral over the inscribed (overscribed) quarter circle of radius $R\left(R\sqrt{2}\right)$; (ii) if the integrand decays asymptotically fast enough as $R \to \infty$, the latter integrals coincide, and evaluate also the former integral over the square.

poles are the same with equal residues on both sides of (9.752c); thus (v) (9.752c) holds in the whole complex plane (9.752a, b) including poles. The proof of (9.752c) is similar to the calculation of the Gaussian integral (subsection III.1.1) with extra factors leading to the gamma and beta functions. Both proofs involve (Figure 9.14) the integral of a positive functions over a square with: (i) the interior (exterior) quarter circle as the lower (upper) bound; and (ii) in the limit of infinite radius the lower and upper bounds coincide, giving a unique value to the integral over the square. The product of the two gamma functions in the r.h.s. of (9.752c) is given (9.431a, b) by (9.754a–c):

$$\mathrm{Re}(\alpha) > 0 < \mathrm{Re}(\beta): \quad \Gamma(\alpha)\Gamma(\beta) = \left(\int_0^\infty u^{\beta-1} e^{-u}\, du\right) \times \left(\int_0^\infty v^{\alpha-1} e^{-v}\, dv\right) = \lim_{A\to\infty} I(A), \tag{9.753a–d}$$

as the limit (9.753d) of the integral (9.754c) ≡ (9.754d) where are made the changes of variable (9.754a, b):

$$u = x^2,\ v \equiv y^2:\ I(A) \equiv \int_0^A du \int_0^A dv\, u^{\beta-1} v^{\alpha-1} e^{-u-v} = 4\int_0^{\sqrt{A}} dx \int_0^{\sqrt{A}} dy\, x^{2\beta-1} y^{2\alpha-1} e^{-x^2-y^2}. \tag{9.754a–d}$$

The integrand in (9.754d) is positive and thus the integral over the square of sides A has for lower (upper) bound (9.755a) the integral over the quarter circle in the first quadrant (9.755b) with radius $A\left(A\sqrt{2}\right)$ equal to the side (diagonal) of the square:

$$J(A) \le I(A) \le J\left(A\sqrt{2}\right): \quad J(A) \equiv \int dx \int\limits_{\substack{x^2+y^2 \le A^2 \\ x>0<y}} dy\, x^{2\alpha-1} y^{2\beta-1} e^{-x^2-y^2}, \qquad \text{(9.755a, b)}$$

as illustrated in Figure 9.14 (≡ Figure III.1.2).

Changing from Cartesian (x, y) to polar (r, ϕ) coordinates (9.756a–d):

$$\{x, y\} = r\{\cos\phi, \sin\phi\}, \qquad x^2 + y^2 = r^2, \qquad dx\, dy = r\, dr\, d\phi, \qquad \text{(9.756a–d)}$$

the integral (9.755b) becomes (9.757):

$$J(A) = 4\int_0^{\pi/2} \cos^{2\beta-1}\phi \sin^{2\alpha-1}\phi\, d\phi \int_0^A r^{2\alpha+2\beta-1} e^{-r^2}\, dr. \qquad \text{(9.757)}$$

The first factor on the r.h.s. of (9.757) is (9.738a–c) the beta function in (9.758c) and in the second factor is made the change of variable (9.758a, b) leading to (9.758d):

$$t \equiv r^2, \quad dr = \frac{dt}{2\sqrt{t}}; \quad J(A) = 2B(\alpha,\beta)\int_0^A r^{2\alpha+2\beta-1} e^{-r^2} dr = B(\alpha,\beta)\int_0^{A^2} t^{\alpha+\beta-1} e^{-t} dt. \qquad \text{(9.758a–d)}$$

Taking in (9.758d) the limit (9.759b) shows that the second factor is (9.431a, b) ≡ (9.759a, b) a gamma function:

$$\begin{aligned} \operatorname{Re}(\alpha+\beta) > 0: \quad B(\alpha,\beta)\Gamma(\alpha,\beta) &= B(\alpha,\beta)\int_0^{\infty} t^{\alpha+\beta-1} e^{-t}\, dt \\ &= B(\alpha,\beta) \lim_{A\to\infty} \int_0^{A^2} t^{\alpha+\beta-1} e^{-t}\, dt = \lim_{A\to\infty} J(A) \\ &= \lim_{A\to\infty} J\left(2\sqrt{A}\right) = \lim_{A\to\infty} I(A) = \Gamma(\alpha)\Gamma(\beta), \end{aligned} \qquad \text{(9.759a–g)}$$

where: (i) from the definition of gamma function (9.431a, b) follows (9.759a, b), that coincides with the limit (9.759c); (ii) using (9.758d) in (9.758c) proves the coincidence of the limits (9.759d) ≡ (9.759e); and (iii) from (9.755a) follows the limit (9.759f) ≡ (9.753d) proving (9.759g). The restrictions (9.753a, b) are shown next to be unnecessary for the validity of (9.752c) although they apply to specific integrals (subsection 9.8.4).

9.8.4 Evaluation of Integrals via Gamma and Beta Functions

The relation (9.752c) between the gamma and beta functions: (i) can be extended from (9.753a, b) by analytic continuation of the gamma (9.434a, b) [beta (9.743a–d; 9.748a–d)] functions to the whole complex-α, β planes, except possibly at the poles; (ii) moreover the poles on the l.h.s. and r.h.s. of (9.752c) are the same at α or β non-positive integers; and (iii) the residues at the poles coincide. For example, the gamma function has a pole for variable a non-positive integer (9.435a, b) with residue (9.435c); using (9.752c) it follows that the beta function also has a pole at the same location, with residue (9.760a, b):

$$\lim_{\alpha\to-m}(\alpha+m)B(\alpha,\beta) = \lim_{\alpha\to-m}(\alpha+m)\frac{\Gamma(\alpha)\Gamma(\beta)}{\Gamma(\alpha+\beta)} = \frac{\Gamma(\beta)}{\Gamma(\beta-m)}\lim_{\alpha\to-m}(\alpha+m)\Gamma(\alpha);$$

$$= \frac{\Gamma(\beta)}{\Gamma(\beta-m)}\Gamma_{-1} = \frac{(-)^m}{m!}\frac{\Gamma(\beta)}{\Gamma(\beta-m)} = A_{-1}(\beta), \tag{9.760a–e}$$

leading (9.760c, d) to (9.760e) ≡ (9.749d) that coincides with the residue of the beta function.

The gamma function (subsection 9.5.14, note III.1.8) can be used to evaluate: (i) directly generalized Gaussian integrals (notes III.1.9–III.1.12); and (ii) through the relation (9.752c) with the beta function integrals of the types (9.738a–e). Using the changes of variable (9.761a–c)

$$\{p,q\} = \{2\alpha-1, 2\beta-1\}, \{-\alpha-\beta, \beta-1\}, \{2\alpha-1, 1-2\alpha-2\beta\}, \tag{9.761a–c}$$

$$\{\alpha,\beta\} = \frac{1}{2}+\frac{1}{2}\{p,q\}, \{-1-p-q, 1+q\}, \frac{1}{2}\{1+p, -p-q\}, \tag{9.762a–c}$$

that are inverted (9.762a–c), leads from (9.738a–e) to:

$$\mathrm{Re}(p) > -1 < \mathrm{Re}(q): \quad 2\int_0^{\pi/2}\sin^p\phi\cos^q\phi\, d\phi = B\left(\frac{1+p}{2}, \frac{1+q}{2}\right)$$

$$= \frac{\Gamma(1/2+p/2)\Gamma(1/2+q/2)}{\Gamma(1+p/2+q/2)}. \tag{9.763a–d}$$

$$\mathrm{Re}(p+q) < -1 < \mathrm{Re}(q): \quad \int_1^\infty s^p(s-1)^q\, ds = B(-1-p-q, 1+q) = \frac{\Gamma(-1-p-q)\Gamma(1+q)}{\Gamma(-p)}, \tag{9.764a–d}$$

$$\mathrm{Re}(p+q)<0, \quad \mathrm{Re}(p)>-1: \quad 2\int_0^\infty \sinh^p \psi \cosh^q \psi \, d\psi$$

$$= B\left(\frac{1+p}{2}, -\frac{p+q}{2}\right) = \frac{\Gamma(1/2+p/2)\Gamma(-p/2-q/2)}{\Gamma(1/2-q/2)}, \tag{9.765a–d}$$

respectively (9.763a–d/(9.764a, d/9.765a–d).

Thus *the gamma (9.431a, b; 9.434a, b) [beta (9.735a–c; 9.745a–d; 9.748a–d)] functions provide (standard CCCLXVI) equivalent (9.752a–c) alternative methods to respectively evaluate the integrals (9.763c/9.764c/9.765c) [(9.763d/9.764d/9.765d)] subject to the conditions (9.763a, b/9.764a, b/9.765a, b).* Some of these integrals will be used to relate the alternative expressions of special functions (Bessel, Neumann, and Hankel functions) that are solutions of singular linear differential equations (the generalized Bessel differential equation) obtained by two methods: (a) analytic/regular/irregular integrals (sections 9.4/9.5/9.6–9.7) leading to power series, possibly with power and logarithmic factors; and (b) the integral transforms (section 9.8) that lead to parametric integral representations.

9.8.5 Kernel and Path of a General Integral Transform

The solution of a linear differential equation with variable coefficients (9.766a):

$$\sum_{n=0}^{N} A_n(x)\, y^{(n)}(x) = B(x): \qquad y(x) = \int_L K(x,s)\, v(s)\, ds, \tag{9.766a, b}$$

may be sought as **a parametric path integral representation** (9.766b) that involves: (i) a linear dependence on the **integral transform** v that depends on the integration variable s; (ii) the product by a **kernel** that depends $K(x,s)$ both on the integration variable s and the independent variable x of the differential equation; and (iii) an integration over a regular path L in the complex s-plane specifies the dependent variable y of the differential equation via the integral (9.766b) where the independent variable x is a parameter. The simplest integral transforms are (1.549a–c) ≡ (9.767b) [(1.569) ≡ (9.767c)] the **Fourier (Laplace) transform**:

$$\sum_{n=0}^{N} A_n\, y^{(n)}(x) = B(x): \; y(x) = \int_{-\infty}^{+\infty} \tilde{v}(s)\, e^{ixs}\, ds, \;\; y(x) = \int_0^\infty \bar{v}(s)\, e^{-sx}\, dx, \tag{9.767a–c}$$

that are solution [notes 1.11–1.14 (1.15–1.28)] of a linear differential equation with constant coefficients (9.767a): (i) because the kernel in (9.766b) is an imaginary (real) exponential in (9.768a) [(9.768b)] and the exponential is (chapter I) a solution of an unforced linear differential equation with constant coefficients:

$$K(x,s) = e^{ixs}, \quad e^{-xs}; \qquad L \equiv (-\infty,+\infty), (0,+\infty), \tag{9.768a–d}$$

(ii) the path of integration is the whole (positive half) real axis (9.768c) [(9.768d)]; and (iii) in the complex s-plane the change of kernel (9.768a, b) corresponds $s \to -is$ to a rotation $-i = \exp(-i\pi/2)$ of 90 degrees in the positive or counterclockwise direction.

A linear differential equation whose variable coefficients (9.766a) are linear functions of the independent variable (9.769a):

$$\sum_{n=0}^{\infty} (p_n + q_n x)\, y^{(n)}(x) = 0: \qquad y(x) = \int_L e^{xs}\, v(s)\, ds, \tag{9.769a, b}$$

has solution (subsection 9.8.6) as a **generalized Laplace transform** (9.769b) with integration along a path L in the complex s-plane instead of the positive real axis for the original Laplace transform (9.768d). The change of sign in the kernel from (9.768b) to (9.769b) is of no consequence in the complex s-plane because it just reverses the coordinate axis $s \to -s$. In the case of linear coefficients (9.769a) the integral transform $v(s)$ satisfies a linear unforced first-order differential equation (subsection 9.8.6) that can always be solved; this no longer applies if the coefficients in (9.769a) were polynomials of degree M, in which case the integral transform would satisfy a linear unforced differential equation of order M. In the case of a linear differential equation with variable coefficients (9.766a) whose coefficients are not of the form (9.769a) an **general integral transform (Bateman 1909)** may be needed (9.766b) with a non-exponential kernel, for example:

$$K(x,s) = K(xs): \quad K(x,s) \equiv x^s, (1 - xs)^a, J_n(xs), P_n^m(xs), F(a,b;c;xs), \tag{9.770a–f}$$

the: (i/ii) **Mellin** (1896) **[Euler** (1778)**] transforms** using powers (9.770b) [(9.770c)]; (iii/iv) the **Hankel** (1869) **[Kontorovich-Lebedev** (1938)**] transforms** using Bessel (9.770d) [associated Legendre (9.770e)] functions [subsection 9.5.21 (note 9.21)]; and (v) the **Fox transform** (9.770f) using Gaussian hypergeometric function (note 9.14). All of the preceding integral transforms (9.767b, c; 9.769b; 9.770c, d, e, f) except the Mellin transform (9.770b) have **product kernels** that depend only (9.770a) on the product of the variables. The generalized Laplace transform (9.769b) will be applied (subsection 9.8.6) to the solution of the generalized (original) Bessel differential equation [subsections 9.8.7–9.8.9 (9.8.10–9.8.11)]; a general integral transform (9.766b) with kernel distinct from (9.768a, b; 9.770b–f) will be used (subsection 9.8.12) to obtain alternative integral representations for the Bessel, Neumann, and Hankel functions (subsections 9.8.13–9.8.16).

9.8.6 Generalized Laplace Transform in the Complex Plane

Substituting the generalized Laplace transform (9.769b) in a linear unforced differential equation (9.769a) whose coefficients are linear functions of the independent variable leads to (9.771c):

$$\{P(s),Q(s)\}=\sum_{n=0}^{N}s^n\{p_n,q_n\}:\quad 0=\int_L v(s)e^{xs}\left\{\sum_{n=0}^{N}s^n(p_n+q_n x)\right\}ds$$
$$=\int_L v(s)e^{xs}\left[P(s)+xQ(s)\right]ds, \qquad (9.771\text{a–d})$$

where appear (9.771d) **two characteristic polynomials** (9.771a, b) whose degree N equals at most the order N of the differential equation (9.769a). The second term in (9.771d) may be integrated by parts (9.772a):

$$\int_L v(s)e^{xs}Q(s)x\,ds=\int_L v(s)Q(s)d\left(e^{xs}\right)=\left[v(s)\,Q(s)\,e^{xs}\right]_{\partial L}-\int_L e^{xs}d\left[v(s)Q(s)\right], \qquad (9.772\text{a, b})$$

and substitution of (9.772b) back in (9.771d) leads to (9.773a):

$$\left[v(s)Q(s)e^{xs}\right]_{\partial L}=\int_L e^{xs}\left\{\frac{d}{ds}\left[v(s)Q(s)\right]-P(s)v(s)\right\}ds=0. \qquad (9.773\text{a, b})$$

The r.h.s. (l.h.s.) of (9.773a) is an integral over a path (a difference at the end points of the path) and it can be satisfied by the vanishing of both (9.773b). Thus *a linear unforced differential equation of order N whose coefficients are linear functions of the independent variable (9.769a) has (standard CCCLXVII) the generalized Laplace transform (9.769b) as solution where: (i) the transform satisfies the differential equation (9.774a):*

$$P(s)\,v(s)=\frac{d}{ds}\left[v(s)\,Q(s)\right];\qquad \left[v(s)Q(s)e^{xs}\right]_{\partial L}=0, \qquad (9.774\text{a, b})$$

and (ii) the path of integration L is such that the function in square brackets in (9.774b) takes the same value at the two ends ∂L, for example vanishes at both ends.

To complete the method it is necessary to solve the differential equation (9.774a) ≡ (9.775a) for the transform:

$$\frac{dv}{ds}=\frac{P(s)-Q'(s)}{Q(s)}v(s),\qquad \frac{dv}{v}=\left[\frac{P(s)}{Q(s)}-\frac{Q'(s)}{Q(s)}\right]ds, \qquad (9.775\text{a, b})$$

that is separable (9.775b) and can be integrated (9.776a) leading to (9.776b) where the constant of integration (9.776c):

$$\log[v(s)] = \log C - \log[Q(s)] + \int^s \frac{P(\zeta)}{Q(\zeta)}\, d\zeta, \qquad C = 1, \tag{9.776a–c}$$

is omitted in (9.777a–c):

$$X(s) = \exp\left\{\int^s \frac{P(\zeta)}{Q(\zeta)} d\zeta\right\}: \qquad v(s) = \frac{X(s)}{Q(s)}, \qquad \left[X(s)e^{sx}\right]_{\partial L} = 0. \tag{9.777a–c}$$

The exponential in (9.777a) ≡ (9.778a) involves the integral of a rational function (9.778c) that is the ratio (9.771a, b) ≡ (9.778d) of two polynomials of degrees (9.778b) that may be less than N if some coefficients p_n or q_n vanish (9.778e):

$$X(s) = \exp\left\{\int^s R(\zeta) d\zeta\right\}; \quad \alpha \le N \ge \beta: \quad R(\zeta) = \frac{P(\zeta)}{Q(\zeta)} = \frac{\sum_{n=0}^{N} p_n \zeta^n}{\sum_{n=0}^{N} q_n \zeta^n} = \frac{P_\alpha(\zeta)}{Q_\beta(\zeta)}. \tag{9.778a–e}$$

The integral of a rational function (sections I.31.8–I.31.9) can have three types of terms: (i) a simple zero of the denominator (9.779a, b) is a simple pole of the rational function (9.779c) and leads to the integral (9.779d) with a power type branch-point (9.253a–e); (ii) a zero (9.780b) of multiplicity (9.780a) of the denominator leads to a pole of order k of the rational function with term (9.780c) whose integral is (9.780d):

$$Q(a) = 0 \ne Q'(a): \qquad R_1(\zeta) = \frac{\sigma}{\zeta - a}, \quad X_1(s) = \exp[\sigma \log(s-a)] = (s-a)^\sigma, \tag{9.779a–d}$$

$$k = 2, \cdots; \quad Q(b) = Q'(b) = \cdots = Q^{(k-1)}(b) = 0 \ne Q^{(k)}(b):$$

$$R_2(\zeta) = \sum_{m=1}^{k} \frac{\sigma_m}{(\zeta - b)^m}, \quad X_2(s) = (s-b)^{\sigma_1} \exp\left\{-\sum_{m=2}^{k} \frac{\sigma_m (s-b)^{1-m}}{m-1}\right\}; \tag{9.780a–d}$$

$$\alpha - \beta = \gamma = 1, 2, \cdots: \quad R_3(\zeta) = \sum_{j=0}^{\gamma} f_j \zeta^j, \quad X_3(s) = \exp\left(\sum_{j=0}^{\gamma} f_j \frac{s^{j+1}}{j+1}\right); \tag{9.781a–c}$$

and (iii) if the polynomial in the numerator (9.771a) is of higher degree (9.781a) than the polynomial in the denominator (9.771b) the rational function (9.778d) involves powers (9.781b) leading to the integral (9.781c). The integral transform (9.777b) is typically (9.782a) a product of terms (9.782b) of the form (9.779d; 9.780d; 9.781c):

$$v(s) = \frac{X_1(s)+X_2(s)+X_3(s)}{Q(s)} = \frac{(s-a)^{\sigma}(s-b)^{\sigma_1}}{Q(s)} \exp\left\{-\sum_{m=2}^{k} \frac{\sigma_m}{m-1}(s-b)^{1-m} + \sum_{m=2}^{k} f_j \frac{s^{j+1}}{j+1}\right\}. \tag{9.782a, b}$$

Thus *the linear differential equation (9.766a) of order N, whose coefficients are linear functions of the independent variable (9.769a), with two characteristic polynomials (9.771a, b) has solution (standard CCCLXVIII) as a generalized Laplace parametric integral (9.769b) with: (i) integral transform (9.777a, b); and (ii) path of integration L such that the function in square brackets in (9.777c) takes the same value at the two ends. The factor (9.777a) is the exponential of the integral (9.778a) of the rational function (9.778b) that is the ratio (9.778c–e) of the two characteristic polynomials. It has terms typically of the forms (9.782a, b).* This will be shown next in the cases of the generalized (original) Bessel differential equation [subsections 9.8.7 (9.8.11)]; the coefficients are quadratic rather than linear functions, requiring a depression of their degree.

9.8.7 Depression of the Degree of the Coefficients of a Differential Equation

If a linear differential equation (9.702a) of order N has coefficients (9.718a) that are polynomials of order M:

$$0 = \sum_{n=0}^{N} y^{(n)}(x)\left\{\sum_{m=0}^{M} a_{n,m}\, x^m\right\}: \qquad \sum_{m=0}^{N} B_m(s)\, v^{(m)}(s) = 0, \tag{9.783a, b}$$

then (standard CCCLXIX) the generalized Laplace transform (9.770b) satisfies a differential equation (9.783b) of order M, because *M* integration by parts like (9.772a, b) are needed. If the differential equation for the transform (9.783b) is less simple than the original differential equation (9.783a) the method loses interest, unless the degree of the polynomial can be depressed, as shown next. The generalized Bessel differential equation (9.428a–f) has cubic coefficients, and the presence of squares of the independent variable suggests the change of variable (9.784a–c):

$$\eta \equiv x^2, \qquad y(x) = \Phi(\eta): \qquad \frac{d}{dx} = \frac{d\eta}{dx}\frac{d}{d\eta} = 2x\frac{d}{d\eta} = 2\sqrt{\eta}\,\frac{d}{d\eta}, \tag{9.784a–c}$$

leading to (9.785a):

$$0=\left\{4\eta\sqrt{\eta}\frac{d}{d\eta}\sqrt{\eta}\frac{d}{d\eta}+\sqrt{\eta}\left(1-\frac{\mu\eta}{2}\right)2\sqrt{\eta}\frac{d}{d\eta}+\eta-v^2\right\}\Phi$$
$$=4\eta^2\Phi''+\eta(4-\mu\eta)\Phi'+(\eta-\nu^2)\Phi, \qquad (9.785a, b)$$

that has quadratic coefficients (9.785b) ≡ (9.785a) instead of cubic in (9.428f).

A further change of variable, this time the dependent variable (9.786a), with arbitrary constant a leads (9.516a–c) to (9.786b, c):

$$\Phi(\eta)=\eta^a\Psi''(\eta):$$
$$0=4\left[\eta^2\Psi''+2a\eta\Psi'+a(a-1)\Psi\right]+(4-\mu\eta)(\eta\Psi'+a\Psi)+(\eta-\nu^2)\Psi$$
$$=4\eta^2\Psi''+\eta(4+8a-\mu\eta)\Psi'+\left[\eta(1-\mu a)+4a^2-\nu^2\right]\Psi. \qquad (9.786a\text{–}c)$$

The choice (9.787a) for the arbitrary constant a cancels the last coefficient in square brackets in (9.786c), that can be divided through by η, depressing the degree of the coefficients from two in (9.786c) to one in (9.787b):

$$a=\pm\frac{\nu}{2}: \qquad \eta\Psi''_\pm+\left(1\pm\nu-\frac{\mu\eta}{4}\right)\Psi'_\pm+\frac{2\mp\mu\nu}{8}\Psi_\pm=0. \qquad (9.787a, b)$$

Thus *the coefficients of the generalized Bessel differential equation (9.428a–f) can be depressed (standard CCCLXX) from cubic to quadratic (9.786c) [linear (9.787b)] via successive changes of independent (9.784a, b) ≡ (9.788a) [dependent (9.786a; 9.787a) ≡ (9.788b)] leading to (9.788c):*

$$y_\pm(x)=\Phi_\pm(x^2)=x^{2a}\Psi_\pm(x^2)=x^{\pm\nu}\Psi_\pm(x^2). \qquad (9.788a\text{–}c)$$

The linear differential equation (9.787b) with variable coefficients linear functions of the independent variable can be solved (subsection 9.8.8) using (9.769b) the generalized Laplace transform (subsection 9.8.6).

9.8.8 Application to the Generalized Bessel Differential Equation

The linear second-order differential equation (9.787b) has coefficients that are linear functions of the independent variable (9.769a) leading (9.771a, b) to the characteristic polynomial (9.789a) [(9.789b)] of degree 2(1):

$$Q(s)=s^2-\frac{\mu s}{4}, \quad P(s)=(1\pm\nu)s+\frac{1}{4}\mp\frac{\mu\nu}{8}, \quad R(s)=\frac{(1\pm\nu)s+1/4\mp\mu\nu/8}{s(s-\mu/4)}, \qquad (9.789a\text{–}c)$$

implying that the rational function (9.778c) has (9.789c); (i) no power terms like (9.781a–c); (ii) no multiple poles like (9.780a–d); and (iii) only two simple poles (9.790a) with residues (9.790b, c):

$$Q(s)=\frac{A_{-1}}{s}+\frac{B_{-1}}{s-\mu/4}:\quad A_{-1}=\lim_{s\to 0} s\,R(s)=\pm\frac{\nu}{2}-\frac{1}{\mu},$$

$$B_{-1}=\lim_{s\to\mu/4}\left(s-\frac{\mu}{4}\right)R(s)=1\pm\frac{\nu}{2}+\frac{1}{\mu}. \tag{9.790a–c}$$

Substitution of (9.790b, c) in (9.790a) leads to (9.791a) that is similar to (9.779c, d) for simple poles (9.779a, b) and leads (9.778a) to (9.791b) thus:

$$R(s)=\frac{\pm\nu/2-1/\mu}{s}+\frac{1\pm\nu/2+1/\mu}{s-\mu/4};\quad X(s)=s^{\pm\nu/2-1/\mu}\left(s-\mu/4\right)^{1\pm\nu/2+1/\mu}. \tag{9.791a, b}$$

From (9.791a, b) follows (9.789a; 9.777b) the integral transform (9.792):

$$v(s)=s^{-1\pm\nu/2-1/\mu}\left(s-\mu/4\right)^{\pm\nu/2+1/\mu}; \tag{9.792}$$

the integral of the generalized Bessel differential equation (9.428a–f) is specified by (9.788c) ≡ (9.793a):

$$y_\pm(x)=x^{\pm\nu}\,\Psi\left(x^2\right)=x^{\pm\nu}\int_L v(s)\,e^{x^2 s}\,ds$$

$$=x^{\pm\nu}\int_L e^{x^2 s}\,s^{-1\pm\nu/2-1/\mu}\left(s-\mu/4\right)^{\pm\nu/2+1/\mu}ds, \tag{9.793a–c}$$

using the generalized Laplace transform (9.769b) ≡ (9.793b) of the variable (9.784a) and the function (9.792) in (9.793b, c).

The path of integration L in (9.793a–c) must be such that the function in square brackets in (9.774b) ≡ (9.794a) takes the same value at the two ends (9.794b, c):

$$0=\left[e^{\eta s}\,v(s)Q(s)\right]_{\partial L}=\left[e^{x^2 s}\,X(s)\right]_{\partial L}=\left[e^{x^2 s}\,s^{\pm\nu/2-1/\mu}\left(s-\mu/4\right)^{1\pm\nu/2+1/\mu}\right]_{\partial L}, \tag{9.794a–c}$$

for example, vanishes at the two ends. The integrand in (9.793c) and the function in square brackets in (9.794c) are single-valued in the complex s-plane with (Figure 9.15) a branch-cut joining the branch-points at $s=0$ and $s=\mu/4$.

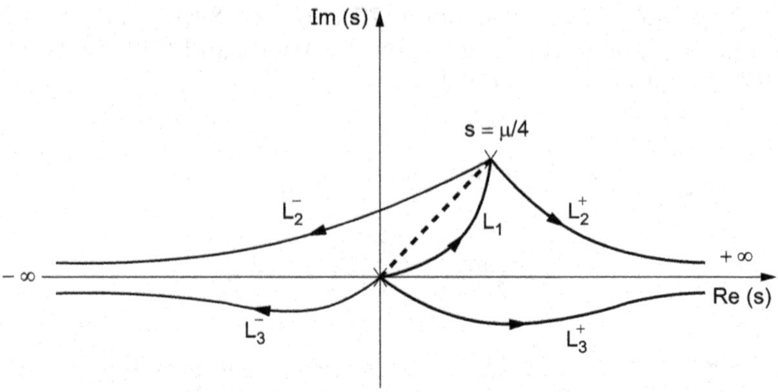

FIGURE 9.15
The solution of the generalized Bessel differential equation using the generalized Laplace transform involves the same integrand along paths in the complex s-plane joining the points $s = 0, \mu/4, \infty$, and not crossing the branch-cut $(0, \mu/4)$. Since the differential equation is of the second-order only two paths lead to linearly independent particular integrals of the generalized Bessel differential equation.

The function in square brackets in (9.794c) vanishes: (i/ii) at the branch-point (9.795b) [(9.796b)] if the condition (9.795a) [(9.796a)] is met:

$$\operatorname{Re}\left(\pm\frac{v}{2}-\frac{1}{\mu}\right)>0: \lim_{s\to 0} e^{x^2 s}\, X(s)=0; \quad \operatorname{Re}\left(x^2\right)>0: \lim_{s\to -\infty} e^{x^2 s}\, X(s)=0, \qquad (9.795\text{a–d})$$

$$\operatorname{Re}\left(\pm\frac{v}{2}+\frac{1}{\mu}\right)>-1: \lim_{s\to \mu/4} e^{x^2 s}\, X(s)=0; \quad \operatorname{Re}\left(x^2\right)<0: \lim_{s\to +\infty} e^{x^2 s}\, X(s)=0, \qquad (9.796\text{a–d})$$

and (iii/iv) at infinity along the negative (9.795d) [positive (9.796d)] real axis if the condition (9.795c) [(9.796c)] is met. From (9.795a–d; 9.796a–d) follow five paths of integration: (i) one (9.797a) valid for all x; (ii/iii) depending on the value of x one more (9.797b, d); (iv/v) the remaining two are unions of the preceding (9.797c, e):

$$L_1 \equiv \left(0, \frac{\mu}{4}\right); \quad \operatorname{Re}\left(x^2\right) >< 0: \quad L_2^{\pm} \equiv \left(\frac{\mu}{4}, \pm\infty\right), \quad L_3^{\pm} \equiv \left(0, \pm\infty\right) = L_1 + L_2^{\pm}. \qquad (9.797\text{a–e})$$

Since the generalized Bessel differential equation (9.428a–f) is of the second-order there can be only two linearly independent particular integrals, for example (9.797a, b) or (9.797a, d) as summarized next (subsection 9.8.9).

9.8.9 Integral Representation for the Generalized Bessel Function

Thus *the generalized Bessel differential equation (9.428a–f) has (standard CCCLXXI) solutions as parametric integrals (9.793c), that are linearly independent*

(Figure 9.15) for the path (9.797a) and for one of the paths (9.797b, c) [(9.797d, e)] if $\operatorname{Re}(x^2) > (<) 0$. The regular integral solutions (subsection 9.5.15) and parametric integrals (subsection 9.8.8) may be related as shown next. As a first example is considered the first path (9.797a) in (9.293c) ≡ (9.798a):

$$y_\pm(x) = x^{\pm\nu} \int_0^{\mu/4} e^{x^2 s} s^{-1\pm\nu/2-1/\mu} (s - \mu/4)^{\pm\nu/2+1/\mu} ds, \tag{9.798a}$$

valid for (9.795a) ≡ (9.798b) and (9.796a) ≡ (9.798c):

$$\operatorname{Re}(\pm\nu) > 2\operatorname{Re}\left(\frac{1}{\mu}\right), -2 - 2\operatorname{Re}\left(\frac{1}{\mu}\right): \quad J^\mu_{\pm\nu}(x) = C(\mu, \pm\nu)\, y_\pm(x). \tag{9.798b–d}$$

The functions (9.798a) must be linear combinations of generalized Bessel functions (9.448) of orders $\pm\nu$, suggesting that they are constant multiples (9.798d) where the coefficient may depend on the order ν and degree μ but not on the variable x. The integral representation for the generalized Bessel function (9.798a, d) will be proved, and the coefficient determined, by expanding the integral (9.798a, d) ≡ (9.799a):

$$J^\mu_\nu(x) = C(\mu, \nu)\, x^\nu \int_0^{\mu/4} e^{x^2 s} s^{-1+\nu/2-1/\mu} (s - \mu/4)^{\nu/2+1/\mu} ds, \tag{9.799a}$$

in power series, after the change of variable (9.799b):

$$s = \frac{\mu t}{4}: \quad J^\mu_\nu(x) = C(\mu, \nu)\left(\frac{\mu x}{4}\right)^\nu \int_0^1 e^{\mu t x^2/4} t^{-1+\nu/2-1/\mu} (t-1)^{\nu/2+1/\mu} dt, \tag{9.799b, c}$$

that uses the unit interval for integration (9.799c).

Using the power series (9.7b) for the exponential in (9.799c) leads to (9.800a):

$$J^\mu_\nu(x) = C(\mu, \nu)\left(\frac{\mu x}{4}\right)^\nu \sum_{k=0}^\infty \frac{(\mu x^2/4)^k}{k!} (-)^{\nu/2+1/\mu} \int_0^1 t^{k-1+\nu/2-1/\mu} (1-t)^{\nu/2+1/\mu} dt, \tag{9.800a}$$

where the integral may be evaluated (9.800d) in terms of the beta function (9.735a–c) for (9.800b, c):

$$\operatorname{Re}(\nu/2 - 1/\mu) > -k, \quad \operatorname{Re}(\nu/2 + 1/\mu) > -1:$$

$$J^\mu_\nu(x) = C(\mu, \nu)\left(\frac{\mu x}{4}\right)^\nu \sum_{k=0}^\infty \frac{(\mu x^2/4)^k}{k!} e^{i\pi\nu/2 + i\pi/\mu} B(k + \nu/2 - 1/\mu, 1 + \nu/2 + 1/\mu). \tag{9.800b–d}$$

Using the relation (9.752a–c) between the beta and gamma functions in (9.735d) leads to (9.801):

$$J_\nu^\mu(x) = C(\mu,\nu)\left(\frac{\mu x}{4}\right)^\nu e^{i\pi\nu/2+i\pi/\mu}\Gamma(1+\nu/2+1/\mu)\sum_{k=0}^{\infty}\frac{\left(\mu x^2/4\right)^k}{k!}\frac{\Gamma(k+\nu/2-1/\mu)}{\Gamma(1+k+\nu)}. \tag{9.801}$$

The series (9.801) coincides with (9.450a, b) for the generalized Bessel function choosing the coefficient to satisfy (9.802):

$$1 = \Gamma\left(\frac{\nu}{2}-\frac{1}{\mu}\right)C(\mu,\nu)\left(\frac{\mu}{2}\right)^\nu e^{i\pi\nu/2+i\pi/\mu}\,\Gamma\left(1+\frac{\nu}{2}+\frac{1}{\mu}\right). \tag{9.802}$$

Substituting (9.802) that is valid for (9.798b, c) ≡ (9.803a, b) in (9.799a) leads to (9.803c):

$$\operatorname{Re}(\nu) > 2\operatorname{Re}\left(\frac{1}{\mu}\right), -2-\operatorname{Re}\left(\frac{1}{\mu}\right):\quad J_\nu^\mu(x) = \frac{(x/2)^\nu}{\Gamma(\nu/2-1/\mu)\Gamma(1+\nu/2+1/\mu)}$$
$$\int_0^{\mu/4} e^{x^2 s}\, s^{-1+\nu/2-1/\mu}\,(\mu/4-s)^{\nu/2+1/\mu}\,ds, \tag{9.803a–c}$$

that is *the representation (standard CCCLXXII) of the generalized Bessel function as a parametric integral (9.803c) valid for order* ν *and degree* μ *satisfying (9.803a, b)*. The conditions (9.803a, b) are not met for zero degree $\mu = 0$, and thus the integral representation (9.803c) for the generalized Bessel functions does not include the original Bessel functions (subsection 9.8.11) that require separate treatment (subsection 9.8.10).

9.8.10 Application to the Original Bessel Differential Equation

In the case (9.804a) ≡ (9.430a) of the original Bessel differential equation (9.430b) ≡ (9.804c) the coefficients are quartic instead of cubic in (9.428a–f), and thus: (i) the change (9.784a–c) of independent variable is not necessary; and (ii) only the change of dependent variable (9.786a) ≡ (9.804b) is used:

$$\mu = 0;\qquad y(x) = x^a z(x):\qquad x^2 y'' + xy' + \left(x^2-\nu^2\right)y = 0, \tag{9.804a–c}$$

leading (9.516a–c) on substitution in (9.804c) to (9.805a):

$$\begin{aligned} 0 &= x^2 z'' + 2axz' + a(a-1)z + xz' + az + \left(x^2-\nu^2\right)z \\ &= x^2 z'' + x(1+2a)\,z' + \left(x^2+a^2-\nu^2\right)z. \end{aligned} \tag{9.805a, b}$$

Choosing (9.806a) that implies (9.804b) that (9.806b) leads in (9.805b) to a linear second-order differential equation (9.806c) whose coefficients are linear functions instead of quadratic in (9.804c):

$$a = \pm\nu; \qquad y_\pm(x) = x^{\pm\nu} z_\pm(x): \qquad x z''_\pm + (1 \pm 2\nu) z'_\pm + x z_\pm = 0. \tag{9.806a–c}$$

The linear differential equation (9.806c) has coefficients that are linear functions of the independent variable (9.769a) leading (9.771a, b) to the characteristic polynomials (9.807a) [(9.807b)] of degree 1(2) and (9.777a, b) to the integral transform (9.807c–e):

$$P_\pm(s) = (1 \pm 2\nu)s, \qquad Q(s) = 1 + s^2:$$

$$v_\pm(s) = \frac{1}{1+s^2} \exp\left[(1 \pm 2\nu)\int^s \frac{\zeta\, d\zeta}{1+\zeta^2}\right] \tag{9.807a–e}$$

$$= \frac{1}{1+s^2} \exp\left[\frac{1 \pm 2\nu}{2} \log(1+s^2)\right] = (1+s)^{\pm\nu-1/2}.$$

Substituting (9.807e) in the generalized Laplace transform (9.769b) for $z_\pm(x)$ in (9.806b) leads to (9.808a, b):

$$x^{\mp\nu} y_\pm(x) = z_\pm(x) = \int_{L_\pm} (1+s^2)^{\pm\nu-1/2} ds; \quad J_{\pm\nu}(x) = C(\pm\nu) y_\pm(x), \tag{9.808a–c}$$

the original Bessel differential equation (9.804c) has solutions $J_{\pm\nu}(x)$, suggesting that they are constant multiples of (9.806b) and implying (9.808c); using the change of variable (9.808d) leads to (9.808e, f):

$$s = it: \qquad J_\nu(x) = x^\nu C(\nu) \int_L (1+s^2)^{\nu-1/2} ds = iC(\nu)\, x^\nu \int_{-iL} (1-t^2)^{\nu-1/2} dt. \tag{9.808d–f}$$

The path of integration must satisfy (9.774b) ≡ (9.809a) leading by (9.807b, e) to (9.809b):

$$0 = \left[e^{sx} v(s) Q(s)\right]_{\partial L} = \left[e^{sx}(1+s^2)^{\nu+1/2}\right]_{\partial L} = \left[e^{ixt}(1-t^2)^{\nu+1/2}\right]_{-i\partial L}, \tag{9.809a–c}$$

and to (9.809c) using (9.808d). The integral representation (9.808f) for the Bessel function is valid for a suitable choice of path of integration (subsection 9.8.11) satisfying (9.809c).

9.8.11 Integral Representation for the Bessel Function

The function in square brackets in (9.809c) vanishes at the points (9.810b) if the condition (9.810a) is met:

$$\mathrm{Re}(\nu) > -\frac{1}{2}: \quad \lim_{t\to\pm1}\left(1-t^2\right)^{\nu+1/2} = 0; \quad J_\nu(x) = i x^\nu C(\nu)\int_{-1}^{+1}\left(1-t^2\right)^{\nu-1/2} e^{ixt}\,dt, \tag{9.810a–c}$$

the integrand in (9.810c) has branch-points at $t = \pm1$ and is single valued in the complex t-plane with (section I.7.8) two semi-infinite branch-cuts (Figure 9.16) joining $t = \pm1$ to $t = \pm\infty$. The integration may be performed between the branch-points in (9.810c) since the primitive converges (9.810b) at the branch-points if (9.810a) is met. Splitting the path of integration (9.811a) the Bessel function can be expressed as a parametric integral (9.811b) over the unit interval:

$$\frac{x^{-\nu}}{iC(\nu)}J_\nu(x) = \left(\int_0^1 + \int_{-1}^0\right)\left(1-t^2\right)^{\nu-1/2} e^{ixt}\,dt = \int_0^1\left(1-t^2\right)^{\nu-1/2}\left(e^{ixt}+e^{-ixt}\right)dt, \tag{9.811a, b}$$

that is equivalent to (9.811c):

$$J_\nu(x) = 2ix^\nu\, C(\nu)\int_0^1\left(1-t^2\right)^{\nu-1/2}\cos(xt)\,dt, \tag{9.811c}$$

using the circular cosine (II.5.3a).

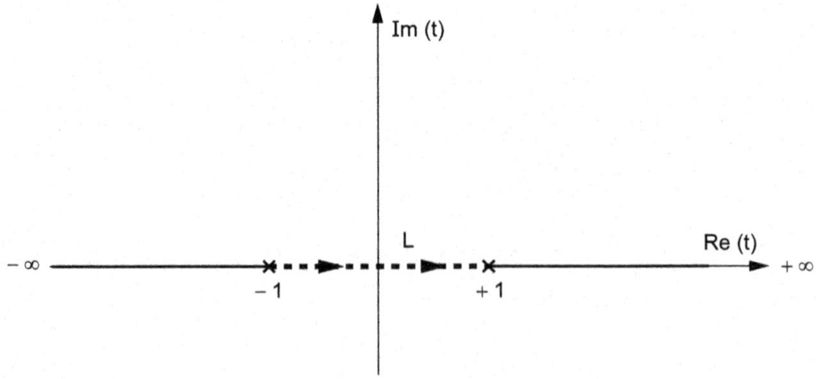

FIGURE 9.16
The solution of the original Bessel differential equation using the generalized Laplace transform involves the same integrand along paths in the complex s-plane with two semi-infinite branch-cuts joining the points $s = \pm1$ to the point at infinity. A possible path of integration joins the branch-points with an integrability restriction on the exponents at each of them.

The proof of (9.811c) and the determination of the coefficient $C(\nu)$ is made expanding the integral in power series and comparing with the power series (9.510a) for the Bessel function. The starting point is the substitution in (9.811c) of the power series (II.7.12a, b) ≡ (9.236a) for the circular cosine leading to (9.812):

$$y_+(x) = 2ix^\nu C(\nu)\sum_{k=0}^{\infty}\frac{(-)^k x^{2k}}{(2k)!}\int_0^1\left(1-t^2\right)^{\nu-1/2} t^{2k}\,dt. \tag{9.812}$$

The change of variable (9.813a) transforms the integral in (9.812) to (9.813b):

$$t^2 \equiv \xi: \qquad \int_0^1\left(1-t^2\right)^{\nu-1/2} t^{2k}\,dt = \frac{1}{2}\int_0^1 (1-\xi)^{\nu-1/2}\,\xi^{k-1/2}\,d\xi$$
$$= \frac{1}{2}B\left(\nu+\frac{1}{2}, k+\frac{1}{2}\right) = \frac{\Gamma(\nu+1/2)\Gamma(k+1/2)}{2\,\Gamma(1+k+\nu)}, \tag{9.813a–d}$$

that can be evaluated using the beta (9.735a–c) [gamma (9.752a–c)] function in (9.813c) [(9.813d)]. When substituting (9.813d) in (9.812) is used (9.814a–d):

$$\frac{\Gamma(k+1/2)}{(2k)!} = \frac{(k-1/2)(k-3/2)\ldots(1/2)\Gamma(1/2)}{(2k)!}$$
$$= \frac{(2k-1)(2k-3)\ldots.1\sqrt{\pi}}{(2k)!2^k} = \frac{2^{-k}\sqrt{\pi}}{(2k)!!} = \frac{2^{-2k}\sqrt{\pi}}{k!}, \tag{9.814a–d}$$

leading to (9.815a):

$$y_+(x) = i\sqrt{\pi}\,C(\nu)x^\nu\,\Gamma(\nu+1/2)\sum_{k=0}^{\infty}\frac{\left(-x^2/4\right)^k}{k!\Gamma(1+\nu+k)} = J_\nu(x); \tag{9.815a, b}$$

the coincidence of (9.815a) with the Bessel function (9.510a) requires that $C(\nu)$ satisfies (9.815c):

$$2^{-\nu} = i\sqrt{\pi}\,C(\nu)\Gamma(\nu+1/2). \tag{9.815c}$$

Substituting (9.815c) in (9.811c) leads to (9.816b) valid for (9.810a) ≡ (9.816a):

$$\mathrm{Re}(\nu) > -\frac{1}{2}: \qquad J_\nu(x) = \frac{2}{\sqrt{\pi}}\frac{(x/2)^\nu}{\Gamma(1/2+\nu)}\int_0^1\left(1-t^2\right)^{\nu-1/2}\cos(xt)\,dt; \tag{9.816a, b}$$

$$t=\cos\phi:\quad J_\nu(x)=\frac{1}{\sqrt{\pi}}\frac{(x/2)^\nu}{\Gamma(1/2+\nu)}\int_0^\pi \sin^{2\nu}\phi\cos(x\cos\phi)\,d\phi, \tag{9.817a, b}$$

$$t=\sin\phi:\quad J_\nu(x)=\frac{2}{\sqrt{\pi}}\frac{(x/2)^\nu}{\Gamma(1/2+\nu)}\int_0^{\pi/2} \cos^{2\nu}\phi\cos(x\sin\phi)\,d\phi, \tag{9.817c, d}$$

the change of variable (9.817a) [(9.817c)] leads from (9.816b) to (9.817b) [(9.817d)]. Thus the *Bessel function of order (9.816a) has (standard CCCLXXIII) the equivalent parametric integral representations (9.816b) ≡ (9.817b) ≡ (9.817b).* Alternative integral representations for the Bessel (also Neumann and Hankel) functions [subsections 9.8.10–9.8.11 (9.8.14–9.8.16)] can be obtained using the generalized Laplace (Bateman) transform [subsection(s) 9.8.6 (9.8.12–9.8.13)].

9.8.12 Partial Differential Equation for the Bateman (1909) Kernel

The linear differential equation (9.818b) with operator (9.818a) has solution as a general integral transform (9.766b) ≡ (9.818c):

$$0=\left\{L\left(\frac{d}{dx}\right)\right\}y(x)\equiv\sum_{n=0}^{N}A_n(x)\frac{d^ny}{dx^n}:\qquad y(x)=\int_L v(s)K(x,s)\,ds, \tag{9.818a–c}$$

where the kernel satisfies the partial differential equation (9.819b) involving another linear differential operator (9.819c):

$$\sum_{n=0}^{N}A_n(x)\frac{d^nK}{dx^n}\equiv\left\{L\left(\frac{d}{dx}\right)\right\}K(x,s)=\left\{M\left(\frac{d}{ds}\right)\right\}K(x,s)=\sum_{m=1}^{M}B_m(s)\frac{\partial^mK}{\partial s^m}. \tag{9.819a–c}$$

Substituting (9.818c) in (9.818a) leads to (9.820a) where may be substituted (9.819b) yielding (9.820b):

$$0=\int_L v(s)\left\{L\left(\frac{d}{dx}\right)\right\}K(x,s)ds=\int_L v(s)\left\{M\left(\frac{d}{ds}\right)\right\}K(x,s)ds. \tag{9.820a, b}$$

Given a linear differential operator M there exists (chapter III.7) an adjoint operator $\bar{M}$ and bilinear concomitant T satisfying (III.7.82) ≡ (9.821):

$$v(s)\left\{M\left(\frac{d}{ds}\right)\right\}K(x,s)-K(x,s)\left\{\bar{M}\left(\frac{d}{ds}\right)\right\}v(s)=\frac{d}{ds}\left[T(K,v)\right]. \tag{9.821}$$

Substituting (9.821) in (9.820b) gives (9.822a):

$$\int_L K(x,s)\left\{\bar{M}\left(\frac{d}{ds}\right)\right\}v(s)\,ds$$
$$= -\int_L dT(x,s) = -\left[T(K,v)\right]_{\partial L} = 0, \tag{9.822a–c}$$

where (9.822b) is a boundary term that can equal the integral only if both vanish (9.822c).

Thus *the linear differential equation (9.818b) with operator (9.818a) has solution (standard CCCLXXIV) as an integral transform (9.818c) where: (i) the kernel satisfies the partial differential equation (9.819b) that involves another operator (9.819c); (ii) the transform is a solution of the ordinary differential equation (9.823b) specified by the adjoint operator (9.823a) in (9.821):*

$$0 = \left\{\bar{M}\left(\frac{d}{ds}\right)\right\}v(s) = \sum_{m=0}^{M} C_m(s)\,\frac{d^m v}{ds^2}; \qquad \left[T(K,v)\right]_{\partial L} = 0, \tag{9.823a–c}$$

and (iii) the path of integration L is such that the bilinear concomitant in (9.821) takes the same value at the two ends (9.823c), for example vanishes at both ends. Although involving a partial differential equation (9.819a–c) may appear to be a complication, actually any particular solution will do, the simpler the better. In the case of the Fourier (9.767b) [Laplace (9.767c)] transform the kernel (9.768a) [(9.768b)] is an exponential, like (9.824a) for the generalized Laplace transform (9.769b) and satisfies (9.824b) the partial differential equation (9.824c):

$$K(x,s) = e^{xs}: \qquad \frac{1}{s}\frac{\partial K}{\partial x} = e^{xs} = K = \frac{1}{x}\frac{\partial K}{\partial s}, \qquad x\frac{\partial K}{\partial x} = s\frac{\partial K}{\partial s}. \tag{9.824a–c}$$

The solution of linear differential equations by power series (integral transforms) differs [sections 9.5–9.9.7 (9.8)] in that: (i) it is systematic (optional) in that the form of the solution is known to within coefficients (depends on the choice of a "suitable" kernel); (ii) distinguishes (does not distinguish) *a priori* the type of singularity; and (iii) there is only one set (may be several sets) of power series (integral representations). As an example, the Bessel differential equation (9.430b) may be solved [subsections 9.8.10 (9.8.13) by the generalized Laplace (Bateman) transform (subsection 9.8.6 (9.8.12)] leading to distinct integral representation (subsections 9.8.11 (9.8.14–9.8.16)].

9.8.13 Adjoint Operator and Bilinear Concomitant

The original Bessel differential operator (9.430b) ≡ (9.825b) applied to the kernel (9.825a) yields (9.825c, d):

$$\left\{L_1\left(\frac{d}{dx}\right)\right\}e^{i\,x\sin s}=\left\{x^2\frac{d^2}{dx^2}+x\frac{d}{dx}+\left(x^2-\nu^2\right)\right\}e^{i\,x\sin s}$$
$$=e^{ix\sin s}\left[x^2\left(1-\sin^2 s\right)+ix\sin s-\nu^2\right] \tag{9.825a–d}$$
$$=e^{ix\sin s}\left(x^2\cos^2 s+ix\sin s-\nu^2\right);$$

$$\left\{L_2\left(\frac{d}{dx}\right)\right\}e^{i\,x\sin s}=-\left(\frac{d^2}{ds^2}+\nu^2\right)e^{ix\sin s}=\left(-\nu^2-\frac{d}{ds}ix\cos s\right)e^{ix\sin s}$$
$$=e^{ix\sin s}\left(ix\sin s-\nu^2+x^2\cos^2 s\right); \tag{9.826a–c}$$

minus the linear harmonic operator with natural frequency ν applied (9.826b) to the same kernel (9.826a) leads to the same result (9.826c) ≡ (9.825d). If follows $L_1=L_2$ that the kernel (9.827a) satisfies (9.825b) ≡ (9.820b) the linear partial differential equation (9.827b):

$$K(x,s)=\exp(ix\sin s):\qquad x^2\frac{\partial^2 K}{\partial x^2}+x\frac{\partial K}{\partial x}+\left(x^2-\nu^2\right)K=-\frac{\partial^2 K}{\partial s^2}-\nu^2 K. \tag{9.827a, b}$$

Thus substituting the general integral transform (9.818c) in the original Bessel differential equation (9.430b) leads to (9.828a):

$$0=\int_L v(s)\left[\left(x^2\frac{\partial^2}{\partial x^2}+x\frac{\partial}{\partial x}+x^2-\nu^2\right)e^{ix\sin s}\right]ds=-\int_L v(s)\left[\left(\frac{\partial^2}{\partial s^2}+\nu^2\right)e^{ix\sin s}\right]ds, \tag{9.828a, b}$$

where the derivatives of the kernel with regard to the independent variable in (9.828a) may be replaced (9.827b) by derivatives with regard to the variable of integration in (9.828b).

Next, the derivatives with regard to the variable of integration are passed from the kernel to the transform using (9.821) the adjoint operator and bilinear concomitant. The second-order derivative is (subsection III.7.7.2) a self-adjoint operator (III.7.92), as follows from (9.829a, b) in the form (9.829c):

$$vK''=(vK')'-v'K'=(vK')'-(v'K)'+v''K:\quad vK''-Kv''=(vK'-v'K)'. \tag{9.829a–c}$$

Comparing (9.829c) with (9.821) it follows that: (i) the operator (9.830a) is self-adjoint (9.830b); and (ii) the bilinear concomitant is (9.830c):

$$M\left(\frac{d}{ds}\right) \equiv \frac{d^2}{ds^2} = \bar{M}\left(\frac{d}{ds}\right), \qquad T(v,k) = vK' - v'K. \tag{9.830a–c}$$

Substituting (9.829c) in (9.828b) allows separation (9.831a) of integral and boundary terms in (9.831b), so that the equation can be satisfied setting both to zero (9.831c):

$$\int_L e^{ix\sin s}\left(\frac{d^2v}{ds^2} + \nu^2 v\right) ds = \left[v\left(e^{ix\sin s}\right)' - e^{ix\sin s}\, v'\right]_L = -\int_L dT(v,k) = 0. \tag{9.831a–c}$$

The same result can be obtained substituting the commutation relation (9.830a) in (9.828b) and integrating twice by parts (9.832a–c) where all derivatives are with regard to s:

$$\begin{aligned}\int_L \nu^2 K(x,s)v(s)ds &= -\int_L K''(x,s)v(s)ds = -\left[K'(x,s)v(s)\right]_{\partial L} + \int_L K'(x,s)v'(s)ds \\ &= \left[K(x,s)v'(x;s) - K'(x,s)v(s)\right] - \int_L K(x,s)v''(s)ds.\end{aligned} \tag{9.832a–c}$$

The coincidence of (9.832c) ≡ (9.831c) shows that *the original Bessel differential equation (9.430b) has (standard CCCLXXV) solution as a general integral transform (9.818c) with: (i) kernel (9.827a); (ii) transform (9.833b) satisfying (9.833a):*

$$v'' + \nu^2 v = 0: \qquad v(s) = e^{\pm i\nu s}; \qquad \left[(\pm\nu - \cos s)e^{\pm i\nu s + ix\sin s}\right]_{\partial L} = 0, \tag{9.833a–c}$$

and (iii) path of integration such that the function in square brackets in (9.831c; 9.833b) ≡ (9.833c) takes the same value at both ends. Use of (9.827a; 9.833b, c) in the integral transform (9.818c) leads to integral representations for Bessel, Neumann, and Hankel functions (subsection 9.8.13).

9.8.14 Integral Representations for the Two Hankel Functions

Assuming (9.834a) the function in square brackets in (9.833c) is dominated by the kernel (9.827a) and vanishes at infinity: (i) along the positive imaginary axis (9.834b–e):

$$\operatorname{Re}(x) > 0; \quad s = it: \qquad \lim_{s\to i\infty} e^{ix\sin s} = \lim_{t\to\infty} e^{ix\sin(it)} = \lim_{t\to\infty} e^{-x\sinh t} = 0; \tag{9.834a–e}$$

$$\begin{aligned} s = u \pm \pi = \pm\pi + it: \quad \lim_{s\to\pm\pi - i\infty} e^{ix\sin s} &= \lim_{u\to -i\infty} e^{ix\sin(u\pm\pi)} = \lim_{u\to -i\infty} e^{-ix\sin u} \\ &= \lim_{t\to-\infty} e^{-ix\sin(it)} = \lim_{t\to-\infty} e^{x\sinh t} = 0,\end{aligned} \tag{9.835a–g}$$

and (ii) along a line parallel to the negative imaginary axis at a distance $\pm\pi$ in (9.835a–g). In (9.834d) and (9.835f) was used (II.5.6b) = (9.836a–c):

$$\sin(it) \equiv \frac{e^{i^2t} - e^{-i^2t}}{2i} = -i\frac{e^{-t} - e^{t}}{2} = i\sinh t, \tag{9.836a–c}$$

that will be re-used in the sequel.

Since the function in square brackets in (9.833c) vanishes at $s = i\infty, \pm\pi - i\infty$, two paths $L_+ (L_-)$ of integration joining these three points (Figure 9.17) lead (9.818c, 9.827a; 9.833b) to (9.837a) [(9.837b)]:

$$y_-(x) = \int_{+i\infty}^{\pm\pi - i\infty} \exp(-i\nu s + ix\sin s)\, ds, \tag{9.837a, b}$$

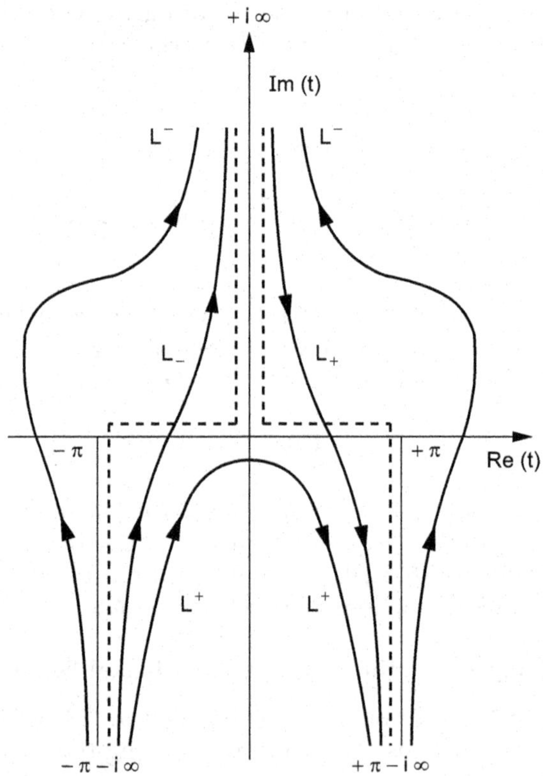

FIGURE 9.17
The solution of the original Bessel differential equation by means of Hilbert transforms involves the same integrand along paths in the complex s-plane joining the points $+i\infty$ and $\pm\pi - i\infty$. The paths $L_\pm$ symmetric relative to the imaginary axis lead to the two Hankel functions that are complex conjugate for real variable and order. The path $L^+(L^-)$ leads to the Bessel (Neumann) function that is real for real variable and order. Since the original Bessel differential equation is linear of the second-order only two paths lead to linearly independent solutions, for example either the Bessel and Neumann functions or the two Hankel functions.

choosing the – sign in (9.833b); this choice of sign does not affect the solution of the Bessel differential equation (9.430b) but is needed for agreement with the usual definitions of Hankel/Neumann/Bessel functions (subsections 9.8.14/9.8.15/9.8.16). The change of integration variable (9.838a) is applied (9.838b–e) to the limits of integration in (9.838a, b):

$$s = -it: \qquad s = i\infty \Rightarrow t = -\infty; \qquad s = \pm\pi - i\infty \Rightarrow t = \infty \pm i\pi, \qquad (9.838\text{a–e})$$

and shows that (9.839b, c) are complex conjugates (9.839d):

$$\operatorname{Re}(x) > 0: \qquad H_\nu^{(1,2)}(x) = \pm\frac{1}{i\pi}\int_{-\infty}^{\infty\pm i\pi} \exp(-\nu t + x\sinh t)\,dt = \left\{H_\nu^{(2,1)}(x)\right\}^*; \qquad (9.839\text{a–d})$$

since (9.839b, c) are complex conjugate (9.839d) solutions of the Bessel differential equation (9.430b) they must coincide to within a multiplying factor with the first and second Hankel function (9.571a) valid for (9.839a) ≡ (9.834a). The constant factors in (9.839b, c) will be confirmed by calculating the Bessel function (subsection 9.8.15) and showing that it agrees with previous results (subsection 9.8.11). Using the variable *s* in (9.838a) instead of *t* in (9.839b) leads to (9.839e, f):

$$H_\nu^{(1,2)}(x) = \pm\frac{1}{\pi}\int_{i\infty}^{-i\infty\pm\pi} \exp(-i\nu s + ix\sin s)\,ds, \qquad (9.839\text{e, f})$$

that coincides with (9.837a, b) apart from the factor $\pm 1/\pi$. Thus *the Hankel function of the first (second) kind and positive real variable (9.839a) are (standard CCCLXXVI) complex conjugates (9.839d) with equivalent integral representations (9.839b) ≡ (9.839e) [(9.839c) ≡ (9.839f)].* From the integral representations for the Hankel functions follow those for the Neumann (Bessel) functions [subsections 9.8.15 (9.8.16)].

9.8.15 Integral Representation for the Neumann Function

The Hankel functions (9.839e, f) specify (9.571d) the Neumann function (9.840a):

$$Y_\nu(x) = \frac{1}{2i}\left[H_\nu^{(1)}(x) - H_\nu^{(2)}(x)\right] = \frac{1}{2\pi i}$$
$$\times\left(\int_{i\infty}^{0} + \int_{0}^{\pi} + \int_{\pi}^{\pi-i\infty} + \int_{i\infty}^{0} + \int_{0}^{-\pi} + \int_{-\pi}^{-\pi-i\infty}\right)\exp(-i\nu s + ix\sin s)\,ds. \qquad (9.840\text{a, b})$$

where the path of integration (Figure 9.17) in (9.840b) is $L_+ - L_- = -2L^-$ implying that the integrals along: (i) the real axis (9.841a) add to (9.841b, c):

$$s=\phi: \quad \frac{1}{2\pi i}\int_0^\pi \left(e^{-i\nu s+ix\sin s} - e^{i\nu s-ix\sin s}\right)ds = \frac{1}{\pi}\int_0^\pi \sin\left(x\sin\phi - \nu\phi\right)d\phi; \quad (9.841a–c)$$

(ii) along the positive imaginary axis are equal (9.842b) leading to the double value (9.842a–c):

$$s=it: \quad \frac{1}{\pi i}\int_{i\infty}^0 \exp\left(-i\nu s+ix\sin s\right)ds = -\frac{1}{\pi}\int_0^\infty \exp\left(\nu t - x\sinh t\right)dt; \quad (9.842a–c)$$

and (iii) along the lines at distances $\pm\pi$ from the negative imaginary axis (9.843b) add to (9.843a, c) that simplify to (9.843d, e):

$$\begin{aligned} s=\pm\pi - it: \quad & \frac{1}{2\pi i}\left(\int_\pi^{\pi-i\infty} + \int_{-\pi}^{-\pi-i\infty}\right)\exp\left(-i\nu s + ix\sin s\right)ds \\ &= -\frac{1}{2\pi}\int_0^\infty \left\{\exp\left[-i\nu(\pi-it)+ix\sin(\pi-it)\right]\right. \\ &\quad \left.+\exp\left[-i\nu(-\pi-it)+ix\sin(-\pi-it)\right]\right\} \\ &= -\frac{1}{2\pi}\int_0^\infty \left(e^{-i\nu\pi}+e^{i\nu\pi}\right)\exp\left[-\nu t - ix\sin(-it)\right]dt \\ &= -\frac{1}{\pi}\cos\left(\nu\pi\right)\int_0^\infty \exp\left(-\nu t - x\sinh t\right). \end{aligned} \quad (9.843a–e)$$

The integral (9.840b) is the sum of (9.841c; 9.842c; 9.843e) showing that *with the condition (9.834a) ≡ (9.844a) the Neumann function has (standard CCCLXXVII) the parametric integral representation (9.844b):*

$$\begin{aligned} \mathrm{Re}(x)>0: \quad \pi Y_\nu(x) &= \int_0^\pi \sin\left(x\sin\phi - \nu\phi\right)d\phi \\ &\quad -\int_0^\infty \left[e^{\nu t} + e^{-\nu t}\cos(\nu\pi)\right]\exp\left(-x\sinh t\right)dt, \end{aligned} \quad (9.844a, b)$$

$$\begin{aligned} n\in|N_0: \quad Y_{2n,2n+1}(x) &= \frac{1}{\pi}\int_0^\pi \sin\left[x\sin\phi - \{2n,2n+1\}\phi\right]d\phi \\ &= -\frac{2}{\pi}\int_0^\infty \{\cosh,\sinh(\nu t)\}\exp\left(-x\sinh t\right)dt, \end{aligned} \quad (9.845a–c)$$

that simplifies to (9.845b) [(9.845c)] for even (odd) integer (9.845a) order.

9.8.16 Second Integral Representation for the Bessel Function

The Hankel functions (9.839e, f) also specify (9.571c) the Bessel function (9.846a):

$$J_\nu(x) = \frac{1}{2}\left[H_\nu^{(1)}(x) + H_\nu^{(2)}(x)\right]$$

$$= \frac{1}{2\pi}\left(\int_{i\infty}^{0} + \int_{0}^{\pi} + \int_{\pi}^{\pi-i\infty} - \int_{i\infty}^{0} - \int_{0}^{-\pi} - \int_{-\pi}^{-\pi-i\infty}\right)\exp(-i\nu s + ix\sin s)\,ds, \tag{9.846a, b}$$

where the path of integration (Figure 9.17) in (9.781b) is $L_+ + L_- = L^+$, implying that the integrals along: (i) the real axis (9.847b) add to (9.847a, c):

$$s \equiv \phi: \frac{1}{2\pi}\int_0^\pi \left[\exp(-i\nu s + ix\sin s) + \exp(i\nu s - ix\sin s)\right]ds$$

$$= \frac{1}{\pi}\int_0^\pi \cos(x\sin\phi - \nu\phi)\,d\phi; \tag{9.847a–c}$$

(ii) along the positive imaginary axis cancel; and (iii) along the lines at distance $\pm\pi$ from the negative imaginary axis (9.848b) add to (9.848a, c) that simplifies to (9.848d, e):

$$s = \pm\pi - it: \qquad \frac{1}{2\pi}\left(\int_{\pi}^{\pi-i\infty} - \int_{-\pi}^{-\pi-i\infty}\right)\exp(-i\nu s + ix\sin s)\,ds$$

$$= -\frac{i}{2\pi}\int_0^\infty \left\{\exp\left[-i\nu(\pi - it) + ix\sin(\pi - it)\right]\right.$$

$$\left. - \exp\left[-i\nu(-\pi - it) + ix\sin(-\pi - it)\right]\right\}dt$$

$$= \frac{1}{2\pi i}\int_0^\infty \left(e^{-i\nu\pi} - e^{i\nu\pi}\right)e^{-\nu t}e^{-ix\sin(-it)}\,dt = -\frac{1}{\pi}\sin(\nu\pi)\int_0^\infty e^{-\nu t}\,e^{-x\sinh t}\,dt. \tag{9.848a–e}$$

The integral (9.846b) is the sum of (9.847c; 9.848e) showing that *with the condition (9.834a) ≡ (9.849a) the Bessel function has (standard CCCXXVIII) a second parametric integral representation (9.849b):*

$$\operatorname{Re}(x) > 0: \qquad \pi J_\nu(x) = \int_0^\pi \cos(x\sin\phi - \nu\phi)\,d\phi$$

$$- \sin(\pi\nu)\int_0^\pi \exp(-\nu t - x\sinh t)\,dt, \tag{9.849, b}$$

$$n \in |N: \qquad J_n(x) = \frac{1}{\pi}\int_0^\pi \cos(x\sin\phi - n\phi)\,d\phi, \tag{9.850a, b}$$

that simplifies to (9.850b) for integer order (9.850a).

The example of the Bessel function of general (integer) order shows that: (i) the power series representation is unique (9.510a) [(9.510b)]; and (ii) there may be alternative parametric integral representations such as (9.817a–c; 9.849a, b) [(9.850a, b; 9.851a, b)].

$$\begin{aligned} J_n(x) &= \frac{2}{\sqrt{\pi}}\frac{(x/2)^n}{\Gamma(1/2+n)}\int_0^{\pi/2} \cos^{2n}\phi\,\cos(x\sin\phi)\,d\phi \\ &= \frac{2}{\pi}\frac{x^n}{(2n-1)!!}\int_0^{\pi/2} \cos^{2n}\phi\,\cos(x\sin\phi)\,d\phi; \end{aligned} \tag{9.851a, b}$$

(9.851a) follows from (9.817d) for positive integer order (9.850a), and in (9.851b) was used (9.852c):

$$\begin{aligned} \Gamma\left(n+\frac{1}{2}\right) &= \left(n-\frac{1}{2}\right)\left(n-\frac{3}{2}\right)\cdots\frac{1}{2}\Gamma\left(\frac{1}{2}\right) \\ &= \frac{(2n-1)\,(2n-3)\cdots 1}{2^n}\sqrt{\pi} = (2n-1)!!\,2^{-n}\sqrt{\pi}. \end{aligned} \tag{9.852a–c}$$

that follows (9.852a, b) from (9.432b; 9.524a). The Bessel function of order zero is given by (9.850b) [(9.851b)] as (9.853a) [(9.853b)]:

$$J_0(x) = \frac{1}{\pi}\int_0^\pi \cos(x\sin\phi)\,d\phi = \frac{2}{\pi}\int_0^{\pi/2} \cos(x\sin\phi)\,d\phi; \tag{9.853a, b}$$

the coincidence of (9.853a) ≡ (9.853b) obtained by different methods confirms the choice of coefficient $1/\pi$ in (9.839a, b). *The* **Bessel coefficients,** *that is Bessel functions of integer order (9.850a), are given (standard CCCLXXXIX) equivalently by (9.850b) ≡ (9.851a, b) and simplify to (9.853a, b) for zero order.* The solution of linear differential equations by the first (second) method of power series (integral transforms) applies to any order [sections 9.4–9.7 (9.8)] whereas a third method of continued fractions (section 9.9) applies only to linear differential equations of the second order.

9.9 Continued Fractions as Solutions of Differential Equations

The first (second) method I (II) of the power series (integral transforms) applies [sections 9.4–9.7 (9.8)] to the solution of linear differential equations of any order. Method III of continued fractions (section 9.9) applies only to second-order linear differential equations (subsection 9.9.1) that can be treated (subsection 9.9.2) as triple recurrence relations (sections II.1.6–II.1.9). Method III expresses the logarithmic derivative of the solution of a linear second-order differential equation as a continued fraction (subsection 9.9.2) that may: (i) terminate (subsection 9.9.3), corresponding to a rational function and implying that the solution of the differential equation is a polynomial; (ii) be non-terminating or infinite (subsection 9.9.4), specifying a transcendental function in the case of convergence, that can be considered for real (complex) variable and parameters [subsections 9.9.5–9.9.6 (9.9.13–9.9.15)]. The confluent hypergeometric and generalized Bessel differential equations can be transformed into each other (subsections 9.9.7–9.9.8), leading to a continued fraction for (subsection 9.9.9) the logarithmic derivative of the generalized Bessel function. If instead of the logarithmic derivative of the solution of a linear second-order differential equation (subsections 9.9.1–9.9.9), what is sought is a continued fraction for the solution (subsections 9.9.12), then the starting point can be a recurrence formula (subsection 9.9.11) obtained from an integral or power series representation (subsection 9.9.10).

9.9.1 Continued Fraction Associated with a Differential Equation

A linear second-order differential equation with variable coefficients (9.854a) can be written in the form (9.854b):

$$y(x) = a_0(x)\,y'(x) + b_1(x)\,y''(x): \qquad \frac{y(x)}{y'(x)} = a_0(x) + \frac{b_1(x)}{y'(x)/y''(x)}, \tag{9.854a, b}$$

that suggests the following recurrence method: (i) differentiating (9.854a) leads to (9.855):

$$y'(x)\left[1 - a_0'(x)\right] = \left[a_0(x) + b_1'(x)\right] y''(x) + b_1(x)\,y'''(x), \tag{9.855}$$

that can be rewritten (9.856a):

$$\frac{y'(x)}{y''(x)} = a_1(x) + \frac{b_2(x)}{y''(x)/y'''(x)}: \qquad \{a_1(x), b_2(x)\} \equiv \frac{\{a_0(x) + b_1'(x),\, b_1(x)\}}{1 - a_0'(x)}, \tag{9.856a–c}$$

with coefficients (9.856b, c); and (ii) it follows by recurrence that the ratio of the n-th to the $(n+1)$-th derivative of the solution of the linear second-order differential equation (9.854a) satisfies (9.857a):

$$\frac{y^{(n)}(x)}{y^{(n+1)}(x)} = a_n(x) + \frac{b_{n+1}(x)}{y^{(n+1)}(x)/y^{(n+2)}(x)}, \tag{9.857a}$$

$$\{a_n(x), b_{n+1}(x)\} = \frac{\{a_{n-1}(x) + b_n'(x), b_n(x)\}}{1 - a_{n-1}'(x)}, \tag{9.857b, c}$$

with coefficients (9.857b, c).

Successive substitution of (9.856a–c; 9.857a–c) in (9.854b) leads to (subsections II.1.6–II.1.9) the continued fraction (9.858):

$$\frac{y(x)}{y'(x)} = a_0(x) + \frac{b_1(x)}{a_1(x)+}\frac{b_2(x)}{a_2(x)+}\cdots\frac{b_{n-1}(x)}{a_{n-1}(x)+}\frac{b_n(x)}{a_n(x) + y^{(n+1)}(x)/y^{(n+2)}(x)}. \tag{9.858}$$

The inverse (II.1.108) is the continued fraction (9.859a):

$$\frac{1}{a_0(x)+}\frac{b_1(x)}{a_1(x)+}\frac{b_2(x)}{a_2(x)+}\cdots\frac{b_{n-1}(x)}{a_{n-1}(x)+}\frac{b_n(x)}{a_n(x)+r_n(x)} = \frac{y'(x)}{y(x)} = \frac{d}{dx}\{\log[y(x)]\}, \tag{9.859a, b}$$

that specifies the logarithmic derivative of the solution of the linear second-order differential equation (9.854a).

9.9.2 Logarithmic Derivative of the Solution of a Differential Equation

It has been shown that *the logarithmic derivative of a solution of the linear second-order differential equation (9.854a) can be expressed (standard CCCLXXX) as a* ***continued fraction*** *(9.859a, b) with: (i)* ***coefficients*** *(9.856b, c; 9.857b, c) and* ***remainder*** *(9.860a) after n terms:*

$$r_n(x) = \frac{b_{n+1}(x)}{y^{(n+1)}(x)/y^{(n+2)}(x)} = \begin{cases} 0 & \text{for} \quad n = N \quad \text{terminating} \\ 0 & \text{as} \quad n \to \infty \quad \text{converging} \end{cases}, \tag{9.860a–c}$$

(ii) if the remainder vanishes after N terms (9.860b) the continued fraction is ***terminating*** *(9.861a) and specifies a* ***rational function*** *(9.860c):*

$$\frac{d}{dx}\{\log[y(x)]\} = \frac{1}{a_0(x)+}\frac{b_1(x)}{a_1(x)+}\cdots\frac{b_N(x)}{a_N(x)} = \frac{p_N(x)}{q_N(x)} = X_N(x), \tag{9.861a–c}$$

whose ***numerators*** $p_N(x)$ *and* ***denominators*** $q_N(x)$ *are polynomials (9.861b); and (iii) if the remainder never vanishes but tends to zero for large order (9.860c) the non-terminating or* ***infinite continued fraction*** *converges and specifies (9.862) a non-rational or* ***transcendental function:***

$$\frac{d}{dx}\{\log[y(x)]\} = \frac{1}{a_0(x)+}\ \frac{b_1(x)}{a_1(x)+}\ \cdots\ \frac{b_n(x)}{a_n(x)+}\ \cdots, \tag{9.862}$$

and its truncation specifies the ***continuants*** *(9.861a–c), that are its rational approximations of order N.* Next are given examples of the solution of a linear second-order differential equation by means of a terminating (infinite) continued fraction [subsections 9.9.3–9.9.5 (9.9.6–9.9.7)].

9.9.3 Solution as a Terminating Continued Fraction

Consider the linear second-order differential equation (9.863b) with positive integer parameter (9.863a) for which (9.864a) the coefficients are (9.863c, d):

$$m \in |N; \qquad y = \frac{x}{m}y' + \frac{y''}{m}: \qquad a_0(x) = \frac{x}{m}, \qquad b_1 \equiv \frac{1}{m}. \tag{9.863a–d}$$

Differentiating (9.863b) less (9.864a) than m times leads to (9.864b) ≡ (9.864c):

$$n = 1,2,\ldots,m-1: \qquad y^{(n)} - \frac{y^{(n+2)}}{m} = \frac{d^n}{dx^n}\left(\frac{x}{m}y'\right) = \frac{x}{m}y^{(n+1)} + \frac{n}{m}y^{(n)}; \tag{9.864a–c}$$

rewriting (9.864c) ≡ (9.865a) and comparing with (9.857a) specifies the coefficients (9.865b, c):

$$\frac{y^{(n)}}{y^{(n+1)}} = \frac{x}{m-n} + \frac{y^{(n+2)}/y^{(n+1)}}{m-n}: \qquad a_n(x) = \frac{x}{m-n}, \qquad b_{n+1} = \frac{1}{m-n}. \tag{9.865a–c}$$

The m-th derivative of (9.863b) is (9.864c) with $n = m$ leading to (9.866a) that compared with (9.857a) specifies the coefficients (9.801b, c):

$$0 = xy^{(m+1)} + y^{(m+2)}: \qquad a_m = x, \qquad b_{m+1} = 0. \tag{9.866a–c}$$

Substitution of (9.865b, c; 9.866b, c) in (9.861a) leads to (9.867):

$$\frac{d}{dx}\{\log[y(x)]\} = \frac{1}{\frac{x}{m}+}\ \frac{\frac{1}{m}}{\frac{x}{m-1}+}\ \frac{\frac{1}{m-1}}{\frac{x}{m+2}+}\ \cdots\ \frac{1}{x}, \tag{9.867}$$

that simplifies to (9.868):

$$\frac{y'(x)}{y(x)}=\frac{m}{x+}\,\frac{m-1}{x+}\,\frac{m-2}{x+}\,\ldots\,\frac{1}{x}. \tag{9.868}$$

Thus *a solution of the linear second-order differential equation (9.863b) with positive integer parameter (9.863a) has (standard CCCLXXXI) logarithmic derivative given by the terminating continued fraction (9.868), corresponding to a rational function.* An infinite continued fraction is considered next (subsection 9.9.4).

9.9.4 Confluent Hypergeometric Differential Equation (Kummer 1830)

The confluent hypergeometric differential equation (9.869c) has for solutions (note 9.29) the confluent hypergeometric function that may be [subsection(s) 9.5.8 (9.5.9–9.5.10)] of the first (9.869a) [second (9.869b)] kinds:

$$y(x)={}_1F_1(\alpha;\gamma;x),\,{}_1G_1(\alpha;\gamma;x): \qquad xy''+(\gamma-x)y'-\alpha y=0. \tag{9.869a–c}$$

Differentiating n times yields (9.870a, b):

$$\alpha y^{(n)}=\frac{d^n}{dx^n}\left[xy''+(\gamma-x)y'\right]=xy^{(n+2)}+(\gamma-x+n)y^{(n+1)}-ny^{(n)}; \tag{9.870a, b}$$

re-writing (9.869b) [(9.870b)] in the form (9.871a) [(9.871b)]:

$$\frac{y}{y'}=\frac{\gamma-x}{\alpha}+\frac{x}{\alpha}\frac{y''}{y'}, \qquad \frac{y^{(n)}}{y^{(n+1)}}=\frac{\gamma-x+n}{\alpha+n}+\frac{x}{\alpha+n}\frac{y^{(n+2)}}{y^{(n+1)}}, \tag{9.871a, b}$$

leads to the continued fraction:

$$\frac{y}{y'}=\frac{\gamma-x}{\alpha}+\frac{\frac{x}{\alpha}}{\frac{y'}{y''}}=\frac{\gamma-x}{\alpha}+\frac{\frac{x}{\alpha}}{\frac{\gamma-x+1}{\alpha+1+}}\,\frac{\frac{x}{\alpha+1}}{\frac{y''}{y'''}}=\frac{\gamma-x}{\alpha}+\frac{\frac{x}{\alpha}}{\frac{\gamma-x+1}{\alpha+1+}}\,\frac{\frac{x}{\alpha+1}}{\frac{\gamma-x+2}{\alpha+2+}}\cdots\frac{\frac{x}{\alpha+n-1}}{\frac{\gamma-x+n}{\alpha+n+}}\cdots \tag{9.872}$$

The inversion (II.1.108) of (9.872) gives (9.873):

$$\frac{y'}{y}=\frac{1}{\frac{\gamma-x}{\alpha}+}\,\frac{\frac{x}{\alpha}}{\frac{\gamma-x+1}{\alpha+1+}}\,\frac{\frac{x}{\alpha+1}}{\frac{\gamma-x+2}{\alpha+2+}}\cdots\frac{\frac{x}{\alpha+n-1}}{\frac{\gamma-x+n}{\alpha+n+}}\cdots \tag{9.873}$$

that simplifies to (9.874):

$$\frac{d}{dx}\left\{\log\left[{}_1F_1(\alpha;\gamma;x)\right]\right\} = \frac{\alpha}{\gamma - x +}\,\frac{(\alpha+1)x}{\gamma - x + 1 +}\,\frac{(\alpha+2)x}{\gamma - x + 2 +}\cdots\frac{(\alpha+n)x}{\gamma - x + n +}\cdots \tag{9.874}$$

Any other solution of the confluent hypergeometric differential equation (9.869c), for example a function of the second kind (9.869b), would satisfy the same continued fraction (9.873) for its logarithmic derivative. Thus *the logarithmic derivative of the confluent hypergeometric function (9.869a) that is a solution of the confluent hypergeometric differential equation (9.869c) has (standard CCCLXXXII) the representation (9.874) as the infinite continued fraction.* This assumes that the continued fraction (9.872) ≡ (9.874) converges, which can be proved rather simply (in a slightly more elaborate way) for real (complex) coefficients [subsections 9.9.5–9.9.6 (9.9.13–9.9.15)].

9.9.5 Convergence of Simple Infinite Continued Fractions

It can be shown (subsection II.1.7.1) that *a* ***simple continued fraction*** *(9.858) whose coefficients (standard CCCLXXXIII) are all real and positive (9.875a, b) ≡ (II.1.113a, b): (i) has its even (odd) continuants in a decreasing (9.875c) [increasing (9.875e)] sequence:*

$$a_n > 0 < b_n: \qquad X_{2n} > X_{2n+2} > \ldots > X > \ldots > X_{2n+1} > X_{2n-1} > \ldots; \tag{9.875a–e}$$

and (ii) all continuants of even order are larger than those of odd order. Thus the limit of the continued fraction has for upper (lower) bound the limit of the continuants of even (odd) order (9.876a) [(9.876b)]:

$$\lim_{n\to\infty} X_{2n} \geq X \geq \lim_{n\to\infty} X_{2n+1}; \qquad \lim_{n\to\infty} X_{2n} = \lim_{n\to\infty} X_{2n+1} = X. \tag{9.876a–d}$$

If the continuants of even (odd) order have the same limit (9.876c), their common value is the unique limit of the infinite continued fraction (9.876d) ≡ (9.875c) that is thus convergent.

In order to apply the preceding convergence theorem, it is noted that (subsection II.1.6.4) for any continued fraction (9.858) *the difference of the successive continuants is (standard CCCLXXXIV) given by (II.1.107a, b) ≡ (9.877a, b):*

$$X_n - X_{n-1} = (-)^n \frac{b_n \ldots . b_2}{q_n\, q_{n-1}}, \qquad X_n - X_{n-2} = (-)^{n-1} \frac{a_n b_{n-1} \ldots . b_2}{q_n\, q_{n-2}}. \tag{9.877a, b}$$

It can also be shown (subsection II.1.6.3) that *the numerators and denominators (9.861c) satisfy (standard CCCLXXXVI) the recurrence formulas (II.1.102a, b) ≡ (9.878a, b):*

$$p_n = a_n\, p_{n-1} + b_n\, p_{n-2}, \quad q_n = a_{n-1}\, q_{n-1} + b_n\, q_{n-2}. \tag{9.878a, b}$$

Also, (subsection I.1.6.5) the *inverse continued fractions (9.793) [(9.797)] interchange (standard CCCLXXXVI) the numerators and denominators (9.814a, b):*

$$a_0 + \frac{b_1}{a_1 +} \frac{b_2}{a_2 +} \cdots \frac{b_n}{a_n} = \frac{p_n}{q_n}, \qquad \frac{1}{a_0 +} \frac{b_1}{a_1 +} \frac{b_2}{a_2 +} \cdots \frac{b_n}{a_n} = \frac{q_n}{p_n}. \tag{9.879a, b}$$

The results (9.875a–e; 9.876a–d; 9.877a, b; 9.878a, b; 9.879a, b) can be used to prove (subsection 9.9.6) the convergence (subsection 9.9.5) of the continued fraction for the logarithmic derivative of the confluent hypergeometric function (subsection 9.9.4) for some combinations of real variable and parameters.

9.9.6 Continued Fraction for the Confluent Hypergeometric Function

In the continued fraction (9.858) for the inverse of the logarithmic derivative of the confluent hypergeometric function (9.872) it is assumed that the variable and parameters are real and satisfy (9.880a–c) so that all coefficients (9.880d, e) are positive:

$$\gamma > x > 0 < \alpha: \qquad a_n = \frac{\gamma - x + n}{\alpha + n} > 0, \qquad b_n = \frac{x}{\alpha + n - 1} > 0, \tag{9.880a–e}$$

from which follows that: (i) the coefficients (9.880d) [(9.880e)] have the limit (9.881a) [(9.881b)] as $n \to \infty$; (ii) the numerators (9.878a) [(9.878b)] thus scale as (9.881c) [(9.881d)]:

$$\lim_{n\to\infty} a_n = 1, \qquad \lim_{n\to\infty} b_n = 0: \qquad p_n \sim O(n) \sim q_n; \tag{9.881a–d}$$

(iii) the continued fractions for the logarithmic derivative of the confluent hypergeometric function (9.874) and its inverse (9.872) interchange the numerators (9.879a, b) in (9.881c, d) but this does not affect (9.881a, b), that holds in both cases; (iv) substituting (9.881a–d) in (9.877a, b) leads to (9.882a, b):

$$X_n - X_{n-1} \sim O\left(n^{-2}\right) \sim X_n - X_{n-2}, \tag{9.882a, b}$$

and (v) since both (9.882a, b) vanish as $n \to \infty$ then (9.876c, d) are satisfied and the limit is unique. It has been shown that *the continued fraction for the logarithmic derivative of the confluent hypergeometric function (9.809) converges (standard CCCLXXXVII) for real positive (9.880a–c) [general complex (subsection 9.9.13)] values of the parameters.* The generalized Bessel differential equation can be transformed to the confluent hypergeometric differential equation (subsection 9.9.7) leading (subsection 9.9.8) to a continued fraction for the logarithmic derivative of the generalized (original) Bessel function (subsection 9.9.9).

9.9.7 Generalized Bessel and Confluent Hypergeometric Differential Equations

The generalized Bessel differential equation (9.428a–f) can be reduced through the changes of dependent and independent variable (9.788c) to the differential equation (9.787b). The change of independent variable (9.883a) transforms (9.883b) the differential equation (9.787b) to (9.883c):

$$\zeta = \frac{\mu\eta}{4}, \qquad \Theta(\zeta) \equiv \Psi(\eta): \qquad \zeta\Theta'' + (1+\nu-\zeta)\Theta' - \left(\frac{\nu}{2} - \frac{1}{\mu}\right)\Theta = 0. \qquad (9.883\text{a–c})$$

The differential equation (9.883c) is of the confluent hypergeometric type (9.869b) with parameters (9.884a, b) leading to (9.884c):

$$\alpha = \frac{\nu}{2} - \frac{1}{\mu}, \qquad \gamma = 1+\nu: \qquad \Theta(\zeta) = {}_1F_1\left(\frac{\nu}{2} - \frac{1}{\mu}; 1+\nu; \zeta\right). \qquad (9.884\text{a–c})$$

Substitution of (9.884c) in (9.788b) leads to (9.885a):

$$J_\nu^\mu(x) = x^\nu \Psi(x^2) = D(\mu,\nu)\, x^\nu\, {}_1F_1\left(\frac{\nu}{2} - \frac{1}{\mu};\ 1+\nu;\ \frac{\mu x^2}{4}\right); \qquad (9.885\text{a, b})$$

since the solution of a linear differential equation is not affected by multiplication by a constant; in (9.885b) has been introduced a factor $D(\mu,\nu)$ that can depend on the degree ν and order μ but not on the variable x. This factor can be determined by comparing power series (or parametric integral representations) of the generalized Bessel and confluent hypergeometric functions (subsection 9.9.8).

9.9.8 Confluent Hypergeometric Series

The confluent hypergeometric differential equation (9.869c) has a regular singularity at the origin and the only other singularity is the point at infinity. Thus the regular integral (9.377b) converges in the finite x-plane and substitution in (9.869c) leads to (9.886):

$$0 = \sum_{n=0}^{\infty} c_n(a)(n+a)(n+a-1+\gamma)x^{n+a-1} - \sum_{k=0}^{\infty} c_k(a)(k+a+\alpha)x^{k+a}. \qquad (9.886)$$

The coefficient (9.887b) of the lowest power (9.887a) leads to the quadratic indicial equation (9.822c) whose roots are the indices (9.887d, e):

$$x^{a-1}: \qquad 0 = c_0(a)a\,(a-1+\gamma); \quad c_0(a) \neq 0, \quad a_{1,2} = 0, 1-\gamma. \qquad (9.887\text{a–e})$$

The change of index of summation (9.888a) in (9.887) leads to (9.888b):

$$k = n-1: \qquad 0 = \sum_{n=0}^{\infty} x^n \left[(n+a)(n+a-1+\gamma) c_n(a) - (n+a-1+\alpha) c_{n-1}(a) \right], \tag{9.888a, b}$$

that implies the recurrence relation for the coefficients:

$$c_n(a) = \frac{n+a-1+\alpha}{(n+a)(n+a-1+\gamma)} c_{n-1}(a), \tag{9.889}$$

to be applied to both indices (9.887d, e).

The first-index (9.887d) leads (9.890a) in (9.889) to the coefficients (9.890b):

$$c_0(0) = 1: \qquad c_n(0) = \frac{(n+\alpha-1)(n+\alpha-2)\cdots\alpha}{n!(n+\gamma-1)(n+\gamma-2)\cdots\gamma}. \tag{9.890a, b}$$

The corresponding regular integral (9.377b) is the **confluent hypergeometric series** (I.30.116a) ≡ (II.3.124a, b) ≡ (9.891a, b, d) with variable x and parameters α, β:

$$\begin{aligned} y_1(x) &= 1 + \frac{\alpha}{\gamma} x + \frac{\alpha(\alpha+1)}{\gamma(\gamma+1)} \frac{x^2}{2!} + \cdots + \frac{\alpha\cdots(\alpha+n-1)}{\gamma\cdots(\gamma+n-1)} \frac{x^n}{n!} + \cdots \\ &= 1 + \sum_{n=1}^{\infty} \frac{\alpha\cdots(\alpha+n-1)}{\gamma\cdots(\gamma+\tilde{n}-1)} \frac{x^n}{n!} = \frac{\Gamma(\gamma)}{\Gamma(\alpha)} \sum_{n=0}^{\infty} \frac{\Gamma(\alpha+n)}{\Gamma(\gamma+n)} \frac{x^n}{n!} \equiv {}_1F_1(\alpha;\gamma;x), \end{aligned} \tag{9.891a–c}$$

where was introduced (9.890c) the gamma function (9.432b). The second index (9.887e) leads (9.889) to (9.892e):

$$\alpha \to \alpha+1-\gamma, \gamma \to 2-\gamma; \quad c_0(1-\gamma) = 1: \quad c_n(1-\gamma) = \frac{(n+\alpha-\gamma)\cdots(1+\alpha-\gamma)}{n!(n+1-\gamma)\cdots(2-\gamma)}, \tag{9.892a–d}$$

that coincides with (9.890b) with the substitutions (9.892a–c). Using (9.887e; 9.892a, b) in (9.891b) the second regular integral (9.377b) is (9.893b):

$$\gamma \notin | N_0: \qquad y(x) = x^{1-\gamma}\, {}_1F_1(\alpha+1-\gamma; 2-\gamma; x), \tag{9.893a, b}$$

that is linearly independent from the first (9.891b) provided that (9.893a) the indices (9.887d, e) do not differ by an integer. It has been shown that *the general integral of the confluent hypergeometric differential equation (9.869b) is (standard*

CCCLXXXVIII) a linear combination (9.894c) with arbitrary constants C_1, C_2 of the linearly independent particular integrals (9.891b; 9.893b):

$$\gamma \notin| Z; \quad |z| < \infty: \qquad y(x) = C_1\, {}_1F_1(\alpha;\gamma;x) + C_2\, x^{1-\gamma}\, {}_1F_1(1+\alpha-\gamma;2-\gamma;x), \tag{9.894a–c}$$

where : (i) appear the confluent hypergeometric series (9.891a–d); (ii) the radius of convergence is infinite (9.894b); and (iii) the parameter γ is not zero or a negative integer (9.894a), otherwise the confluent hypergeometric function of the second kind (note 9.28) is needed.

9.9.9 Continued Fraction for the Generalized Bessel Function

Substituting the confluent hypergeometric series (9.891c) in (9.885c) leads to (9.895):

$$J_\gamma^\mu(x) = D(\mu,\nu)\, x^\nu \frac{\Gamma(1+\nu)}{\Gamma(\nu/2-1/\mu)} \sum_{n=0}^{\infty} \frac{\left(\mu x^2/4\right)^n}{n!} \frac{\Gamma(n+\nu/2-1/\mu)}{\Gamma(1+n+\nu)}. \tag{9.895}$$

Comparison of (9.895) with the series (9.450b) for the generalized Bessel function specifies the coefficient (9.896a):

$$2^{-\nu} = D(\mu,\nu)\Gamma(1+\nu); \qquad J_\nu^\mu(x) = \frac{(x/2)^\nu}{\Gamma(1+\nu)}\, {}_1F_1\left(\frac{\nu}{2}-\frac{1}{\mu};1+\nu;\frac{\mu x^2}{4}\right), \tag{9.896a, b}$$

substitution of (9.896a) in (9.885b) leads to *the relation (9.896b) between (standard CCCLXXXIX) the generalized Bessel function (9.450b) and the confluent hypergeometric function (9.891c), and hence to (standard CCCXC) the continued fraction for the logarithmic derivative of the generalized Bessel function (9.897b):*

$$\mu \neq 0: \quad \frac{d}{dx}\left\{\log\left[J_\nu^\mu(x)\right]\right\} = \frac{\nu}{x} + \frac{\nu/2-1/\mu}{1+\nu-x+} \frac{(\nu/2-1/\mu+1)x}{2+\nu-x} \cdots \frac{(\nu/2-1/\mu+n)x}{n+1+\nu-x+}, \tag{9.897a, b}$$

valid for non-zero degree (9.897a). The proof of (9.897b) follows taking the logarithmic derivative of (9.896b) and using the continued fraction (9.874). The method used was: (i) to transform the generalized Bessel differential equation (9.428a–f) to the confluent hypergeometric differential equation (9.869c); (ii) hence to relate the generalized Bessel function to the confluent hypergeometric function (9.885b) to within a multiplying factor dependent on the parameters and independent of the variable; (iii) the multiplying factor is determined (9.896a) comparing the respective series for the generalized

Bessel (9.450b) and confluent hypergeometric (9.891c) functions; and (iv) logarithmic differentiation of the relation (9.896b) thus obtained and use of (9.874) leads to the continued fraction for the logarithmic derivative of the generalized Bessel function (9.897b) that is not valid for the ordinary Bessel function (9.897a). A continued fraction for the original Bessel function is obtained (subsection 9.9.11) by a different method based on recurrence relations (subsection 9.9.10).

9.9.10 Recurrence and Differentiation Relations for Cylinder Functions

The **cylinder functions** are solutions of the original Bessel differential equation (9.430b), including the Bessel (9.510a, b) ≡ (9.898a), Neumann (9.511; 9.509b) ≡ (9.898b), and Hankel (9.571a, b) ≡ (9.898c, d) functions:

$$C_\nu(x) \equiv \left\{J_\nu(x), \Psi_\nu(x); H_\nu^{(1,2)}(x)\right\}: \qquad C_\nu(x) = i\int_L e^{-i\nu s + ix\sin s}\, ds, \qquad (9.898a\text{–}e)$$

they all have (9.837b) parametric integral representations of the form (9.899e) with distinct paths of integration L in the complex x-plane. Since the following results depend only on the uniform convergence of the integrals (9.899e) and not on the particular path they apply to all cylinder functions. The change of variable (9.899a) implies (9.899b, c):

$$u = e^{is}, \quad du = ie^{is}ds = iu\,ds, \qquad 2i\sin s = e^{is} - e^{-is} = u - \frac{1}{u}, \qquad (9.899a\text{–}c)$$

and leads to the parametric integral representation (9.900) for the cylinder functions (9.899a–e):

$$C_\nu(x) = \int_L u^{-\nu-1} \exp\left[\frac{x}{2}\left(u - \frac{1}{u}\right)\right] du. \qquad (9.900)$$

An integration by parts leads to (9.901a):

$$\begin{aligned} C_\nu(x) &= -\frac{1}{\nu}\int d\left(u^{-\nu}\right)\exp\left[\frac{x}{2}\left(u-\frac{1}{u}\right)\right] = \frac{1}{\nu}\int u^{-\nu}\, d\left\{\exp\left[\frac{x}{2}\left(u-\frac{1}{u}\right)\right]\right\} \\ &= \frac{x}{2\nu}\int\left(u^{-\nu} + u^{-\nu-2}\right)\exp\left[\frac{x}{2}\left(u-\frac{1}{u}\right)\right]du = \frac{x}{2\nu}\left[C_{\nu+1}(x) + C_{\nu-1}(x)\right], \end{aligned}$$

(9.901a–d)

where: (i) a boundary term was omitted in (9.901b) due to the choice of path of integration (subsection 9.8.13); and (ii) in (9.901c) was used (9.900) leading to (9.901d).

Differentiation of (9.900) leads to (9.902a, b):

$$2C'_\nu(x) = \int_L \left(u^{-\nu} - u^{-\nu-2}\right)\exp\left[\frac{x}{2}\left(u - \frac{1}{u}\right)\right]du = C_{\nu-1}(x) - C_{\nu+1}(x). \quad (9.902a, b)$$

Thus *the cylinder functions (9.899a–e) satisfy (standard CCCXCI): (i) the recurrence relation (9.901d) ≡ (9.903a):*

$$\frac{2\nu}{x}C_\nu(x) = C_{\nu+1}(x) + C_{\nu-1}(x); \qquad 2C'_\nu(x) = C_{\nu-1}(x) - C_{\nu+1}(x). \quad (9.903a, b)$$

and (ii) the differentiation formulas (9.902b) ≡ (9.903b) and (9.903c, d):

$$C'_\nu(x) = \frac{\nu}{x}C_\nu(x) - C_{\nu+1}(x) = C_{\nu-1}(x) - \frac{\nu}{x}C_\nu(x). \quad (9.903c, d)$$

The latter (9.903c) [(9.903d)] follow substituting (9.903b) in (9.903a) in different ways (9.904a) [(9.904b)]:

$$2C'_\nu(x) = -C_{\nu+1}(x) - C_{\nu+1}(x) + \frac{2\nu}{x}C_\nu(x), \quad (9.904a)$$

$$2C'_\nu(x) = C_{\nu-1}(x) + C_{\nu-1}(x) - \frac{2\nu}{x}C_\nu(x). \quad (9.904b)$$

From the relations (9.903a–d) can be deduced other differentiation relations (subsection 9.9.11) and a continued fraction (subsection 9.9.12).

9.9.11 Cylinder Functions with Integer Order Difference

The differentiation formula (9.903c) can be written (9.905a):

$$x^{-\nu-1}C_{\nu+1}(x) = -x^{-\nu-1}C'_\nu(x) + \nu x^{-\nu-2}C_\nu(x) = -\frac{1}{x}\frac{d}{dx}\left[x^{-\nu}C_\nu(x)\right], \quad (9.905a, b)$$

that is re-arranged (9.905b). Applying (9.905b) n times leads to the relation between cylinder functions (9.906b) whose orders differ by a positive integer (9.906a):

$$n \in |N: \qquad x^{-\nu-n}C_{\nu+n}(x) = (-)^n\left(\frac{1}{x}\frac{d}{dx}\right)^n\left[x^{-\nu}C_\nu(x)\right]. \quad (9.906a, b)$$

Setting (9.907a) and applying (9.906b) to the spherical Bessel (9.519a) [Neumann (9.519c)] functions leads to (9.907b–e) [(9.908a–d)]:

$$\nu=\frac{1}{2}: \quad j_n(x)=\sqrt{\frac{\pi}{2}}\,x^{-1/2}J_{n+1/2}(x)=\sqrt{\frac{\pi}{2}}(-x)^n\left(\frac{1}{x}\frac{d}{dx}\right)^n\left[x^{-1/2}J_{1/2}(x)\right]$$

$$=(-x)^n\left(\frac{1}{x}\frac{d}{dx}\right)^n j_0(x)=x^n\left(-\frac{1}{x}\frac{d}{dx}\right)^n\frac{\sin x}{x}, \tag{9.907a–e}$$

$$y_n(x)=\sqrt{\frac{\pi}{2}}\,x^{-1/2}Y_{n+1/2}(x)=\sqrt{\frac{\pi}{2}}(-x)^n\left(\frac{1}{x}\frac{d}{dx}\right)^n\left[x^{-1/2}Y_{1/2}(x)\right] \tag{9.908a–d}$$

$$=(-x)^n\left(\frac{1}{x}\frac{d}{dx}\right)^n y_0(x)=-x^n\left(-\frac{1}{x}\frac{d}{dx}\right)^n\frac{\cos x}{x},$$

that provide *an alternate proof (standard CCCXCII) of the Rayleigh formulas (9.530c) ≡ (9.907e) [(9.531c) ≡ (9.908d)] for the spherical Bessel (Neumann) functions* [subsection 9.5.26 (9.5.27)].

9.9.12 A Continued Fraction for Cylinder Functions

From the recurrence relation (9.903a) for the cylinder functions in the form (9.909a, b):

$$\frac{C_{\nu-1}(x)}{C_\nu(x)}=\frac{2\nu}{x}-\frac{C_{\nu+1}(x)}{C_\nu(x)}=\frac{2\nu}{x}-\frac{1}{2(\nu+1)/x-C_{\nu+2}(x)/C_{\nu+1}(x)}, \tag{9.909a, b}$$

follows the continued fraction (9.910a):

$$\frac{C_{\nu-1}(x)}{C_\nu(x)}=\frac{2\nu}{x}-\frac{1}{2(\nu+1)/x-}\,\frac{1}{2(\nu+2)/x-}\cdots\frac{1}{2(\nu+n)/x-C_{\nu+n+1}/C_{\nu+n}}, \tag{9.910a}$$

that is equivalent to (9.910c) with remainder (9.910b):

$$r_n(x)\equiv x\frac{C_{\nu+n+1}(x)}{C_{\nu+n}(x)}: \qquad \frac{C_\nu(x)}{C_{\nu-1}(x)}=\frac{2\nu}{x}-\frac{x}{2(\nu+1)-}\,\frac{x^2}{2(\nu+2)-}\cdots\frac{x^2}{2(\nu+n)-r_n(x)}. \tag{9.910b, c}$$

The continued fraction (9.900b) can be (II.1.108) inverted (9.911):

$$\frac{C_\nu(x)}{C_{\nu-1}(x)}=\frac{1}{2\nu/x-}\,\frac{1}{2(\nu+1)/x-}\,\frac{1}{2(\nu+2)/x-}\cdots\frac{1}{2(\nu+n)/x-r_n(x)}. \tag{9.911}$$

If the remainder tends to zero (9.912a) as $n \to \infty$ the continued fraction (9.911) converges to (9.912b):

$$\lim_{n\to\infty} r_n(x) = 0: \quad \frac{C_\nu(x)}{C_{\nu-1}(x)} = \frac{x/(2\nu)}{1-} \frac{x^2/[4\nu(\nu+1)]}{1-} \frac{x^2/[4(\nu+1)(\nu+2)]}{1-} \cdots \frac{x^2/[4(\nu+n)(\nu+n+1)]}{1-}. \tag{9.912a, b}$$

It can be proved [subsections 9.9.5–9.9.6 (9.9.13–9.9.15)] that the continued fractions (9.909b) ≡ (9.912b) converge for real positive (all complex values) of the parameters. It has been shown that *the cylinder functions (9.898a–d) can be represented by (standard CCCXCIII) the equivalent inverse continued fractions (9.909b) ≡ (9.912b) that: (i) converge for all complex values of the parameters; (ii) imply (standard CCCXCIV) the limit (9.913):*

$$\lim_{n\to\infty} x \frac{C_{\nu+n+1}(x)}{C_{\nu+n}(x)} = 0, \tag{9.913}$$

that corresponds to (9.912a; 9.910b) and follows from the comparison of (9.911) ≡ (9.912b). The earlier results (subsections 9.9.5–9.9.6) prove the convergence of the continued fraction (9.879b) ≡ (9.911) only if the coefficients (9.914a, b) are (9.875a, b) real and positive (9.914c–d):

$$a_n(x) = \frac{2(\nu+n)}{x}, \qquad b_n(x) = 1: \qquad \nu > 0 < x. \tag{9.914a–d}$$

The convergence can be proved both for (9.911) ≡ (9.912b) [(9.872) ≡ (9.874)] with coefficients (9.880d, e) [(9.914a, b)] for all complex values of the variable x and parameters, using the following theorem (subsections 9.9.13–9.9.15) for functional continued fractions.

9.9.13 Special Limit Periodic Continued Fractions

The continued fraction (9.879a) represents a function of the variable x if: (i) the coefficients (a_n, b_n), and hence the numerators p_n and denominators q_n depend (9.915a) on x; and (ii) for x in the domain of the function the continuants converge (9.915b):

$$a_0(x) + \frac{b_1(x)}{a_1(x)+} \frac{b_2(x)}{a_2(x)+} \cdots \frac{b_n(x)}{a_n(x)+} \equiv \frac{p_n(x)}{q_n(x)} \equiv X_n(x), \quad \lim_{n\to\infty} X_n(x) = X(x). \tag{9.915a, b}$$

A continued fraction is **limit periodic** if the coefficients converge for large order (9.916a, b):

$$\lim_{n\to\infty} x_n(x) = a, \qquad \lim_{n\to\infty} b_n(x) = b: \qquad 0 \le |a|, |b| \le \infty, \tag{9.916a–d}$$

where the limit may be (9.916c, d) zero, finite, or infinity. The continued fraction for the logarithmic derivative of the confluent hypergeometric function (9.872) ≡ (9.874) [the cylinder functions (9.910a) ≡ (9.912b)] are limit periodic (9.880d, e) [(9.914a, b)] with (9.916a, b) limits (9.917a) [(9.917b)]:

$$\{a,b\} = \{1,0\}, \{\infty,1\}; \quad \gamma \equiv \{p_n, q_n\}: \quad 0 = \sigma^2 + a\sigma + b = (\sigma - \sigma_+)(\sigma - \sigma_-), \tag{9.917a–e}$$

the recurrence formulas (9.878a, b) for the numerators and denominators (9.917c) suggest the consideration of the quadratic polynomial (9.917d). The roots (9.917e) ≡ (9.918a) of (9.917d) are (9.918b, c) in the case (9.917a):

$$\sigma_\pm = -\frac{a}{2} \pm \frac{1}{2}\sqrt{a^2 - 4b}: \qquad \sigma_+ = 0, \quad \sigma_- = -a; \quad \lim_{n\to\infty} \frac{b_n(x)}{a_n(x)} = \frac{b}{a} = 0, \tag{9.918a–d}$$

both cases (9.917a, b) are instances of a **special** limit periodic continued fraction (9.918d) for which the ratio of the limits (9.916a, b) is zero. It follows that the fractions b_n/a_n in (9.915a) are small for sufficiently high order n and thus the continued fraction should converge (9.915b) for all values of the parameters for which it exists. Thus the convergence of the continued fractions (9.872) ≡ (9.874) [(9.909a) ≡ (9.912b)] for the confluent hypergeometric (cylinder) functions for all complex values of the parameter follows from the **theorem of convergence of special limit periodic continued fractions**: *(standard CCCXCIV) a special (9.918d) limit periodic (9.916a, b) continued fraction (9.915a) converges (9.915b) for all values of the variables and parameters.* This proves the vanishing (9.912a) of the remainder (9.910b) of the continued fraction (9.910c) implying (9.913) that the *cylinder functions; that is, the solutions of the Bessel differential equation (9.430b), including the Bessel (9.899a), Neumann (9.899b), and Hankel (9.899c; d) functions have (standard CCCXCV) the asymptotic property (9.913) for high order.*

9.9.14 Convergence of Complex Continued Fractions

The proof of the convergence theorem for special limit periodic continued fractions starts with the assumption (9.918d) that implies that beyond a certain order the individual fractions are small:

$$\forall_{\varepsilon>0}\, \exists_{m_1 \in |N}: \qquad n \ge m_1 \Rightarrow \left|\frac{b_n(x)}{a_n(x)}\right| < \varepsilon. \tag{9.919}$$

From the recurrence formula for the denominators (9.878b) follows (9.920):

$$|q_n(x)| \geq |a_n(x)| \left(|q_{n-1}(x)| - \left|\frac{b_n(x)}{a_n(x)}\right| |q_{n-2}(x)| \right). \tag{9.920}$$

The limits (9.916a, b) imply that (a_n, b_n) are relatively close to (a, b) for large n:

$$\forall_{\delta_1>0<\delta_2} \exists_{m_2 \in |N} \exists_{n \in |N}: \qquad n \geq m_2 \Rightarrow |a_n| \geq |a|(1+\delta_1), \quad |b_n| \leq |b|(1-\delta_2). \tag{9.921a, b}$$

For (9.922a) the largest of the orders in (9.919) and (9.921a, b) the upper bound (9.920) can be re-stated (9.922b):

$$n \geq m \geq m_1, m_2: \qquad |q_n(x)| \geq |a||1+\delta_1| \left\{ |q_{n-1}(x)| - \varepsilon |q_{n-2}(x)| \right\}. \tag{9.922a, b}$$

All assumptions (9.916a, b) [(9.918d)] have been used (9.919) [(9.921a, b)] to prove (9.922a, b); the latter is sufficient to prove the theorem using the general relations for continued fractions (subsection 9.9.5) in a broadly similar but more detailed sequence than before (subsection 9.9.6).

Using the parameters $\lambda_\pm$ defined by:

$$\lambda \equiv |a|(1+\delta_1): \qquad \lambda_- + \lambda_+ = \lambda, \qquad \lambda_- \lambda_+ = \varepsilon, \tag{9.923a–c}$$

the inequality (9.922b) can be re-written (9.924a, b):

$$|q_n(x)| - \lambda_- |q_{n-1}(x)| \geq \lambda_+ |q_{n-1}(x)| - \lambda_- \lambda_+ |q_{n-2}(x)| = \lambda_+ \left\{ |q_{n-1}(x)| - \lambda_- |q_{n-2}(x)| \right\}. \tag{9.924a, b}$$

The roots of the quadratic expression (9.925a–c):

$$0 = (\xi - \lambda_+)(\xi - \lambda_-) = \xi^2 - (\lambda_+ + \lambda_-)\xi + \lambda_+ \lambda_- = \xi^2 - \lambda\xi + \varepsilon\lambda, \tag{9.925a–c}$$

can be used to invert (9.923b, c), leading to (9.926a, b) that implies (9.926c):

$$\lambda_\pm = \frac{\lambda}{2} \pm \frac{1}{2}\sqrt{\lambda^2 - 4\varepsilon} = \frac{\lambda}{2}\left(1 \pm \sqrt{1 - \frac{4\varepsilon}{\lambda^2}}\right): \qquad \lambda > \lambda_+ > \frac{\lambda}{2} > \lambda_- > 0. \tag{9.926a–c}$$

The relation (9.924b) may be applied iteratively $n - m$ times leading to (9.927):

$$|q_n(x)| - \lambda_- |q_{n-1}(x)| \geq (\lambda_+)^{n-m} \left\{ |q_m(x)| - \lambda_- |q_{m-1}(x)| \right\}. \tag{9.927}$$

The last factor in (9.927) is finite (9.928a) and using (9.927) leads to (9.928b–d):

$$A \equiv |q_m(x)| - \lambda |q_{m-1}(x)|: \quad |q_n(x)| \ge \lambda_- |q_{n-1}(x)| + (\lambda_+)^{n-m} A \ge \left(\frac{\lambda}{2}\right)^{n-m} A, \tag{9.928a–c}$$

that is used to complete the proof of the theorem (subsection 9.9.15).

9.9.15 Convergence of Special Continued Fractions

The difference of continuants (9.877a) in modulus has upper bound (9.929b) where (9.929a) is finite:

$$B \equiv |b_2 \cdots b_m|: \qquad |X_n - X_{n-1}| = \frac{|b_2 \cdots b_n|}{|q_n \, q_{n-1}|} = B \frac{|b_m \cdots b_n|}{|q_n \, q_{n-1}|}. \tag{9.929a, b}$$

For order (9.930a) larger than (9.922a) substitution of (9.921b; 9.928c) in (9.929b) leads to (9.930b):

$$n \ge m: \qquad |X_n - X_{n-1}| \le \frac{B}{A^2} \frac{\left[|b|(1-\delta_2)\right]^{n-m}}{(\lambda/2)^{2n-2m-1}}. \tag{9.930a, b}$$

The upper bound can be rewritten (9.930b) ≡ (9.931b) with finite (9.931a):

$$C \le \frac{2B}{\lambda A^2}: \quad |X_n - X_{n-1}| \le C \eta^{n-m}, \quad \eta = \frac{4|b|(1-\delta_2)}{\lambda^2} \le \frac{4\varepsilon(1-\delta_2)}{|a|(1+\delta_1)^2} < 1, \tag{9.931a–e}$$

and the factor (9.931c) involves (9.921b; 9.919) in (9.931d) and is less than unity in (9.931e) for sufficiently small ε.

From (9.932b) follows (9.932c) with finite (9.932a):

$$D = |X_0| + \sum_{k=0}^{m} |X_k - X_{k-1}|: \qquad X_n = X_0 + \sum_{k=0}^{n} (X_k - X_{k-1}), \tag{9.932a, b}$$

$$|X_n| \le D + \sum_{k=m+1}^{n} |X_k - X_{k-1}|. \tag{9.932c}$$

In the inequality (9.932c) may be used (9.931b) leading to (9.933b) and with the change of summation variable (9.933a) to (9.933c):

$$j = k - m - 1: \qquad |X_n| \le D + C \sum_{k=m+1}^{N} \eta^k = D + C \sum_{j=0}^{N-m-1} \eta^j. \tag{9.933a–c}$$

The condition (9.931e) allows summation of the geometric series (I.21.62a) in (9.934a) leading to the upper bound:

$$|X| = \lim_{n\to\infty}|X_n| \le D + C\sum_{j=0}^{\infty}\eta^j = D + \frac{C}{1-\eta}; \tag{9.934a–c}$$

thus the continuants (9.934a–c) and hence the continued fraction (9.914a) converge (9.914b). QED. The methods of solution of linear differential equations with variable coefficients (notes 9.4–9.9) have been illustrated using the generalized (9.428a–f) [original (9.430b)] Bessel differential equation and associated functions, and apply as well to a variety of other special functions, some of which are mentioned briefly next (notes 9.1–9.47).

NOTE 9.1: Classes of Differential Equations with Exact Analytical Solutions

Exact analytic solutions are available only for a limited set of classes of ordinary differential equations (recollection 10.1), covering only a small part of relevant applications (recollection 10.2). To be more precise: (i) linear ordinary differential equations and simultaneous systems with constant coefficients and without forcing can always be solved subject to the determination of the roots of the characteristic polynomial (sections 1.3 and 7.4); (ii) several methods of solution apply to a variety of forcing terms (sections 1.4–1.5 and 7.5); and (iii) analog methods apply to linear equations with power coefficients (sections 1.6–1.8 and 7.6–7.7) and to finite difference equations (sections 1.9 and 7.8–7.9). Solutions for general forms of forcing terms (note 1.1) can be obtained using: (i) the method of variation of parameters (notes 1.2–1.4); (ii) the Green or influence functions (notes 1.5–1.8); (iii) Fourier series (notes 1.9–1.10); (iv) Fourier integrals (notes 1.11–1.14); and (v) Laplace transforms (notes 1.15–1.28). The latter three are also useful in connection with initial and boundary conditions respectively in (iii) finite, (iv) infinite, and (v) semi-infinite intervals.

Exact analytical solutions of (i) linear differential equations with variable coefficients or (ii) non-linear differential equations are the exception rather than the rule. They apply to a fair number of classes of first-order differential equations and differentials in several variables (chapter 3 and sections 5.1–5.5), and become fewer for higher-order equations (sections 5.6–5.9) and simultaneous systems (section 7.1–7.2). Exact analytical solutions in finite or explicit form are not possible for most linear differential equations with variable coefficients; these lead to special or extended functions (notes 9.6–9.47) expressible as power series (sections 9.4–9.7) or parametric integrals (section 9.8) or continued fractions (section 9.9). The exact analytical solutions, even in non-closed form, are less frequent for non-linear differential or integral equations more so if the coefficients are variable. The present account has included a fair number of non-linear differential equations, and lesser number of linear differential equations with variable coefficients; some of the main methods of solution of the latter have been presented (sections 9.4–9.9) using as example the original and generalized Bessel differential equation and associated functions. Other examples are briefly mentioned in the sequel (note(s) 9.5–9.47). Their relative scarcity makes the exact analytical solutions of differential equations which are available even more valuable, because (i) they demonstrate the detailed properties of solutions applicable to important practical problems; and (ii) they suggest approaches to obtain some properties of more general differential equations, as indicated next.

NOTE 9.2: Existence, Unicity, and Regularity Theorems

When an exact analytical solution of a differential equation is not available in a closed form, or is too cumbersome as a series or integral, approximate methods may be used, either (i) numerical or (ii) analytical. The numerical methods (notes 4.1–4.13) can in principle be applied to any differential equation, and will in most cases (i.e., if they are neither divergent nor unstable) lead to a "result," whose correctness needs to be established, raising four questions: (i) does a solution exist? If not, the result cannot be correct; (ii) is the solution unique? If not, the method could oscillate between several solutions and converge to none of them; (iii/iv) is the solution continuous or differentiable with regard to (iii) initial conditions and/or (iv) parameters of the problem? If not, interpolation between solutions for different initial conditions and/or parameters may be invalid.

Thus a reliable application of a numerical method to the solution of a differential equation requires that: (I) the solution exists (i) and is unique (ii); (II) the method chosen converges to the solution (v) with sufficient accuracy (vi); (III) the proof of the convergence and accuracy of the method may require knowledge of some properties of the solution, like (ii–iv). The theorems on existence, unicity, and regularity of solutions of differential equations fortunately apply to much wider classes of differential equations (sections 9.1–9.3) than those for which solutions are known or can hopefully be found; unfortunately, most of these theorems give no hint of how the solution might be found, so that approximate methods are the only way forward.

The importance of the existence, unicity, and regularity theorems for the solution of differential equations is that: (a) they provide a check on the properties of analytical solutions, when they are available; (b) otherwise, when analytical solutions are not available, they enable approximate solutions. There are several approaches to the proof of theorems of existence, unicity, and regularity of solution of differential approximations and to establish their properties, both in the qualitative (quantitative) theory of differential equations [chapter 4 (9)] that in fact overlap: some methods provide qualitative properties, others quantitative solutions, and still others provide both; for example, a qualitative method may suggest the form of a solution enabling a quantitative method to obtain that solution.

NOTE 9.3: Qualitative Theory of Differential Equations

The existence, unicity, and regularity theorems obtained by the Picard method (section 9.1) may be seen as the "classical" precursors of the "modern" qualitative theory of differential equations, since they have the same objective: to establish some properties of the solution of a differential equation without actually solving it, for example by examining its functional form. The four theorems of Lyapunov are good examples of the qualitative theory of differential equations. The first and third theorems of Lyapunov (section 9.2), which concern the stability of non-linear systems together with the mapping theorems of Poincaré (sections 4.8–4.9), have received most attention due to their application to non-linear dynamical systems (chapter 4). The other two Lyapunov theorems on linear differential equations, with bounded (periodic) coefficients have also been mentioned (section 9.2) as the second and fourth theorems.

Both the Poincare and Lyapunov approaches are relevant and to some extent complementary, to address the problem of stability of systems: (i) an unstable system cannot be expected to be found in nature, because possible environmental perturbations are likely to cause its transition to another state; and (ii) the instability of a device, a structure, or a machine can impair its ability to perform the task it was designed for, or even cause incidents or accidents. The assessment of stability or instability cannot be restricted to differential equations for which analytical solutions are available; the approximate methods considerably enlarge the scope of stability analysis to non-linear and variable systems that may be intractable from the more demanding point-of-view of exact solutions. The key to the Lyapunov method (section 9.2) is the choice of the Lyapunov function, which plays a role similar to the perturbation energy: if it decays (does not decay) to zero an equilibrium position is (cannot be) stable.

The Lyapunov function may be the energy or it may be another function; for example, if there is no energy balance or it does not have the required properties. The key to the Lyapunov method is to find an appropriate Lyapunov function; just as some existence and unicity theorems do not hint at the form of the solution, the Lyapunov method does not hint at the form of the Lyapunov function. Two examples of Lyapunov functions were given in the proof of theorems linear and non-linear differential equation as several examples of linear dynamical systems were given in connection with oscillator with one (chapter 2 and 4) or several (chapter 8) degrees of freedom. The case of linear differential equations with periodic coefficients leads to the Floquet theory (section 9.3) that applies in particular to the Mathieu equation describing single parametric resonance (section 4.3) and to its extension to the Hill equation (section 9.7) applying to multiple parametric resonance.

NOTE 9.4: Approximate Numerical and Analytic Solutions of Differential Equations

The subject of differential (and integral) equations is arguably the most important topic of mathematical physics since the majority of quantitative scientific and technological problems lead to (i) ordinary or (ii) partial differential equations, (iii) integral equations, or (iv) coupled integro-differential systems with suitable (a) boundary and/or (b) initial conditions. The present volume presents mostly methods of analytical solution of ordinary differential equations as an introduction to a subject that will be present in every subsequent volume of the course. There are other analytical methods of solution of differential-integral equations as well as numerical methods and approximate methods (Diagram 9.1). There is a variety of approximate analytical methods of solution of differential equations, of which three were mentioned: (i) perturbation expansions, mostly for non-linear problems, like the free and forced oscillations of anharmonic oscillators (section 4.5), non-linear resonance (section 4.6), and the strong bending and stretching of plates (section 6.9); (ii) the wave envelope technique used to study the parametric resonance of an oscillator with vibrating support (section 4.3); and (iii) the "ray approximation" to linear second-order differential equations with variable coefficients (notes 5.1–5.20).

The linear differential equations with variable coefficients can have "turning points"; that is, points where the nature of the solution changes from

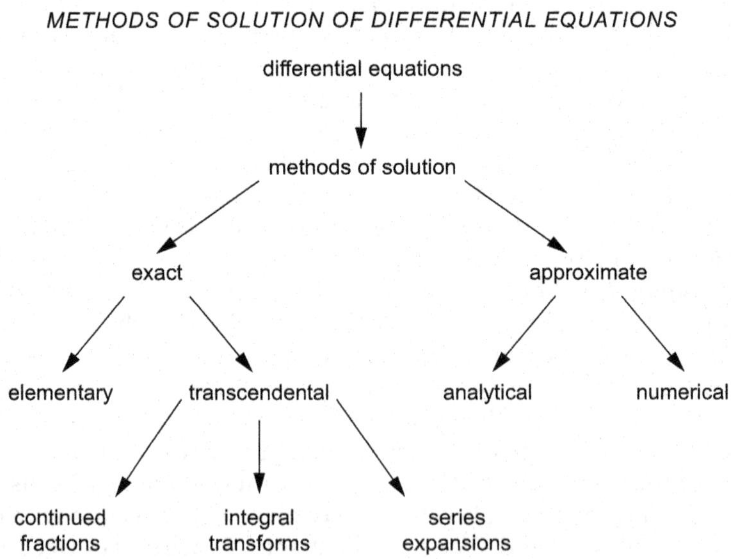

DIAGRAM 9.1
Some possible choices as methods of solution of differential equations and simultaneous systems including linear and non-linear, constant or variable coefficients, and forced and unforced.

monotonic to oscillatory; this could be seen as another aspect of the qualitative theory of differential equations, as it adds an approximate solution (notes 5.1–5.20). The approximate solution was applied to the longitudinal vibrations of a rod of varying cross-section; this "solid displacement amplifier" has a cut-off frequency associated with vibrations with variable amplitude and non-linear phase. There are a number of analogous wave propagation or filtering problems (notes 7.1–7.55): (i/ii) transverse or torsional vibrations of a rod of varying cross section; (iii/v) transverse vibrations of a string, membrane, or plate of varying thickness; (vi) sound propagation in a tube of varying cross-section; (vii) electromagnetic wave propagation in a non-uniform wave guide; (viii/ix) water waves in a basin of variable depth or a channel of variable width. All of these wave problems are described by partial differential equations, in the same cases as the ordinary differential equations: (a/b) linear (non-linear) for small (large) gradients or amplitudes; (α/β) with constant (variable) coefficients for uniform (non-uniform) media.

NOTE 9.5: Ordinary and Partial Differential Equations

The ordinary (partial) differential equations are considered in volume IV (V) of the present series. Two cases when a partial differential equation can be reduced to a set of ordinary differential equations are illustrated: (i) the method of separation of variables for linear differential equations, that in the case of two independent variables always applies for constant coefficients (notes 6.1–6.22); and (ii) the coefficients depend only on one variable (notes 5.1–5.20 and 7.1–7.55). The (ii) approximate methods can be: (ii-1) analytical, in which some terms of the equations are omitted, in cases where they are negligible compared with the terms retained; or (ii-2) numerical when a continuous problem is discretized with a certain error, or the values are taken from measurements with limited accuracy. The (i) exact methods lead to solutions that are expressible (i-1) in finite terms using only elementary functions (chapters 1–8) or (i-2) require infinite or transcendental representations like series, parametric integrals, or continued fractions (chapter 9). The second-order differential equations are an example: (i) in the linear case with constant (homogenous) coefficients the exact solution is elementary (sections 1.3–1.9 and 7.4–7.9); (ii) in the linear case with variable coefficients the JWKB or ray approximation may apply (notes 5.1–5.19); (iii) the exact solution in linear cases with variable coefficients may require non-elementary or higher transcendental functions (sections 9.3–9.9, notes 5.1–5.20, 7.1–7.55, and 9.1–9.47).

NOTE 9.6: Non-Cartesian, Inhomogenous, and Unsteady Problems

The linear unforced differential equations (simultaneous systems) with constant coefficients [sections 1.3–1.5 (7.4–7.5)] can be solved in terms of exponentials possibly with powers, using the (matrix of) characteristic polynomial(s), thus reducing to an algebraic problem of finding roots and solving linear systems. The linear differential equations or simultaneous systems with constant coefficients most often hold only if four conditions are met: (i) small perturbations or slopes to linearize the differential equation; (ii) Cartesian coordinates so that the scale factors are unity in the invariant differential operators like the gradient, curl, divergence, and Laplacian; and (iii–iv) steady, homogenous medium so that the coefficients are constant, that is do not depend on position or time. Even in the linear case (i), the other conditions may not be met, for example: (ii) for a problem with curved boundaries (such as cylindrical/spherical), the use of curvilinear coordinates (cylindrical/spherical) introduces scale factors dependent on position, hence not constant; (iii–iv) if the properties of the medium (or parameters of the system) depend on position and/or time, these dependences may affect the coefficients, that are again not constant. It may be quite useful, even for linear differential equations with variable coefficients, to consider approximations with constant coefficients, that lead to straightforward solutions and simple interpretations as a preliminary step; however, this may not be enough, and the solution of the linear differential equations with variable coefficients may require special functions.

The difference between ordinary (special) functions, that is the elementary (higher) transcendental functions are: (i) they provide the solution of linear (non-linear) differential equations with constant (variable) coefficients; (ii) they have mostly simple (less simple) properties that are straightforward (less straight forward) to prove in many cases; and (iii) the same (different) functions provide solutions for all (distinct) linear (non-linear) differential equations with constant (variable) coefficients. Thus the designation special functions applies to a set of functions with different properties, opening up a vast subject, that can be addressed in three ways: (i) a dedicated monograph for each set of functions demonstrating in detail its properties; (ii) a broader coverage in a volume with a chapter on each function proving the main properties; or (iii) a table of functions listing most known properties with conditions of validity and without proofs. There is some benefit in knowing how to derive the equations and properties: (i) it ensures that all conditions of validity are met; (ii) if one or more are not met, it may suggest either (a) suitable methods of generalization or (b) why such a generalization cannot hold. The purpose of chapter 9 is to indicate some general methods of solution of linear differential equations, illustrating them with the original and generalized Bessel functions. There are many other special functions of frequent use, and some of them are briefly mentioned in the sequel.

NOTE 9.7: Special or Higher Transcendental Functions

There are relations among many special functions, and thus a good starting point is the Gaussian hypergeometric differential equation (note 9.14) that has three regular singularities. The Gaussian hypergeometric functions (notes 9.15–9.19) have three parameters and are equivalent to the hyperspherical associated Legendre functions (note 9.23) that also have three parameters, and include (note 9.24) as particular cases: (i, ii) with two parameters the associated (hyperspherical) Legendre functions [note 9.22 (9.25)]; and (iii) with one parameter the common sub-case of (i, ii) that is the original Legendre functions (note 9.20). The Gaussian hypergeometric functions are equivalent to (include) the Jacobi (ultraspherical Legendre) functions that have three (two) parameters [note 9.26 (9.21)]. The particular one parameter cases of the Gaussian hypergeometric functions include the Chebychev functions of the first (second) type [note 9.27 (9.28)]. The coalescence of two singularities of the Gaussian hypergeometric differential equation leads to the confluent hypergeometric differential equation (note 9.29). The confluent hypergeometric functions (subsection 9.9.6) have two parameters and are equivalent to the generalized Bessel (associated Laguerre) functions [subsection 9.9.8 (note 9.31)] that include as a particular one parameter case the original Bessel (Laguerre) functions [subsection 9.5.22 (note 9.30)]. The confluent hypergeometric functions also include the Hermite functions (note 9.32). The preceding special functions (notes 9.19–9.32) are part of the sub-Gaussian hypergeometric set (note 9.33) that is are all equivalent alternatives or particular cases of the Gaussian hypergeometric functions (notes 9.14–9.18).

The set of super-Gaussian hypergeometric differential equations and special functions (note 9.34) consists of those not reducible to the Gaussian hypergeometric case because they extend it in several possible directions: (I) more than three regular singularities, for example the Heun differential equation; (II) at least one irregular singularity of degree more than unity, for example the Mathieu (Hill) differential equation [subsections 4.3.2–4.3.11 (9.7.11–9.7.16)] that has an irregular singularity of degree two (infinite degree) and are a particular case of the generalized Hill differential equation (note 9.34); and (III) differential equations of higher order, for example the generalized hypergeometric differential equation (notes 9.9–9.13) of order *N*. The singly extended differential equations, for example the extended confluent (Gaussian) hypergeometric [note(s) 9.37 (9.35–9.36)] differential equations differ by allowing the singularity at infinity to be irregular of any degree by modifying only one coefficient. The doubly extended differential equation, which may be designated extended Bessel differential equation (note 9.38) changes two coefficients so that the singularity at the origin (infinity) remains regular (is irregular) of any degree. A linear second-order differential equation can be re-written in self-adjoint (invariant) forms [notes 5.7 (5.8)] leading to transformations of the differential equations associated with special functions (notes 9.39–9.43); for example the invariant form of the confluent hypergeometric differential equations leads to the Whittaker differential equation (notes 9.39–9.41). Two classes of other transformations are applied to the generalized Bessel differential equation, involving changes of variable, either the independent or the dependent variable or both. The special functions are a large and important set of functions (note 9.46) with an extensive theory (note 9.47) of which the present note is a small sample focused on the solution of the corresponding differential equation. Although the generalized hypergeometric differential equation of order N (notes 9.9–9.13) includes most others, its solution is fairly straightforward using a method of two characteristic polynomials (note 9.8).

NOTE 9.8: Methods of One or Two Characteristic Polynomials

The method of one or two characteristic polynomials (Table 9.9) is one of the simplest approaches to solving important classes of ordinary differential or finite difference equations. The characteristic polynomial of a linear differential equation with constant coefficients (sections 1.3–1.5) specifies the solutions through its roots; for example in the unforced (section 1.3) case the solutions are exponentials without (with) power factors for single (multiple) roots. Similar solutions apply for simultaneous systems of linear differential equations with constant coefficients (sections 7.4–7.5), using a matrix of polynomials of ordinary differential operators and its determinant as the characteristic polynomial. In the case of a linear differential equations with variable coefficients that are linear functions of the independent variable (subsections 9.8.5–9.8.11) there are two characteristic polynomials appearing in a parametric integral solution that is a generalized Laplace transform with symmetric exponential kernel and integration along a path in the complex plane.

The method of characteristic polynomials also applies [subsection(s) 1.9 (7.8–7.9)] to linear finite difference equations (simultaneous systems), and to linear differential equations (coupled systems) with homogenous derivatives [sections 1.6–1.8 (7.6–7.7)]. For linear differential equations with power coefficients leading to homogenous derivatives the characteristic polynomial also specifies the solutions (sections 1.6–1.8); for example, in the unforced case (sections 1.6) the solutions are powers without (with) logarithmic factors for single (multiple) roots. Similar solutions apply to a simultaneous system of

TABLE 9.9

Method of Characteristic Polynomials

Derivative	Ordinary	Homogeneous
Linear differential equation	Constant coefficients	Homogeneous coefficients
Operator	One polynomial: sections 1.3–1.6	One polynomial: sections 1.7–1.8
Simultaneous systems of differential equations	Constant coefficients	Homogeneous coefficients
Operator	Matrix of polynomials: sections 7.3–7.5	Matrix of polynomials: sections 7.6–7.8
Linear differential equation	Linear coefficients	Polynomial coefficients
Method	generalized Laplace transform subsections: 9.8.5–9.8.8	Regular integrals of 2 kinds: notes 9.9–9.18

linear differential equations with homogenous derivatives, using a matrix of polynomials of homogenous differential operators and its determinant as "the" characteristic polynomial (sections 9.6–9.7). The method of two characteristic polynomials applies to a differential equation consisting of two sets of linear homogenous derivatives with one set multiplied by the independent variable (note 9.9). This leads to power series solutions with two-term recurrence relations that can be solved explicitly (note 9.10). In other words, the generalized hypergeometric differential equation of order N has explicit solutions in term of generalized hypergeometric functions of two kinds (notes 9.11–9.13). The particular case of a second-order $N=2$ differential equation is the Gaussian hypergeometric differential equation (notes 9.14–9.19) that leads to sub-hypergeometric differential equations (notes 9.20–9.33) but does not include the super-hypergeometric differential equations (notes 9.34–9.39).

NOTE 9.9: Method of Two Polynomials of Homogenous Derivatives

The linear differential equation with homogenous derivatives (sections 1.6–1.8), involves a single characteristic polynomial, and in the unforced case has solutions as single powers (multiplied by logarithms) for single (multiple) roots. The single powers are replaced by power series in the **method of two polynomials of homogenous derivatives**, that applies to the solution of the differential equation (9.935c) consisting of (9.935a, b) the difference of two polynomials of arbitrary degrees N, M, with one multiplied by the independent variable:

$$P_N(a) \equiv \prod_{n=1}^{N}(a-\alpha_n),\; Q_M(a) \equiv \prod_{m=1}^{M}(a-\beta_m):\; \left\{P_N\left(x\frac{d}{dx}\right) - xQ_M\left(x\frac{d}{dx}\right)\right\}y(x) = 0. \tag{9.935a–c}$$

From (1.303a, b) it follows that each of the polynomials of homogenous derivatives in (9.935c) is of the form (9.936a, b), and thus the differential equation (9.935c) can be re-written (9.936c):

$$P_N\left(x\frac{d}{dx}\right) \equiv \sum_{n=0}^{N} A_n\, x^n \frac{d^n}{dx^n},\quad Q_M\left(x\frac{d}{dx}\right) = \sum_{m=1}^{M} B_m\, x^m \frac{d^m}{dx^m}:$$

$$0 = \sum_{n=1}^{N} A_m\, x^n\, y^{(n)}(x) - \sum_{m=1}^{M} B_m\, x^{m+1}\, y^{(m)}(x). \tag{9.936a–c}$$

The cases $N>M$, $N<M$, and $N=M$ are considered separately respectively in the notes 9.9–9.10, 9.11–9.12, and 9.13–9.14. Starting with the first case (9.937a) the leading term of the differential equation (9.936c) is (9.937b)

showing that is has a regular singularity at the origin so a regular integral solution (9.937d) exists:

$$N > M: \quad 0 = x^N y^{(N)} + \cdots; \quad 0 \le |x| < \infty: \qquad y(x) = \sum_{k=0}^{\infty} x^{k+a} c_k(a); \qquad \text{(9.937a–d)}$$

the only other possible singularity of the differential equation is at infinity, and thus the regular integral solution around the origin (9.937d) converges in the finite x-plane (9.937c).

Substituting the regular integral solution (9.937d) in the differential equation (9.935c) leads to (9.938):

$$0 = \sum_{k=0}^{\infty} P_N(k+a)\, c_k(a)\, x^k - \sum_{j=0}^{\infty} Q_M(j+a)\, c_j(a)\, x^{j+1}, \qquad \text{(9.938)}$$

or (9.939b) with the change of variable of summation (9.939a):

$$j = k-1: \qquad c_0(a) P_N(a) + \sum_{k=1}^{\infty} x^k \left[P_N(k+a) c_k(a) - Q_M(k+a-1) c_{k-1}(a) \right]. \qquad \text{(9.939a, b)}$$

The first term in (9.939b) implies (9.940a) that the indices are the roots of the first polynomial (9.940b):

$$P_N(a) = 0: \quad a_n = \alpha_n: \quad c_k(a) = c_{k-1}(a) \frac{Q_M(k+a-1)}{P_N(k+a)} = c_0(a) \prod_{j=1}^{k} \frac{Q_M(j+a-1)}{P_N(j+a)}, \qquad \text{(9.940a–d)}$$

and the second term in (9.939b) leads to the recurrence formula for the coefficients (9.940c) that may be iterated (9.940d). From (9.940c) follows (9.941a) showing that the coefficients decay like (9.941b):

$$\frac{c_k(a)}{c_{k-1}(a)} \sim O\left(k^{M-N}\right), \quad c_k(a) \sim O(k!)^{M-N}; \quad R = \lim_{k\to\infty} \frac{c_{k-1}(a)}{c_k(a)} \sim \lim_{k\to\infty} O\left(k^{M-N}\right) = \infty, \qquad \text{(9.941a–c)}$$

thus (9.937a) implies that the radius of convergence of convergence of the solution (9.937d) is infinite (9.941c) in agreement with (9.937c).

It has been shown that *the differential equation (9.935c) where (standard CCCXCVI) the first polynomial (9.935a) is of higher degree (9.937a) than (9.935b): (i) has indices that are (9.940b) the roots (9.940a) of the polynomial (9.935a) of higher degree; (ii) if the roots are distinct the general integral is a linear combination (9.942b) with arbitrary constants (9.942a) of functions of the first kind:*

$$A_n \equiv c_0(a_n): \qquad y(x) = \sum_{n=1}^{N} A_n \, y_n(x); \tag{9.942a, b}$$

(iii) the functions of the first kind are regular integrals (9.937d) with indices (9.940b) and coefficients (9.940d) leading to (9.943a):

$$y_n(x) = x^{\alpha_n} \left\{ 1 + \sum_{k=1}^{\infty} x^k \left[\prod_{j=1}^{k} \frac{Q_M(\alpha_n + j - 1)}{P_N(\alpha_n + j)} \right] \right\} \tag{9.943a}$$

$$= x^{\alpha_n} \left\{ 1 + \sum_{k=1}^{\infty} x^k \prod_{j=1}^{k} \left[\frac{\prod_{m=1}^{M} (\alpha_n - \beta_m + j - 1)}{\prod_{\ell=1}^{N} (\alpha_n - \alpha_\ell + j)} \right] \right\} \tag{9.943b}$$

$$= x^{\alpha_n} \left\{ 1 + \left[\frac{\prod_{m=1}^{M} \Gamma(1 + \alpha_n - \alpha_\ell)}{\prod_{m=1}^{N} \Gamma(\alpha_n - \beta_m)} \right] \sum_{k=1}^{\infty} x^k \prod_{j=1}^{k} \left[\frac{\prod_{m=1}^{M} \Gamma(\alpha_n - \beta_m + j)}{\prod_{\ell=1}^{N} \Gamma(\alpha_n - \alpha_\ell + j + 1)} \right] \right\} \tag{9.943c}$$

$$= x^{\alpha_n} \, {}_M F_{N-1} \left(\alpha_n - \beta_1, \ldots, \alpha_n - \beta_M; \alpha_n - \alpha_1, \ldots, \alpha_n - \alpha_{n-1}, \alpha_n - \alpha_{n+1}, \ldots, \alpha_n - \alpha_N; x \right), \tag{9.943d}$$

(iv) the polynomials (9.935a, b) were substituted in (9.943b) and the Gamma function (9.432b) was used in (9.943c); and (v) in (9.943d) appear the ***generalized hypergeometric series*** *with variable x and upper (lower) parameters* $(\delta_1, \ldots, \delta_P)[(\gamma_1, \ldots, \gamma_Q)]$ *defined (example I.30) by (9.944):*

$${}_P F_Q(\delta_1, \ldots, \delta_P; \gamma_1, \ldots \gamma_Q; x) \equiv 1 + \sum_{k=1}^{\infty} \frac{x^k}{k!} \frac{\delta_1 \ldots (\delta_1 + k - 1) \ldots \delta_P \ldots (\delta_P + k - 1)}{\gamma_1 \ldots (\gamma_1 + k - 1) \ldots \gamma_Q \ldots (\gamma_Q + k - 1)}, \tag{9.944}$$

The case of indices differing by an integer leads to functions of the second kind (note 9.16). Next is given an example (note 9.10) with $N = 3, M = 2$ leading to generalized hypergeometric functions of type ${}_2F_2$.

NOTE 9.10: Generalized Hypergeometric Functions of Type $_2F_2$

Consider the differential equation:

$$\left\{\left(x\frac{d}{dx}-\alpha_1\right)\left(x\frac{d}{dx}-\alpha_2\right)\left(x\frac{d}{dx}-\alpha_3\right)-x\left(x\frac{d}{dx}-\beta_1\right)\left(x\frac{d}{dx}-\beta_2\right)\right\}y=0. \tag{9.945}$$

If the indices (9.940b) do not differ by an integer (9.946a) three linearly independent solutions are (9.946c):

$$\alpha_1-\alpha_2,\alpha_1-\alpha_3,\alpha_2-\alpha_3\notin Z;\quad \{\text{r,s,t}\}\equiv\text{circular permutation of }\{1,2,3\}:$$

$$y_r(x)=x^{\alpha_r}\left\{1+\frac{\Gamma(1+\alpha_r-\alpha_s)\,\Gamma(1+\alpha_r-\alpha_t)}{\Gamma(\alpha_r-\beta_1)\,\Gamma(\alpha_r-\beta_2)}\right.$$

$$\left.\times\sum_{k=1}^{\infty}\frac{x^k}{k!}\left[\prod_{j=1}^{k}\frac{\Gamma(\alpha_r-\beta_1+j)\,\Gamma(\alpha_r-\beta_2+j)}{\Gamma(\alpha_r-\alpha_s+j+1)\,\Gamma(\alpha_r-\alpha_t+j+1)}\right]\right\}$$

$$=x^{\alpha_r}\,{}_2F_2\left(\alpha_r-\beta_1,-\alpha_r-\beta_2;1+\alpha_r-\alpha_s,1+\alpha_r-\alpha_t;x\right), \tag{9.946a–d}$$

involving generalized hypergeometric functions (9.946d) of type $_2F_2$ with $\{\alpha_r,\alpha_s,\alpha_t\}$ taking distinct values (1, 2, 3) in a circular permutation (9.946b). The general integral is a linear combination (9.947b) of the three linearly independent solutions (9.946c, d):

$$A_{1,2,3}=c_0(\alpha_{1,2,3}):\qquad y_1(x)=A_1\,y(x)+A_2\,y_2(x)+A_3\,y_3(x), \tag{9.947a, b}$$

with arbitrary constants (9.947a).

The differential equation (9.945) uses the difference of the operators (9.948a) and (9.948b):

$$xQ_2\left(x\frac{d}{dx}\right)=x\left(x\frac{d}{dx}-\beta_1\right)\left(x\frac{d}{dx}-\beta_2\right)=x\left[\left(x\frac{d}{dx}\right)^2-(\beta_1+\beta_2)x\frac{d}{dx}+\beta_1\beta_2\right]$$

$$=x\left[x^2\frac{d^2}{dx^2}+(1-\beta_1-\beta_2)x\frac{d}{dx}+\beta_1\beta_2\right], \tag{9.948a}$$

$$
\begin{aligned}
P_3\left(x\frac{d}{dx}\right) &= \left(x\frac{d}{dx}-\alpha_3\right)\left(x\frac{d}{dx}-\alpha_2\right)\left(x\frac{d}{dx}-\alpha_1\right) \\
&= \left(x\frac{d}{dx}-\alpha_3\right)\left[x^2\frac{d^2}{dx^2}+(1-\alpha_1-\alpha_2)\,x\frac{d}{dx}+\alpha_1\alpha_2\right] \\
&= x^3\frac{d^3}{dx^3}+(3-\alpha_1-\alpha_2-\alpha_3)\,x^2\frac{d^2}{dx^2} \\
&\quad +(1-\alpha_1-\alpha_2-\alpha_3+\alpha_1\alpha_2+\alpha_1\alpha_3+\alpha_2\alpha_3)\,x\frac{d}{dx}-\alpha_1\alpha_2\alpha_3\,;
\end{aligned}
\tag{9.948b}
$$

thus the differential equation (9.945) is equivalent to:

$$
\begin{aligned}
0 &= x^3y'''+(3-x-\alpha_1-\alpha_2-\alpha_3)x^2y'' \\
&\quad +\left[1-\alpha_1-\alpha_2-\alpha_3+\alpha_1\alpha_2+\alpha_1\alpha_3+\alpha_2\alpha_3-x(1-\beta_1-\beta_2)\right]xy' \\
&\quad -\left(\alpha_1\,\alpha_2\,\alpha_3+\beta_1\,\beta_2\,x\right)y=0.
\end{aligned}
\tag{9.949}
$$

It has been shown that *the differential equation (9.945) ≡ (9.949) has (standard CCCXCVII) general integral (9.947a, b) as a linear combination of three generalized hypergeometric functions (9.946b–d) provided that* $(\alpha_1,\alpha_2,\alpha_3)$ *do not differ by an integer (9.946a).* The generalized hypergeometric differential equation (9.935a–c) is solved next (note 9.11) in the second case opposite to (9.937a).

NOTE 9.11: Asymptotic Regular Series Solutions

In the case (9.950a) opposite to (9.937a) the solutions (9.943a–d) do not converge because the coefficients in (9.937b) diverge (9.941a). This suggests the change of independent variable (9.950b, c) that leads to (9.950d):

$$
M>N: \qquad \xi=\frac{1}{x}, \qquad w(\xi)=y(x): \qquad x\frac{d}{dx}=-\,\xi\frac{d}{d\xi}. \tag{9.950a–d}
$$

Substitution of (9.950b–d) in (9.935c) leads to the differential equation (9.951):

$$
\left\{Q_M\left(-\xi\frac{d}{d\xi}\right)-\xi\,P_N\left(-\xi\frac{d}{d\xi}\right)\right\}w(\xi)=0, \tag{9.951}
$$

that interchanges the polynomials (9.952a) with reversed sign of the argument in the asymptotic regular integral (9.952b, c):

$$\{P_N(a), Q_M(a)\} \leftrightarrow \{Q_M(-a), P_N(-a)\}: \quad w(\xi) = \xi^a \sum_{k=0}^{\infty} e_n(a)\,\xi^n$$

$$= x^{-a} \sum_{k=0}^{\infty} e_n(a)\, x^{-n} = y(x); \tag{9.952a–c}$$

thus the indices (9.953b) are now the roots of (9.953a) and the coefficients (9.940b, c) are replaced by (9.952c):

$$Q_M(-a) = 0: \qquad a_m = -\beta_m; \qquad e_k(a) = e_0(a) \prod_{j=1}^{k} \frac{P_N(j+a-1)}{Q_M(j+a)}. \tag{9.953a–c}$$

The order of the differential equation is now M, the same as the number of indices (9.953a, b), and the coefficients (9.941a–c) with (N, M) interchanged show that the solutions converge in the whole complex x-plane including the point at infinity and excluding the origin.

It has been shown that *the differential equation (9.935a–c) in the case (9.950a) has (standard CCCXCVIII) general integral (9.954c) valid in the whole complex plane including the point at infinity and excluding the origin (9.954a):*

$$0 < |x| \le \infty; \quad B_m = e_0(-\beta_m): \qquad y(x) = \sum_{m=1}^{M} B_m\, y^m(x), \tag{9.954a–c}$$

that is a linear combination with arbitrary constants of the regular asymptotic series (9.955a):

$$y^{(m)}(x) = x^{-\beta_m} \left\{ 1 + \sum_{k=1}^{\infty} x^{-k} \left[\prod_{j=1}^{k} \frac{P_N(-\beta_m + j - 1)}{Q_M(-\beta_m + j)} \right] \right\}, \tag{9.955a, b}$$

$$= x^{-\beta_m}\, {}_{M-1}F_N\left(-\beta_m - \beta_1, \ldots, -\beta_m - \beta_{m-1}, -\beta_m - \beta_{m+1}, \ldots, -\beta_m - \beta_M; -\beta_m - \alpha_1, \ldots, -\beta_m - \alpha_n; \frac{1}{x}\right),$$

involving generalized hypergeometric functions (9.955b) of variable 1/x. An example with $M = 3, N = 2$ follows, leading to generalized hypergeometric functions of type ${}_2F_2$, this time as asymptotic series (note 9.12).

NOTE 9.12: Generalized Hypergeometric Asymptotic Series

The differential equation (9.956):

$$\left\{\left(x\frac{d}{dx}-\alpha_1\right)\left(x\frac{d}{dx}-\alpha_2\right)-x\left(x\frac{d}{dx}-\beta_1\right)\left(x\frac{d}{dx}-\beta_2\right)\left(x\frac{d}{dx}-\beta_3\right)\right\}y=0, \tag{9.956}$$

is (9.948a, b) equivalent to (9.890):

$$\begin{aligned} 0 &= x^3y''' + \left[(3-\beta_1-\beta_2-\beta_3)x-1\right]x^2y'' \\ &+\left[(1-\beta_1-\beta_2-\beta_3+\beta_1\beta_3+\beta_1\beta_3+\beta_2\beta_3)\,x+\alpha_1+\alpha_2-1\right]xy' \\ &-(\beta_1\,\beta_2\,\beta_3\,x-\alpha_1\,\alpha_2)y. \end{aligned} \tag{9.957}$$

Assuming that the indices do not differ by an integer (9.958a), the three (9.958b) linearly independent asymptotic series (9.958c):

$$\begin{aligned} &\beta_r-\beta_s, \beta_r-\beta_t, \beta_s-\beta_t \notin| Z: \quad \{r,s,t\} = \textit{circular permutations of } \{1,2,3\}; \\ &y^r(x) = x^{-\beta_r}\,{}_2F_2\left(-\beta_r-\beta_s, -\beta_r-\beta_t; -\beta_r-\alpha_1, -\beta_r-\alpha_2; \frac{1}{x}\right). \end{aligned} \tag{9.958a–c}$$

specify the general integral:

$$0<|x|\le\infty; \quad B_{1,2,3}=e_0(-\beta_{1,2,3}); \qquad y(x)=\sum_{m=1}^{3}B_m\,y^m(x). \tag{9.959a–c}$$

It has been shown that *the differential equation (9.956) ≡ (9.957) has (standard CCCXCIX) general integral (9.959c) that is a linear combination of generalized hypergeometric asymptotic series of the type (9.958b, c), valid in the whole complex x-plane including the point at infinity and excluding the origin (9.959a), assuming that the indices do not differ by an integer (9.958a).* The differential equation (9.935a–c) has been considered in the opposite cases (9.936a) and (9.950a), and the third remaining case $M = N$ is considered next (note 9.13), when both solutions are valid in distinct regions.

NOTE 9.13: Analytic Continuation between the Interior and Exterior of the Unit Disk

In the case (9.960a) when the polynomials (9.935a, b) in the differential equation (9.935c) have the same degree, both of the preceding solutions apply, namely in ascending (9.942b) ≡ (9.960c) [descending (9.954c) ≡ (9.960e)] series converging inside (9.966b) [outside (9.960d)] the unit disk:

$$N = M: \quad |x| < 1: \quad y(x) = \sum_{n=1}^{N} A_n \, y_n(x), \quad |x| > 1: y(x) = \sum_{n=1}^{N} B_n \, y^n(x). \qquad (9.960\text{a–e})$$

Concerning the ascending series solutions (9.943a–d) the convergence condition is (I.29.2a–c) ≡ (9.961a):

$$1 > \lim_{k\to\infty} \left| x \frac{c_{k+1}(a)}{c_k(a)} \right| = |x| \lim_{k\to\infty} \left| \frac{Q_N(k+a)}{P_N(k+a+1)} \right| = |x| \lim_{k\to\infty} \left| \frac{(k+a-\beta_1)\cdots(k+a-\beta_N)}{(k+a+1-\alpha_1)\cdots(k+a+1-\alpha_N)} \right|, \qquad (9.961\text{a, b})$$

and using (9.935a, b) leads to (9.961b), that can be evaluated as (9.961c–e):

$$\frac{(k+a-\beta_1)\cdots(k+a-\beta_N)}{(k+a+1-\alpha_1)\cdots(k+a+1-\alpha_N)} = \prod_{n=1}^{N} \frac{1 + \dfrac{a-\beta_n}{k}}{1 + \dfrac{a+1-\alpha_n}{k}}$$

$$= \prod_{n=1}^{N} \left(1 + \frac{a-\beta_n}{k}\right) \left[1 - \frac{a+1-\alpha_n}{k} + O\left(\frac{1}{k^2}\right)\right]$$

$$= 1 - \frac{1}{k} \left[N + \sum_{n=1}^{N} (\beta_n - \alpha_n)\right] + O\left(\frac{1}{k^2}\right). \qquad (9.961\text{c–e})$$

Re-writing (9.961b, e) in the form (9.962a, b):

$$g \equiv N + \sum_{n=1}^{N} (\beta_n - \alpha_n); \qquad 1 > |x| \left[1 - \frac{g}{k} + O\left(\frac{1}{k^2}\right)\right], \qquad (9.962\text{a, b})$$

allows application of the combined convergence test (section I.29.1).

From (9.962a, b) and (I.29.3a–c; I.29.4a–d; I.29.5a–d) it follows that *for the generalized hypergeometric differential equation (9.935a–c) in the case (9.960a) of the solution (9.960c) involving (standard CD) the generalized hypergeometric functions (9.943a–d): (i) converges (Figure 9.18a) absolutely (9.963b) [totally (9.963e)] in the open unit disk (9.963a) [closed unit sub-disk (9.963c, d)]:*

$$|x| < 1 \;\Rightarrow\; A.C.; \qquad 0 < \delta < 1: \qquad |x| \le 1 - \delta \;\Rightarrow\; T.C.; \qquad (9.963\text{a–e})$$

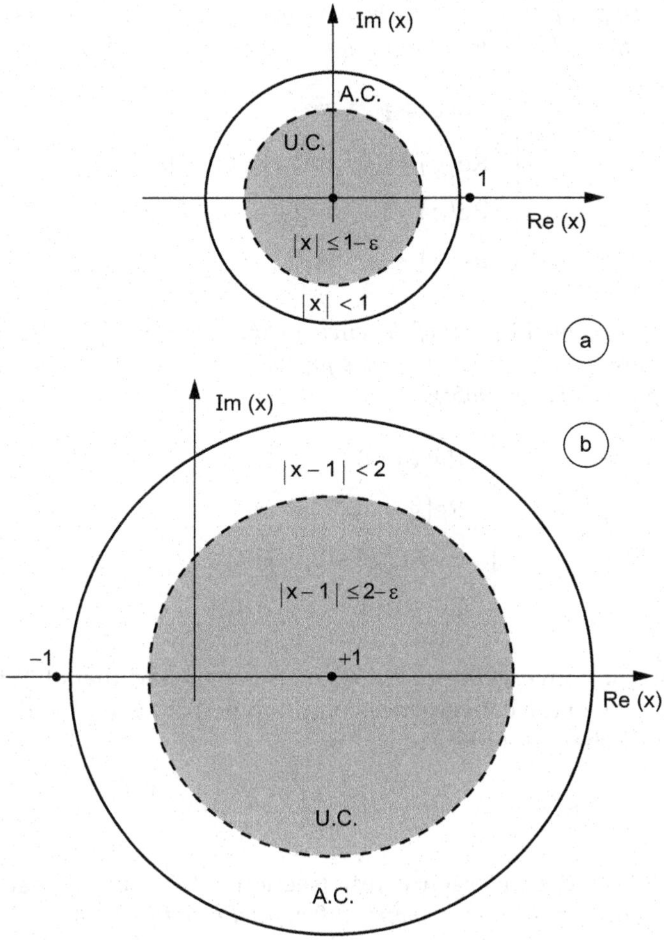

FIGURE 9.18
The region of validity of the solutions of the Gaussian hypergeometric (original, associated, ultraspherical, and hyperspherical Legendre) functions is (a) [(b)] a circle of radius 1 (2) with center at $x = 0(x = 1)$, leading to: (i) absolute convergence in the open interior; also (ii) uniform convergence, hence total convergence (chapter I.21) is a closed sub-disk. The convergence on the boundary circle $|x| = 1\left(|x-1| = 2\right)$ distinguishes the special point $x = 1(x = -1)$ [all other points] and is specified by (9.964a–e) [(9.965a–f)] with g depending on the parameters of the function: (i) Gaussian hypergeometric (9.974c); (ii) Legendre (9.1011f); (iii) ultraspherical Legendre (9.1121f); (iv) associated Legendre (9.1030f); and (v) hyperspherical Legendre (9.1042d). Case (b) also applies to the: (v) Jacobi functions (9.1061d): (vi/vii) Chebychev functions of first (second) type (9.1073g) [(9.1086g)]. Case (b) also applies to the extended Hill differential equation (9.1013e) and case (a) is unchanged (9.974c) for the extended Gaussian hypergeometric functions.

(ii) at the special point (9.964a) in the boundary of convergence the series diverges for (9.964b, c), oscillates for (9.964d) and converges absolutely for (9.964e):

$$x = 1: \quad \begin{cases} \operatorname{Re}(g) < 1: & D. \\ \operatorname{Re}(g) = 1, & \operatorname{Im}(g) = 0: \quad D. \\ \operatorname{Re}(g) = 1, & \operatorname{Im}(g) \neq 0: \quad D. \\ \operatorname{Re}(g) > 1, & A.C.; \end{cases} \tag{9.964a–e}$$

(iii) at the other points (9.965a) of the circle (9.965b) of convergence (dotted curve) the series diverges for (9.965c), oscillates for (9.965d), and converges conditionally (absolutely) for (9.965e) [(9.965f)]:

$$x \neq 1 = |x|: \quad \begin{cases} \operatorname{Re}(g) < 0: & D. \\ \operatorname{Re}(g) = 0: & O. \\ 0 < \operatorname{Re}(g) \leq 1: & C.C. \\ \operatorname{Re}(g) > 1: & A.C. \end{cases} \tag{9.965a–f}$$

Following the convergence of (9.960b, c) is considered that of (9.960d, e). In the case of (9.960e) the convergence condition (9.962b) is replaced by (9.966d) because of the changes (9.966a–c):

$$x \leftrightarrow \frac{1}{x}, \qquad \alpha_n \leftrightarrow \beta_n, \quad g \rightarrow -g: \qquad 1 > \frac{1}{|x|}\left[1 + \frac{g}{k} + O\left(\frac{1}{k^2}\right)\right], \tag{9.966a–d}$$

and the combined convergence test (section I.29.1) applies again stating that *for the generalized hypergeometric differential equation (9.935a–c) in the case (9.960a) the solution (9.960d) involving (standard CDI) the generalized hypergeometric asymptotic series (9.955a, b): (i) converges absolutely (9.967b) outside the unity disk (9.967a) and also uniformly (9.967e) in a closed (9.967d) sub-region (9.967c):*

$$|x| > 1 \;\Rightarrow\; A.C.; \qquad \delta > 0: \qquad |x| \geq 1 + \delta \;\Rightarrow\; T.C.; \tag{9.967a–e}$$

(ii) at the exceptional point (9.968a) on the unit disk there is divergence for (9.968b, c), oscillation for (9.968d), and absolute convergence for (9.968e):

$$x = 1: \quad \begin{cases} \operatorname{Re}(g) > -1: & D. \\ \operatorname{Re}(g) = -1: & \operatorname{Im}(g) = 0: \quad D. \\ \operatorname{Re}(g) = -1: & \operatorname{Im}(g) \neq 0: \quad O. \\ \operatorname{Re}(g) < -1: & A.C.; \end{cases} \tag{9.968a–e}$$

(iii) on the unit disk (9.969a) excluding (9.969b) the exceptional point there is divergence for (9.969c), oscillation for (9.969d), or conditional (absolute convergence for (9.969e) [(9.969f)]:

$$|x| = 1 \neq x: \qquad \begin{cases} \operatorname{Re}(g) > 0: & D. \\ \operatorname{Re}(g) = 0: & O. \\ 0 > \operatorname{Re}(g) \geq -1: & C.C. \\ \operatorname{Re}(g) < -1: & A.C. \end{cases} \tag{9.969a–f}$$

Comparing the two sets of preceding results it follows that *there is (standard CDII) little or no overlap the regions of validity (9.963a–e; 9.964a–e; 9.965a–f) [(9.967a–e; 9.968a–e; 9.969a–f)] of the inner (9.960b, c) [outer (9.960d, e)] solution in ascending (9.943a–d) [descending (9.955a, b)] powers of the generalized hypergeometric differential equation (9.935a–c) in the case (9.960a).* Thus analytic continuation between the interior and exterior of the unit disk requires changes of the independent variable as shown next.

The case (9.960a) of the **generalized hypergeometric differential equation** (9.935a–c) has a regular singularity at $x = 1$, besides the origin and point-at-infinity (9.970a) as in the other cases (9.937a–d; 9.954a–c). The **Schwartz group (1972)** of coordinate transformations (9.970b) interchanges between themselves (9.970c) the regular points (9.970a):

$$x = 0, 1, \infty: \qquad x \to \frac{1}{x}, 1 - x, 1 - \frac{1}{x}, \frac{1}{1-x}, \frac{x}{x-1} \equiv \zeta, \tag{9.970a, b}$$

$$\frac{1}{x} = \infty, 1, 0; \quad 1 - x = 1, 0, \infty; \quad 1 - \frac{1}{x} = \infty, 0, 1; \quad \frac{1}{1-x} = 1, \infty, 0; \quad \frac{x}{x-1} = 0, \infty, 1, \tag{9.970c}$$

and thus: (i) transforms the generalized hypergeometric differential equation (9.935a–c) with variable x to another with variable ζ in (9.970b); and (ii) leads to solutions in terms of generalized hypergeometric functions of the variable ζ in (9.970b), that are valid in overlapping regions $|\zeta| < 1$, thus providing analytic continuation (section I.31.1) over the whose complex x-plane. It has been shown that *the generalized hypergeometric differential equation (9.935a–c) with polynomials of the same degree (9.960a) has (standard CDIII) solutions in terms of: (i/ii) generalized hypergeometric functions (9.942a, b; 9.943a–d) [(9.954a–c; 9.955a, b)] inside (9.963a–e; 9.964a–e; 9.965a, f) [outside (9.967a–e; 9.968a–e; 9.969a–f)] the unit disk; also (iii) in the regions $|\zeta| < 1$ in terms of the variables (9.970b) of the Schwartz group (9.970c) that interchange between themselves the regular singularities (9.970a). This allows several possibilities for analytic continuation over the whole complex x-plane, for example $|\zeta| = |1 - x| < 1$ is (Figure 9.18b)* *the circle of unit radius with center at the unit point and overlaps both with the interior and exterior of unit disk.* The case of three regular singularities (9.970a) for a second-order differential equation leads to the Gaussian hypergeometric functions (note 9.14).

NOTE 9.14: **The Gaussian Hypergeometric Series (Gauss 1812) and Differential Equation**

The **Gaussian hypergeometric series** with variable x and upper (lower) parameters $\alpha, \beta(\gamma)$ is **(Gauss 1812)** defined (section I.29.9) by (I.29.74) ≡ (9.971b):

$$\gamma \neq 0,-1,\ldots: \quad {}_2F_1(\alpha,\beta;\gamma;z) = 1 + \sum_{k=1}^{\infty} \frac{x^k}{k!} \frac{\alpha(\alpha+1)\cdots(\alpha+k-1)\beta(\beta+1)\cdots(\beta+k-1)}{\gamma(\gamma+1)\cdots(\gamma+k-1)}$$

$$= 1 + \frac{\Gamma(\gamma)}{\Gamma(\alpha)\Gamma(\beta)} \sum_{k=1}^{\infty} \frac{x^k}{k!} \frac{\Gamma(\alpha+k)\Gamma(\beta+k)}{\Gamma(\gamma+k)}, \qquad \text{(9.971a–c)}$$

where may be used (9.971c) the gamma function (9.432b) and γ is not zero or a negative integer (9.971a). The Gaussian hypergeometric function is thus specified by a power series (9.971a) ≡ (9.972a) with first coefficient unity (9.972b) and recurrence formula for the coefficients (9.972c):

$${}_2F_1(\alpha,\beta;\gamma;x) = \sum_{k=1}^{\infty} c_k\, x^k: \qquad c_0 = 1, \qquad c_{k+1} = c_k \frac{(\alpha+k)(\beta+k)}{(1+k)(\gamma+k)}. \qquad \text{(9.972a–c)}$$

Comparing (9.972c) ≡ (9.940c), it follows that the two polynomials have roots (9.973a, b) [(9.973d, e)] and hence (9.935a) [(9.935b)] are given by (9.973c) [(9.973f)]:

$$\alpha_1 = 0, \alpha_2 = 1-\gamma: \quad P_2(a) = a(a+\gamma-1);$$
$$\beta_1 = -\alpha, \beta_2 = -\beta: \quad Q_2(a) = (a+\alpha)(a+\beta). \qquad \text{(9.973a–f)}$$

The convergence of the **Gaussian hypergeometric series** (9.971a–c) is thus specified by (9.963a–e; 9.964a–e; 9.965a–f) with g given (9.962a) ≡ (9.974a) by (9.973a, b, d, e) ≡ (9.974b):

$$g = 2 + \beta_1 + \beta_2 - \alpha_1 - \alpha_2 = 1 + \gamma - \alpha - \beta, \qquad \frac{c_{k+1}}{c_k} = 1 - \frac{g}{k} + O\left(\frac{1}{k^2}\right), \qquad \text{(9.974a–c)}$$

in agreement with (9.972c) = (9.974c) ≡ (I.29.80b).

From (9.973c, f) it follows that the Gaussian hypergeometric function (9.971b, c) must satisfy (9.935c) the linear differential equation (9.975):

$$\left\{x\frac{d}{dx}\left(x\frac{d}{dx}+\gamma-1\right)-x\left(x\frac{d}{dx}+\alpha\right)\left(x\frac{d}{dx}+\beta\right)\right\}y(x)=0. \tag{9.975}$$

Omitting the common factor x, in (9.975) appear the operators:

$$\frac{d}{dx}\left(x\frac{d}{dx}+\gamma-1\right)=x\frac{d^2}{dx^2}+\gamma\frac{d}{dx}, \tag{9.976a}$$

$$\left(x\frac{d}{dx}+\alpha\right)\left(x\frac{d}{dx}+\beta\right)=x^2\frac{d^2}{dx^2}+(1+\alpha+\beta)x\frac{d}{dx}+\alpha\beta. \tag{9.976b}$$

Substituting (9.976a, b) in (9.975) leads to the Gaussian hypergeometric differential equation (9.977b) with parameters (α,β,γ):

$$y(x)\equiv{}_2F_1(\alpha,\beta;\gamma;x):\quad x(1-x)y''+\left[\gamma-(\alpha+\beta+1)x\right]y'-\alpha\,\beta y=0. \tag{9.977a, b}$$

It has been shown that *(standard CDIV): the Gaussian hypergeometric differential equation (9.977b) can be derived (9.977a) from the Gaussian hypergeometric series (9.971b, c) for* γ *not zero or a negative integer (9.971a).* It is confirmed next that the Gaussian hypergeometric differential equation (9.977b) is satisfied (9.977a) by the Gaussian hypergeometric function (9.971b), and a second linearly independent solution is obtained as a Gaussian hypergeometric function of the first (second) kind [note(s) 9.15 (9.16–9.18)].

NOTE 9.15: Gaussian Hypergeometric Function of the First Kind

The origin is a regular singularity of the Gaussian hypergeometric differential equation (9.977b), and thus solutions exists as regular integral (9.937d) leading to (9.978):

$$0=\sum_{j=0}^{\infty}c_j(a)x^{a+j-1}(a+j)(a+j+\gamma-1)-\sum_{k=0}^{\infty}c_k(a)x^{a+k}\left[(a+k)(a+k+\alpha+\beta)+\alpha\beta\right], \tag{9.978}$$

or to (9.979b) the change of summation variable (9.979a):

$$j=k+1:\quad 0=x^{-1}a\,(a+\gamma-1)\,c_0(a)$$
$$+\sum_{k=0}^{\infty}x^k\left\{c_{k+1}(a)(a+k+1)(a+k+\gamma)-c_k(a)\left[(a+k)(a+k+\alpha+\beta)+\alpha\beta\right]\right\}. \tag{9.979a, b}$$

The indices are given by (9.980a, b) in agreement with (9.973a, b) and the recurrence formula for the coefficients by (9.980c):

$$a_1 = 0, a_2 = 1-\gamma: \qquad c_{k+1}(a) = c_k(a)\frac{(a+k+\alpha)(a+k+\beta)}{(a+k+1)(a+k+\gamma)}. \tag{9.980a–c}$$

The first index (9.980a) substituted in (9.980c) leads to (9.972c) showing that the Gaussian hypergeometric function (9.971b) is the first solution (9.977a) of the Gaussian hypergeometric differential equation (9.977b).

The second index (9.980b) substituted in (9.980c) is equivalent to the change of parameters (9.981a–c):

$$\begin{gathered}\alpha \to \alpha+1-\gamma, \quad \beta \to \beta+1-\gamma, \quad \gamma \to 2-\gamma; \\ \gamma \neq 1,2,\ldots: \quad x^{1-\gamma} F(\alpha+1-\gamma;\beta+1-\gamma;2-\gamma;x),\end{gathered} \tag{9.981a–e}$$

leading to the solution (9.981e) for (9.981d). It has been shown that *the general integral (standard CDV) of the Gaussian hypergeometric differential equation (9.977b) converging (9.974b) for (9.963a–e; 9.964a–e; 9.965a–f), is a linear combination (9.982c) with arbitrary constants (A,B) of (9.971b; 9.981e) the* **Gaussian hypergeometric functions of the first kind:**

$$\gamma \neq 0,\pm1,\pm2,\ldots; \quad |x|<1: \qquad \begin{aligned} y(x) = {} & A\,F(\alpha,\beta;\gamma;x) + B\,x^{1-\gamma} \\ & F(\alpha+1-\gamma,\beta+1-\gamma;2-\gamma;x), \end{aligned} \tag{9.982a–c}$$

provided that γ is not (9.971a; 9.981d) an integer (9.982a). The case γ an integer leads to the Gaussian hypergeometric functions of the second kind (notes 9.16–9.18).

NOTE 9.16: Gaussian Hypergeometric Function of the Second Kind

The functions of the second kind are needed (subsections 9.5.10–9.5.11) if the difference of exponents (9.973a, b) is an integer; that is, if γ is an integer. For example, (a) for $\gamma = 1$ the two solutions (9.971b) ≡ (9.981e) coincide and (9.982c) cannot be the general integral because it involves only one arbitrary constant $A + B$. If (b) γ is a positive integer larger than unity $\gamma = n \geq 2$, then the second solution (9.981d) has a factor $2-\gamma+k-1 = 1-n+k$ in the denominator that vanishes for $k = n-1$. Thus in both cases (a) and (b) *of γ a positive integer (9.883a, b) the general integral (9.982b) of the Gaussian hypergeometric differential equation (9.977b) is (standard CDVI) replaced by (9.982c):*

$$\gamma = 1,2\ldots,n; \quad n \in |N: \qquad y(x) = A\,F(\alpha,\beta;n;x) + B\,G(\alpha,\beta;n;x), \tag{9.983a–c}$$

where the second solution (9.981d) is replaced (9.409d; 9.980c) the **Gaussian hypergeometric function of the second kind:**

$$\gamma \equiv n \in |N: \quad G(\alpha,\beta;n;x) = \lim_{a\to 1-n} \frac{\partial}{\partial a}\left\{(a+n-1)\, x^a \left[1+\sum_{k=1}^{\infty} x^k \frac{(a+\alpha)...(a+\alpha+k-1)(a+\beta)....(a+\beta+k-1)}{(a+1)...(a+k)(a+n)....(a+n+k-1)}\right]\right\}, \tag{9.984a, b}$$

that is evaluated next.

The factor $a+n-1$ in the numerator cancels with $a+k$ in the denominator for $k=n-1$ that appears for all $k \ge n-1$. Thus for $k \le n-2$ the factor $a+n-1$ leads to zero in the limit $a \to 1-n$ unless it is differentiated, specifying the set of terms:

$$E(\alpha,\beta;n;x) = \lim_{a\to 1-n}\left\{x^a\left[1+\sum_{k=1}^{n-2} x^k \frac{(a+\alpha)...(a+\alpha+k-1)(a+\beta)....(a+\beta+k-1)}{(a+1)...(a+k)(a+n)....(a+n+k-1)}\right]\right\}, \tag{9.985}$$

that form the **preliminary Gaussian hypergeometric function:**

$$E(\alpha,\beta;n;x) = x^{1-n}\left\{1+\sum_{k=1}^{n-2} \frac{x^k}{k!}\frac{(\alpha+1-n)...(\alpha+k-n)(\beta+1-n)....(\beta+k-n)}{(-n)...\,(1-n+k)}\right\}$$

$$= x^{1-n}\left[1+\sum_{k=1}^{n-2}(-x)^k\frac{(n-k-2)!}{k!\,n!}(\alpha+1-n)...(\alpha+k-n)(\beta+1-n)...(\beta+k-n)\right], \tag{9.986a, b}$$

that has a pole of order $n-1$ at the origin. Subtracting the preliminary function (9.985) leaves in (9.984b) only the sum starting with $k=n-1$ leading to:

$$G(\alpha,\beta;n;x) - E(\alpha,\beta;n;x) = \lim_{a\to 1-n}\frac{\partial}{\partial a}\left\{x^a\left[\sum_{k=n-1}^{\infty}\frac{x^k}{(a+1)...(a+n-2)}\frac{(a+\alpha)...(a+\alpha+k-1)(a+\beta)....(a+\beta+k-1)}{(a+n)...(a+k)(a+n)....(a+n+k-1)}\right]\right\}, \tag{9.987}$$

whose evaluation involves a complementary function (note 9.17).

NOTE 9.17: Preliminary and Complementary Gaussian Hypergeometric Functions

The change of index of summation (9.988a) simplifies (9.987) to (9.988b):

$$j = k - n + 1: \qquad G(\alpha,\beta;n;x) - E(\alpha,\beta;n;x) = \lim_{a\to 1-n} \frac{\partial}{\partial a}$$

$$\left\{ x^a \sum_{j=0}^{\infty} \frac{x^{j+n-1}(a+\alpha)...(a+\alpha+j+n-2)(a+\beta)...(a+\beta+j+n-2)}{(a+1)...(a+n-2)(a+n)...(a+n+j-1)(a+n)...(a+2n+j-2)} \right\}. \tag{9.988a, b}$$

Not differentiating the power leads to the **complementary Gaussian hypergeometric function:**

$$H(\alpha,\beta;n;x) = \lim_{a\to 1-n} x^a \frac{\partial}{\partial a}$$

$$\left[\sum_{j=0}^{\infty} \frac{x^{j+n-1}}{(a+1)....(a+n-2)} \frac{\Gamma(a+\alpha+j+n-1)}{\Gamma(a+\alpha)} \frac{\Gamma(a+\beta+j+n-1)}{\Gamma(a+\beta)} \right. \tag{9.989}$$

$$\left. \frac{\Gamma(a+n)}{\Gamma(a+n+j)} \frac{\Gamma(a+n)}{\Gamma(a+2n+j-1)} \right],$$

where was introduced the gamma function (9.432b). The differentiations in (9.920) involve (9.460b, c) the digamma function:

$$H(\alpha,\beta;n;x) = \frac{(-)^n}{n!} \sum_{j=0}^{\infty} x^j \frac{(\alpha+1-n)...(\alpha+j-1)}{j!} \frac{(\beta+n-1)\cdots(\beta+j-1)}{(n+j-1)!}$$

$$\left\{ \psi(\alpha+j) + \psi(\beta+j) + 2\psi(1) - \psi(\alpha+1-n) - \psi(\beta+1-n) - \psi(1+j) - \psi(n+j) \right\}, \tag{9.990}$$

and show that the complementary function is analytic at the origin.

Substituting (9.990) in (9.988b) only one term remains, namely the differentiation of the power, leading to:

$$G(\alpha,\beta;n;x)-E(\alpha,\beta;n;x)-H(\alpha,\beta;n;x)=\lim_{a\to 1-n}$$

$$\left\{x^a\log x\sum_{j=0}^{\infty}\frac{x^{j+n-1}(a+\alpha)...(a+\alpha+j+n-2)(a+\beta)...(a+\beta+j+n-2)}{(a+1)...(a+n-2)(a+n)...(a+n+j-1)(a+n)....(a+2n+j-2)}\right\}$$

$$=\log x\sum_{j=0}^{\infty}\frac{x^j(\alpha+1-n)...(\alpha+j-1)(\beta+1-n)...(\beta+j-1)}{(-n)...(-1)\times 1...j\times 1....(n+j-1)}$$

$$=\frac{(-)^n}{n!}\log x\sum_{j=0}^{\infty}x^j\frac{(\alpha+1-n)...(\alpha+j-1)}{j!}\frac{(\beta+1-n)...(\beta+j-1)}{(n+j-1)!}$$

$$=\frac{(-)^n}{n!}\frac{(\alpha+1-n)...(\alpha-1)(\beta+1-n)...(\beta-1)}{(n-1)!}$$

$$\left\{1+\sum_{j=1}^{\infty}\frac{x^j}{j!}\frac{\alpha....(\alpha+j-1)\,\beta...(\beta+j-1)}{n....(n+j-1)}\right\}$$

$$=C(\alpha,\beta,n)\,F(\alpha,\beta;n;x), \tag{9.991a–e}$$

where in (9.991e): (i) the term in curly brackets is the hypergeometric series (9.971b) with variable x and parameters $(\alpha,\beta;n)$; and (ii) the multiplying factor is independent of the variable and depends only on the parameters:

$$C(\alpha,\beta;n)\equiv(-)^n\frac{(\alpha+1-n)...(\alpha-1)(\beta+1-n)....(\beta-1)}{n!(n-1)!}. \tag{9.992}$$

Thus the *Gaussian hypergeometric function of the second kind is given (standard CDVII) by (9.993):*

$$G(\alpha,\beta;n;x)=C(\alpha,\beta;n;x)\log x\,F(\alpha,\beta;n;x)+E(\alpha,\beta;n;x)+H(\alpha,\beta;n;x), \tag{9.993}$$

involving the preliminary (9.986a, b) and complementary (9.990) functions and the coefficient (9.992) multiplying the logarithm and the Gaussian hypergeometric function of the first kind. The general integral of the Gaussian hypergeometric differential equation (note 9.14) has been obtained for γ not integer (note 9.15) and γ positive integer (note 9.16) so only the case γ non-positive integer remains (note 9.18).

NOTE 9.18: General Integral of the Gaussian Hypergeometric Differential Equation

If γ is zero or a negative integer (9.994a, b) the second integral (9.981e) remains valid but not the first (9.971b) and the general integral (standard CDVIII) of the Gaussian hypergeometric differential equation (9.977b) is (9.994c):

$$\gamma = 0, -1, -2, \ldots, -m, m \in |N_0: \quad y(x) = A\, G(\alpha+m+1, \beta+m+1; 2+m; x) + B\, x^{1+m}\, F(\alpha+m+1, \beta+m+1; 2+m; x), \tag{9.994a–c}$$

involves a Gaussian hypergeometric function of the second kind:

$$G(\alpha+m+1, \beta+m+1; 2+m; x) = \lim_{a\to 0} \frac{\partial}{\partial a}\left\{ a\, x^a \left[1 + \sum_{k=1}^{\infty} x^k \frac{(a+\alpha)\ldots.(a+\alpha+k-1)(a+\beta)\ldots.(a+\beta+k-1)}{(a+1)\ldots.(a+k)(a-m)\ldots.(a-m+k-1)} \right]\right\}, \tag{9.995}$$

that is similar to (9.984b) replacing the index $a_2 = 1-\gamma = 1-n$ by $a_1 = 0$. When $a \to 0$ the term $a-m+k-1$ in the denominator vanishes for $k = m+1$; thus the sum up to $k = m$ is separated, and the derivative applied to a, leading to the preliminary function:

$$E(\alpha+m+1, \beta+m+1; 2+m; x) = 1 + \sum_{k=1}^{m} \frac{x^k}{k!} \frac{\alpha\ldots(\alpha+k-1)}{(-)^k} \frac{\beta\ldots(\beta+k-1)}{m\ldots.(m+1-k)}$$

$$= 1 + \sum_{k=1}^{m} \frac{(-x)^k}{k!} \frac{(m-k)!}{m!} \alpha\ldots(\alpha+k-1)\beta\ldots(\beta+k-1), \tag{9.996a, b}$$

that is finite at the origin. Using the transformations:

$$\alpha \to \alpha+m+1, \qquad \beta \to \beta+m+1, \quad n \to 2+m, \tag{9.997a–c}$$

the preliminary functions (9.986a, b) ≡ (9.996a, b) coincide (9.997d):

$$\alpha + 1 - n \to (\alpha+m+1) + 1 - (m+2) = \alpha,$$

$$\frac{(n-k-2)!}{n!} \to \frac{(m-k)!}{(m+2)!} = \frac{1}{(m+1)(m+2)} \frac{(m-k)!}{m!}, \tag{9.997d, e}$$

apart from: (i) a constant factor in (9.997e); and (ii) the power $x^{1-n} \to x^{-1-m}$ in (9.986a, b) that does not appear in (9.996a, b).

The remaining terms in (9.995) are:

$$G(\alpha+m+1,\beta+m+1;2+m;x)-E(\alpha+m+1,\beta+m+1;2+m;x)$$

$$=\lim_{a\to 0}\frac{\partial}{\partial a}\left\{x^a\left[\sum_{k=m+1}^{\infty}x^k\frac{(a+\alpha)...(a+\alpha+k-1)}{(a+1)...(a+k)}\frac{(a+\beta)...(a+\beta+k-1)}{(a-m)...(a-1)(a+1)...(a-m+k-1)}\right]\right\}. \tag{9.998}$$

Not differentiating the power in (9.998) leads to the complementary function (9.999):

$$H(\alpha+m+1,\beta+m+1;2+m;x)$$

$$=\lim_{a\to 0}\left\{x^a\frac{\partial}{\partial a}\left[\sum_{k=m+1}^{\infty}\frac{x^k}{(a-1)...(a-m)}\frac{\Gamma(a+\alpha+k)}{\Gamma(a+\alpha)}\frac{\Gamma(a+\beta+k)}{\Gamma(a+\beta)}\right.\right. \tag{9.999}$$

$$\left.\left.\frac{\Gamma(a+1)}{\Gamma(a+k+1)}\frac{\Gamma(a+1)}{\Gamma(a-m+k)}\right]\right\}.$$

The change of variable of summation (9.1000a) shows that (9.999) ≡ (9.1000b) is an analytic function at the origin:

$$j=k-m-1:\quad H(\alpha+m+1;\beta+m+1;2+m;x)$$

$$=\frac{(-)^m}{m!}x^{1+m}\sum_{j=0}^{\infty}\frac{x^j}{j!}\frac{\alpha...(\alpha+m+j)\beta...(\beta+m+j)}{(m+j+1)!} \tag{9.1000a, b}$$

$$\left[\psi(\alpha+m+j+1)+\psi(\beta+m+j+1)-\psi(m+j+2)\right.$$

$$\left.-\psi(1+j)-\psi(\alpha)-\psi(\beta)+2\psi(1)\right].$$

The complementary functions (9.990) ≡ (9.1000b) coincide (9.997d) under the transformations (9.997a–c) except for the factor (9.997e). Comparing (9.986b) [(9.990)] with (9.996b) [(9.1000b)] for γ positive (9.983a, b) [non-positive (9.994a, b)] integer the factor $x^{1-n}\left(x^{1+m}\right)$ is suppressed (inserted). Differentiation of the power in (9.998) adds to (9.1000b) a term with a logarithm:

$$\begin{aligned} G(\alpha+m+1,\beta+m+1;2+m;x) &= E(\alpha+m+1,\beta+m+1;2+m;x) \\ &+C(\alpha+m+1,\beta+m+1;2+m)\log x\, F(\alpha+m+1,\beta+m+1;2+m;x) \\ &+H(\alpha+m+1,\beta+m+1;2+m;x), \end{aligned} \tag{9.1001}$$

and a constant factor (9.992) multiplying the Gaussian hypergeometric function of the first kind. Thus *the Gaussian hypergeometric functions of the second kind (9.993) [(9.1001)] that appear in the general integral (9.983c) [(9.994a)] of the Gaussian hypergeometric differential equation (9.977b) for $\gamma = n$ positive (9.983a, b) [non-positive $\gamma = -m$ (9.994a, b)] integer consists [standard CDVII (CDIX)] of two sets related by (9.997a–c; 9.998a, b) of the sum of: (i) a preliminary function (9.986b) [(9.996b)] that has a pole of order $1-n$ (is analytic) at the origin; (b) a complementary function (9.990) [(9.1000b)] that is finite (has a zero of order $1+m$); and (c) the product of a logarithm by the function of the first kind with a constant factor (9.992).* The solutions of the Gaussian hypergeometric differential equation (9.977b) have been obtained (notes 9.15–9.17) for all values of γ, allowing the identification of analytic cases including polynomials and singular cases including logarithms and poles (note 9.18).

NOTE 9.19: Analytic and Logarithmic Cases, Poles, and Polynomials

In the particular case (9.1002a) when the particular integrals in (9.982c) coincide (9.971b) ≡ (9.981e) as an hypergeometric series, a second linearly independent solution is specified by the Gaussian hypergeometric function of second kind (9.993) whose (9.1002b) preliminary function (9.986a, b) reduces to unity (9.1002b):

$$\gamma = 1: \quad E(\alpha,\beta;1;x) = 1; \qquad \gamma = 0: \quad E(\alpha+1,\beta+1;2;x) = 1. \tag{9.1002a–d}$$

in the particular case (9.1002c) the preliminary function (9.996a, b) in (9.1001) is also unity (9.1002d). For (9.1002a) setting (9.1002b; 9.983a, b) ≡ (9.1003a, b) in (9.991c) leads to (9.1003c):

$$\begin{aligned} \gamma = n = 1: \quad & G(\alpha,\beta;1;x) - E(\alpha,\beta;1;x) - H(\alpha,\beta;1;x) \\ &= -\log x \sum_{j=0}^{\infty} \frac{x^j}{(j!)^2}\alpha\ldots(\alpha+j-1)\beta\ldots(\beta+j-1) \\ &= -\log x\, F(\alpha,\beta;1;x), \end{aligned} \tag{9.1003a–d}$$

involving the Gaussian hypergeometric function of the first kind (9.971b) with $\gamma = 1$ and showing that in this case the coefficient (9.992) in (9.993) is –1. Substituting the preliminary (9.1002b) [complementary (9.990)] functions for (9.1003a, b) in (9.1003d) specifies *the Gaussian hypergeometric function of the second kind (9.1004) for (standard CDX) the case* $\gamma = 1$*:*

$$G(\alpha,\beta;1;x) = 1 - \log x\, F(\alpha,\beta;1;x) - \frac{1}{\Gamma(\alpha)\Gamma(\beta)} \sum_{j=0}^{\infty} \frac{x^j}{(j\,!)^2} \Gamma(\alpha+j)\Gamma(\beta+j)$$
$$\left[\psi(\alpha+j)+\psi(\beta+j)+2\psi(1)-\psi(\alpha)-\psi(\beta)-2\psi(1+j)\right]. \tag{9.1004}$$

In (9.1004) as *in (9.990) [(9.1001b)], the terms in square brackets in the complementary functions that do not involve the summation variably may (standard CDX1) be omitted since they are multiples of the Gaussian hypergeometric series, and can be included in the arbitrary constant A in (9.983c) [(9.994c)], with the exception of the case* α *or* β *a negative integer.* There is *a double exception (standard CDXII) in the case* α *or* β *a negative integer because: (i) the Gaussian hypergeometric series (9.971b) terminates as polynomial (9.1005a–c):*

$$q \in |N: \quad F(-q;\beta;\gamma;x) = 1 + \sum_{k=1}^{q} \frac{x^k}{k!}(-q)....(-q+k-1)\frac{\beta...(\beta+k-1)}{\gamma...(\gamma+k-1)}$$
$$= 1 + \sum_{k=1}^{q} \frac{(-x)^k}{k!} \frac{q!}{(q-k)!} \frac{\beta...(\beta+k-1)}{\gamma...(\gamma+k-1)}; \tag{9.1005a–c}$$

(ii) some digamma functions in (9.990, 9.1000b, 9.1004) diverge, but they always appear in finite pairs, for example for α a non-positive integer (9.100d, e) the difference is finite (9.1005f):

$$\alpha = -p, p \in |N_0: \quad \psi(\alpha+j) - \psi(\alpha) = \psi(j-p) - \psi(-p) = -\frac{1}{p} - \frac{1}{p-1} .... - \frac{1}{p+1-j}, \tag{9.1005d–f}$$

as follows using (9.466a) with $\nu = -p, n = j$.

In conclusion, *the general integral (standard CDXIII) of the Gaussian hypergeometric differential equation (9.977b) is a linear combination with arbitrary constants (A,B) of: (i) the Gaussian hypergeometric series (9.971a–c) or functions of the first kind (9.982c) if* γ *is not an integer (9.982a, b); (ii/iii) in the remaining cases of* γ *a positive (9.983a, b) [non-positive (9.994a, b)] integer appear the Gaussian hypergeometric function of the second kind (9.983c) [(9.994c)] that has three terms (9.993) [(9.1001)], namely: (iv) a logarithm multiplying the function of the first kind; (v) a preliminary function (9.986a, b) [(9.996a, b)] that is unity (9.1002b) [(9.1002d)] for*

(9.1002a) [(9.1002c)] and otherwise has a pole (is analytic); (vi) a complementary function (9.990) [(9.1000b)] where the terms in square brackets not involving the variable of summation j may be omitted if (α,β) *are not negative integers; (vii) if* α *(or* β*) is a negative integer then the pairs of terms are evaluated as in (9.1005a–d); (viii) if* α *or* β *are negative integers all the sums like the Gaussian hypergeometric series (9.971a–c) terminate as polynomials (9.1005a–c) of degree q that is the smallest of the integers* $-\alpha$ *and* $-\beta$*. The series solutions (i–vii): (ix) converge absolutely (9.963b) [also uniformly, that is totally (9.963e)] in the open unit disk (9.963a) [a closed sub-disk (9.963c, d)]; and (x) the convergence (Figure 9.18a) on the boundary, that is the unit circle, is specified by (9.964a–e) [(9.965a–f)] at the special point (all other points) in terms of the parameter (9.974b).* The preceding solutions (i-x) valid in the unit disk (Figure 9.18a) can be continued analytically to the whole complex x-plane via the changes of variable (9.970b) of the Schwartz group that all lead to Gaussian hypergeometric differential equations with modified parameters $(\bar{\alpha},\bar{\beta},\bar{\gamma})$. The Gaussian hypergeometric differential equation (notes 9.14–9.17) include as equivalent or particular cases the Legendre/Jacobi/Chebychev differential equations (notes 9.20–9.25/9.26/9.27–9.28).

NOTE 9.20: Legendre (1785) Differential Equation

The multipoles in three-dimensions have angular dependences specified by Legendre polynomials (section III.8.3) that satisfy the **Legendre differential equation** (8.359a) of degree ν with $m=0$, that is (9.1006b, c):

$$w(\theta)=P_\nu(\cos\theta):\quad 0=\frac{1}{\sin\theta}\frac{d}{d\theta}\left(\sin\theta\frac{dw}{d\theta}\right)+\nu(\nu+1)w=w''+\cot\theta\, w'+\nu(\nu+1)w, \tag{9.1006a–c}$$

where the degree ν may take complex values in the Legendre functions (9.1006a). The change of independent variable:

$$y(x)\equiv w(\theta),\quad x\equiv\cos\theta:\quad \frac{d}{d\theta}=\frac{dx}{d\theta}\frac{d}{dx}=-\sin\theta\frac{d}{dx}=-\sqrt{1-x^2}\,\frac{d}{dx},$$

$$\frac{d^2}{d\theta^2}=\sqrt{1-x^2}\,\frac{d}{dx}\left(\sqrt{1-x^2}\,\frac{d}{dx}\right)=\left(1-x^2\right)\frac{d^2}{dx^2}-x\frac{d}{dx}, \tag{9.1007a–d}$$

leads to the Legendre differential equation with polynomial coefficients (9.1008b) ≡ (III.9.191b):

$$y(x)=P_\nu(x):\qquad \left(1-x^2\right)y''-2xy'+\nu(\nu+1)y=0, \tag{9.1008a, b}$$

that has regular singularities at the points (9.1009a):

$$x=1,-1,\infty;\quad \xi=0,1,\infty:\qquad \xi=\frac{1-x}{2},\quad x=1-2\xi,\quad z(\xi)=y(x). \tag{9.1009a–e}$$

the points (9.1009a) are mapped to the regular singularities (9.970a) ≡ (9.1009b) of the Gaussian hypergeometric differential equation by the change of independent variable (9.1009c–e) that leads to the differential equation (9.1010):

$$\xi\left(1-\xi\right) z'' + \left(1-2\xi\right) z' + \nu(\nu+1)\, z = 0. \qquad (9.1010)$$

The differential equation (9.1010) is of the Gaussian hypergeometric type (9.977b) with parameters satisfying (9.1011a–c):

$$\gamma = 1, \qquad \alpha+\beta = 1, \qquad \alpha\beta = -\nu(\nu+1): \quad \alpha = -\nu, \qquad \beta = 1+\nu, \quad g = 1, \qquad (9.1011\text{a–f})$$

and leading to (9.1011d, e) and also (9.974b) to (9.1011f).

Thus *the general integral (9.983a–c) of the Legendre differential equation (9.1008b) is (standard CDXIV) a linear combination (9.1012a) with arbitrary constants (A,B):*

$$y(x) = A\,P_\nu(x) + B\,Q_\nu(x): \qquad P_\nu(x) = F\left(-\nu, 1+\nu; 1; \frac{1-x}{2}\right),$$

$$Q_\nu(x) = G\left(-\nu, v+1; 1; \frac{1-x}{2}\right), \qquad (9.1012\text{a–c})$$

of the **Legendre functions of the first (second) kind** *(9.1012b) [(9.1012c)] and degree ν specified (standard CDXV) by the Gaussian hypergeometric functions of the first (second) kind (9.971a–c) [(9.993)] kind with parameters (9.1011a, d, e) and variable (9.1009c). The (Figure 9.18b) solution (9.1012a–c): (i) converges absolutely (9.1013c) in the disk (9.1013a, b) of radius 2 and center at x = 1:*

$$|\xi| < 1 \Leftrightarrow |1-x| < 2: \quad \text{A.C.}, \quad 0 < \delta < 1: \quad |\xi| < 1-\delta \Leftrightarrow |1-x| < 2-2\delta: \quad \text{T.C.} \qquad (9.1013\text{a–f})$$

(ii) converges also uniformly hence totally (9.1013g) in a closed sub-disk (9.1013d–f); (iii/iv) at the special point (9.1014a, b) [other points (9.1014d, e) on the boundary of convergence (9.1014f, g)] three is:

$$\xi = 1 \quad \Leftrightarrow \quad x = -1: \quad \text{D.}; \quad \xi \neq 1 = |\xi| \Leftrightarrow \quad x \neq 1 = \frac{|1-x|}{2}: \text{C.C.}, \qquad (9.1014\text{a–h})$$

(9.1011f) divergence (9.964c) ≡ (9.1014c) [conditional convergence (9.965e) ≡ (9.1014h)].

The solution of the Legendre differential equation (9.1006b, c) finite (9.1015b) on a sphere (9.1015a) is (standard CDXVI) a constant multiple (9.1015d) of the Legendre function of integer order (9.1015c):

$$0 \le \theta \le \pi; \qquad w(\theta) < \infty: \qquad n \in |N_0: \quad w(\theta) = A\,P_n\left(\cos\theta\right), \qquad (9.1015\text{a–d})$$

that is the **Legendre polynomial** *(9.1016a) of degree n corresponding to a terminating (9.1016b) Gaussian hypergeometric series (9.971a, b):*

$$P_n(\cos\theta) = F(-n,1+n;1;(1-\cos\theta)/2)$$

$$= 1 + \sum_{k=1}^{n} \left(\frac{1-\cos\theta}{2}\right)^k \frac{(-n)...(-n+k-1)(1+n)....(n+k)}{k!(1...k)}$$

$$= 1 + \sum_{k=1}^{n} \left(\frac{\cos\theta - 1}{2}\right)^k \frac{n...(n+1-k)\,(n+1)....(n+k)}{(k!)^2} \qquad (9.1016a\text{–}d)$$

$$= 1 + \sum_{k=1}^{n} \left(\frac{\cos\theta - 1}{2}\right)^k \frac{(n+k)!}{(n-k)!}\frac{1}{(k!)^2}.$$

The first three Legendre polynomials are:

$$P_0(\cos\theta) = 1, \qquad P_1(\cos\theta) = \cos\theta, \qquad P_2(\cos\theta) = \frac{3\cos^2\theta - 1}{2}, \qquad (9.1017a\text{–}c)$$

in agreement with (III.8.75a–c) ≡ (9.1017a–c). The result (9.1015a–d) can be proved from (9.1012a–c) as follows: (i) at the north pole $\theta = 0, x = 1, \xi = 0$ the Legendre function of the second kind (9.1012c) has a logarithmic singularity, and (9.1012a) cannot be finite (9.1015b) unless $B = 0$; (ii) this leaves the first term in (9.1012a) that is (9.1015d) a constant multiple of the Legendre function of the first kind (9.1012b); and (iii) the Legendre function of the first kind diverges (9.1014a–c) at the south pole $\theta = \pi, x = -1, \xi = 1$, unless the series terminates, that is, ν is a non-negative integer (9.1015c). The ultraspherical Legendre functions are a two-parameter generalization (note 9.21) of the Legendre functions that have one parameter.

NOTE 9.21: Ultraspherical Legendre Differential Equation

The angular dependence of multipoles in spaces of any dimension (section III.9.4) is specified by the ultraspherical Legendre polynomials of variable x, degree ν, and dimension λ that satisfy the differential equation (III.9.190) ≡ (9.1018c):

$$\lambda \equiv N - 3; \quad y(x) = P^{\nu,\lambda}(x): \qquad \left(1-x^2\right)y'' - (2+\lambda)xy' + \nu(\nu+1+\lambda)y = 0; \qquad (9.1018a\text{–}c)$$

the (9.1018a) three-dimensional case $N = 3$ reduces (9.1018b, c) with $\lambda = 0$ to the original Legendre differential equation (9.1008a, b). Using the inverse of the change of variable (9.1007a–d) it follows that the ultraspherical generalization of (9.1006a–c) is (9.1019a, b):

$$w(\theta) = P^{\nu,\lambda}(\cos\theta): \qquad w'' + (1+\lambda)\cot\theta\, w' + \nu(\nu+1+\lambda)\, w = 0. \tag{9.1019a, b}$$

The change of independent variable (9.1009c, d) leads from (9.1018c) to (9.1020):

$$\xi(1-\xi)z'' + (1+\lambda/2)(1-2\xi)\, z' + \nu(\nu+1+\lambda)z = 0, \tag{9.1020}$$

that is a Gaussian hypergeometric differential equation (9.977b) with parameters (9.1021a–c):

$$\gamma = 1+\lambda/2, \quad \alpha+\beta = 1+\lambda, \alpha\beta = -\nu(\nu+1+\lambda): \quad \alpha = -\nu, \quad \beta = 1+\nu+\lambda,$$
$$g = 1-\lambda/2, \tag{9.1021a–f}$$

leading to (9.1021d, e) and (9.974b) also to (9.1021f). The parameter $\lambda/2 = k$ is a non-negative integer only for spaces (9.1018a) of odd dimension $N = 3+\lambda = 3+2k$.

Thus the general integral of the **ultraspherical Legendre differential equation** *(9.1018c) of degree* ν *and dimension* λ *is: (i) in (standard CDXVII) the case (9.1022a) a linear combination (9.1022b) with arbitrary constants (A,B) of* **ultraspherical Legendre functions of the first (second) kind** *(9.1022c) [(9.1022d)] for spaces of odd dimension (9.1022a):*

$$\lambda = 0,2,4,\ldots: \qquad y(x) = A\, P^{\nu,\lambda}(x) + BQ^{\nu,\lambda}(x), \tag{9.1022a, b}$$

$$P^{\nu,\lambda}(x) = F(-\nu, 1+\nu+\lambda; 1+\lambda/2; (1-x)/2), \tag{9.1022c}$$

$$Q^{\nu,\lambda}(x) = G(-\nu, 1+\nu+\lambda; 1+\lambda/2; (1-x)/2); \tag{9.1022d}$$

(ii) otherwise (standard CDXVII) for (9.1023a) a linear combination (9.1023b):

$$\lambda \neq 0, \pm 2, \pm 4, \ldots: \qquad y(x) = A\,P^{\nu,\lambda}(x) + B\,R^{\nu,\lambda}(x), \tag{9.1023a, b}$$

of (9.982a–c) **first (second) ultraspherical Legendre functions of the first kind** *(9.1022c) [(9.1024a, b)]:*

$$\begin{aligned} R^{\nu,\lambda}(x) &= (1-x)^{1-\gamma} F(\alpha+1-\gamma, \beta+1-\gamma; 2-\gamma; (1-x)/2) \\ &= (1-x)^{-\lambda/2} F(-\nu-\lambda/2, 1+\nu+\lambda/2; 1-\lambda/2; (1-x)/2), \end{aligned} \tag{9.1024a, b}$$

except for $\lambda/2$ a negative integer; (iii) for $\lambda/2$ a negative integer the (standard CDXIX) general integral derives from (9.994a–c) with (9.1021a, d, e); (iv) the region of convergence is the same (9.1013a–f) as for the Legendre differential equation; and (v) the convergence on the boundary (Figure 9.18b) at the special (9.1014a, b) [other (9.1014d, e)] points is specified by (9.964a–e) [(9.965a–f)] with (9.1021f). Since (9.964b) hold for (9.1025a) *the finite (standard CDXX) solution (9.1025c) of the ultraspherical Legendre differential equation (9.1019a, b) in a sphere (9.1025b) is a constant multiple of the* ***ultraspherical Legendre polynomial*** *(9.1025d, e):*

$$\mathrm{Re}(\lambda) > 0, \quad 0 \le \theta \le \pi, \quad w(\theta) < \infty, \quad n \in |N_0: \quad w(\theta) = A\, P^{n,\lambda}(\cos\theta). \qquad \text{(9.1025a–e)}$$

Two distinct generalizations of the Legendre differential equation (note 9.19) are the ultraspherical (associated) Legendre differential equation [note 9.21 (9.22)].

NOTE 9.22: Associated Legendre Differential Equation

The separation of variables in the Laplace operator in spherical coordinates (note 8.5) leads to the associated Legendre differential equation (8.359a) ≡ (9.1026a, b) of degree ν and order μ:

$$w(\theta) = P_\nu^\mu(\cos\theta): \qquad 0 = w'' + \cot\theta\, w' + \left[\nu(\nu+1) - \mu^2 \csc^2\theta\right] w. \qquad \text{(9.1026a, b)}$$

The change of variable (9.1007a–d) leads to:

$$y(x) = P_\nu^\mu(x): \quad \left(1-x^2\right)y'' - 2xy' + \left[\nu(\nu+1) - \mu^2/\left(1-x^2\right)\right]y = 0. \qquad \text{(9.1027a, b)}$$

The differential equation (9.1027b) is simplified by the change of dependent variable (9.1028a) that leads from (9.1027b) to (9.1028b):

$$y(x) = \left(\frac{x+1}{x-1}\right)^{\mu/2} h(x): \qquad \left(1-x^2\right)h'' + 2(\mu - x)\, h' + \nu(\nu+1)h = 0. \qquad \text{(9.1028a, b)}$$

Next is performed the change of independent variable (9.1009c, d) leading to (9.1029b):

$$h(x) = z(\xi): \qquad \xi(1-\xi)\, z'' + (1-\mu-2\xi)z' + \nu(\nu+1)z = 0. \qquad \text{(9.1029a, b)}$$

The differential equation (9.1029b) is of the Gaussian hypergeometric type (9.977b) with parameters (9.1030a–c):

$$\gamma = 1-\mu, \quad \alpha+\beta = 1, \quad \alpha\beta = -\nu(\nu+1): \quad \alpha = -\nu, \quad \beta = 1+\nu, \quad g = 1-\mu, \qquad \text{(9.1030a–f)}$$

leading to (9.1030d, e) and (9.974b) also (9.1030f).

From (9.1027a, 9.1028a) and (9.1030a, d, e) follows that **second associated Legendre function of the first kind** (9.1031a) with variable x, degree ν, and order μ:

$$R_\nu^\mu(x) = \frac{1}{\Gamma(1-\mu)}\left(\frac{x+1}{x-1}\right)^{\mu/2} F(-\nu, 1+\nu; 1-\mu; (1-x)/2)$$

$$= \frac{1}{\Gamma(-\nu)\Gamma(1+\nu)}\left(\frac{x+1}{x-1}\right)^{\mu/2}\left\{1+\sum_{k=1}^{\infty}\left(\frac{1-x}{2}\right)^k \frac{\Gamma(k-\nu)\Gamma(1+k+\nu)}{k!\,\Gamma(1+k-\mu)}\right\}, \tag{9.1031a, b}$$

where: (i) the factor $\Gamma(1-\mu)$ in the denominator of (9.1031a) cancels the pole of the Gaussian hypergeometric series (9.971c) when μ is a positive integer; and (ii) in the denominator of (9.1031b) may be used the symmetry formula (9.440a–c) for the Gamma function. A particular integral linearly independent from (9.1031a, b) for μ not a negative integer (9.1032a) is (9.1032b) that follows from (9.981e) the **first associated Legendre function of the first kind:**

$$\mu \neq 0, -1, -2, \ldots: \quad P_\nu^\mu(x) = e^{i\pi\mu/2}\left(\frac{x+1}{x-1}\right)^{\mu/2}(1-x)^{1-\gamma} F\left(\alpha+1-\gamma, \beta+1-\gamma; 2-\gamma; \frac{1-x}{2}\right)$$

$$= e^{i\pi\mu/2}\left(\frac{x+1}{x-1}\right)^{\mu/2}(1-x)^{\mu} F\left(-\nu+\mu, \nu+1+\mu; 1+\mu; \frac{1-x}{2}\right)$$

$$= (1-x^2)^{\mu/2} F(\mu-\nu, 1+\mu+\nu; 1+\mu; (1-x)/2), \tag{9.1032a–d}$$

using (9.1030a, d, e) in (9.1032c, d). Thus *the general integral of the associated Legendre differential equation (9.1027b) is (standard CDXXI) a linear combination (9.1033c) with arbitrary constants (A, B) of the first (9.1032b–d) and second (9.1031a, b) associated Legendre functions of the first kind valid for (9.1033a, b):*

$$\mu \neq 0, \pm 1, \pm 2 \ldots: \qquad (1-x) < 2: \qquad y(x) = A\,P_\nu^\mu(x) + B\,R_\nu^\mu(x), \tag{9.1033a–c}$$

with convergence given (Figure 9.18b) by (9.1013a–f) and (9.964a–e; 9.965a–f; 9.1030f).

In the case of **spherical harmonics**, that is order a positive integer (9.1034a) the solution (9.1031a, b) has a singular factor at $x = 1, \theta = 0$ and involves a function of the second kind, and must be suppressed by setting $B = 0$ in (9.1033b) to have a finite result (9.1034d). The remaining particular integral (9.1032d) diverges (9.965b) [oscillates (9.965c)] at $x = -1, \theta = \pi$ because $g = 1 - m$ in (9.1030f) is $g < 0$ for $m \geq 2$ ($g = 0$ for $m = 1$). Hence a finite solution requires that the series (9.1032d) terminates; that is, the degree is an integer (9.1034e) larger than the order (9.1034f). Thus *the spherical harmonics as solutions (standard*

CDXXII) of the associated Legendre differential equation (9.1027b) [(9.1026b)] with positive integer order (9.1034a) are finite (9.1034d) in the interval (9.1034b) [sphere (9.1034c) only for larger (9.1034f) integer degree (9.1034e) when they are given (9.1032d) by (9.1034g) [(9.1034h)]:

$$\mu \equiv m \in |N, -1 \le x \le +1 \Leftrightarrow 0 \le \theta \le \pi, \quad y(x) = w(\theta) < \infty: \nu \equiv n \in |N, \quad n > m: \tag{9.1034a–f}$$

$$y(x) = P_n^m(x) = \left(1 - x^2\right)^{m/2} F\left(m - n, m + n + 1; 1 + m; (1 - x)/2\right), \tag{9.1034g}$$

$$w(\theta) = P_n^m(\cos\theta) = \sin^m\theta\, F\left(m - n, m + n + 1; 1 + m; (1 - \cos\theta)/2\right). \tag{9.1034h}$$

The associated Legendre differential equation (9.1027b) [(9.1026b)] is (standard CDXXIII) unaffected changing the sign of the order $\mu \to -\mu$, and thus (9.1034g) [(9.1034h)] hold for negative integer order $\mu = -m, m \in |N$, that is are finite (9.964e) [(9.965f)] at $x = 1(x = -1)$ because $g = 1 + m > 1$ in (9.1030f) and are singular, instead of vanishing, at $x = \pm 1(\theta = 0, \pi)$. The only finite non-vanishing solution at $x = \pm 1(\theta = 0, \pi)$ is the case $m = 0$ of the original Legendre polynomials (9.1016a–d). A further generalization is the hyperspherical associated Legendre differential equation (note 9.22).

NOTE 9.23: Hyperspherical Associated Legendre Differential Equation

In the separation of variables of the Laplace operator in hyperspherical coordinates (note 8.13) appears the **hyperspherical associated Legendre differential equation** (8.391b) ≡ (9.1035b) of order ν, degree μ, and dimension λ:

$$w(\theta) = A_{\nu,\lambda}^{\mu}(\cos\theta): \quad w'' + (1 + \lambda)\cot\theta\, w' + \left[\nu(\nu + 1) - \mu^2 \csc^2\theta\right] w = 0, \tag{9.1035a, b}$$

that: (i/ii) includes the associated (original) Legendre differential equation (9.1026b) [(9.1006c)] for $\lambda = 0$ (and $\mu = 0$); and (iii) for $\mu = 0$ does not reduce to the ultraspherical (9.1018c) but rather to an **hyperspherical Legendre differential equation** of degree ν and dimension λ:

$$w(\theta) = A_{\nu,\lambda}(\cos\theta): \qquad w'' + (1 + \lambda)\cot\theta\, w' + \nu(\nu + 1) w = 0, \tag{9.1036a, b}$$

that is considered subsequently (note 9.25) as a particular case of (9.1035a, b). The change of independent variable (9.1007a–d) in (9.1035a, b) leads to the hyperspherical associated Legendre differential equation with polynomial coefficients:

$$y(x) = A_{\nu,\lambda}^{\mu}(x): \quad \left(1 - x^2\right) y'' - (2 + \lambda)\, x\, y' + \left[\nu(\nu + 1) - \mu^2/\left(1 - x^2\right)\right] y = 0. \tag{9.1037a, b}$$

The change of independent variable (9.1009c–e) is not useful to reduce (9.1037b) to a Gaussian hypergeometric differential equation and is replaced by the change of independent variable (9.1038a–d):

$$\zeta \equiv x^2: \qquad \frac{d}{dx} = \frac{d\zeta}{dx}\frac{d}{d\zeta} = 2x\frac{d}{d\zeta} = 2\sqrt{\zeta}\frac{d}{d\zeta}, \tag{9.1038a–d}$$

$$y(x) = h(\zeta): \qquad \frac{d^2}{dx^2} = 4\sqrt{\zeta}\frac{d}{d\zeta}\sqrt{\zeta}\frac{d}{d\zeta} = 4\zeta\frac{d^2}{d\zeta^2} + 2\frac{d}{d\zeta}, \tag{9.1038c, d}$$

that leads to the differential equation (9.1039):

$$4\zeta(1-\zeta)h'' + 2\left[1-(3+\lambda)\zeta\right]h' + \left[\nu(\nu+1) - \frac{\mu^2}{1-\zeta}\right]h = 0, \tag{9.1039}$$

with coefficients of h'' and h' similar to those of y' in the Gaussian hypergeometric differential equation (9.977b).

Instead of (9.1028a) is made the change of dependent variable (9.1040a) leading (9.516a–c) to (9.1040b):

$$h(\zeta) = (1-\zeta)^{\vartheta} g(\zeta): \qquad 4\zeta(1-\zeta)\, g'' + 2\left[1-(3+\lambda+4\vartheta)\,\zeta\right] g'$$
$$+\left[\nu(\nu+1) - 4\vartheta^2 - 2\vartheta - 2\lambda\vartheta + \left(4\vartheta^2 + 2\lambda\vartheta - \mu^2\right)/(1-\zeta)\right] g = 0. \tag{9.1040a, b}$$

Choosing ϑ to be a root of (9.1041a):

$$4\vartheta^2 + 2\lambda\vartheta - \mu^2 = 0:$$
$$\zeta(1-\zeta)\, g'' + \frac{1}{2}\left[1-(3+\lambda+4\vartheta)\right] g' + \left[\frac{\nu(\nu+1)}{4} - \vartheta^2 - \frac{\vartheta}{2} - \frac{\lambda\vartheta}{2}\right] g = 0. \tag{9.1041a, b}$$

simplifies the differential equation (9.1040b) to (9.1041b) that is of the Gaussian hypergeometric type (9.977b) with parameters (9.1042a–c) leading (9.974b) to (9.1042d):

$$\gamma = \frac{1}{2}, \; \alpha+\beta = 2\vartheta + \frac{\lambda+1}{2}, \; \alpha\beta = \vartheta^2 + \frac{\vartheta}{2}(1+\lambda) - \frac{\nu(\nu+1)}{4} \equiv c, \; g = 1 - 2\vartheta - \frac{\lambda}{2}. \tag{9.1042a–d}$$

The roots of (9.1041a) specify two possible values (9.1043a) of the parameter in (9.1040a):

$$\vartheta_\pm = -\frac{\lambda}{4} \pm \frac{1}{4}\sqrt{\lambda^2+\mu^2}; \quad (X-\alpha)(X-\beta) = X^2 - \left(2\vartheta + \frac{\lambda+1}{2}\right)X + c, \qquad (9.1043a–c)$$

the parameters α, β in (9.1042b, c) are the roots of (9.1043b, c) and are thus given by:

$$\alpha,\beta = \vartheta_\pm + \frac{\lambda+1}{4} \pm \sqrt{\left(\vartheta_\pm^2 + \frac{\lambda+1}{4}\right)^2 - c} = \vartheta_\pm + \frac{\lambda+1}{4} \pm \frac{1}{2}\sqrt{\left(\frac{\lambda+1}{2}\right)^2 + \nu(\nu+1)}, \qquad (9.1044a, b)$$

completing the transformation into the Gaussian hypergeometric differential equation of the hyperspherical associated Legendre differential equation that tops the hierarchy of Legendre functions (note 9.24).

NOTE 9.24: A Hierarchy of Legendre Functions and Differential Equations

Two linearly independent solutions of the hyperspherical associated Legendre differential equation (9.1037b) follow (9.1038a, c; 9.1040a; 9.1042a) from (9.971b) [(9.981e)] leading to the first (9.1045a) [second (9.1045b)] **modified hyperspherical associated Legendre functions:**

$$A_{\nu,\lambda}^{\mu}(x) = \left(1-x^2\right)^{\vartheta} F\left(\alpha,\beta;1/2;x^2\right), \qquad (9.1045a)$$

$$B_{\nu,\lambda}^{\mu}(x) = \left(1-x^2\right)^{1/2+\vartheta} F\left(\alpha+\frac{1}{2},\beta+\frac{1}{2};\frac{3}{2};x^2\right). \qquad (9.1045b)$$

The notation $A_{\nu,\lambda}^{\mu}\left(B_{\nu,\lambda}^{\mu}\right)$ is used in (9.1045a) [(9.1045b, c)] because although $A_{\nu,0}^{\mu}\left(B_{\nu,0}^{\mu}\right)$ is a solution (9.1035b) of the associated Legendre differential equation (9.1027b) it need not coincide with (9.1031a, b) or (9.1032a–d), as it is generally a linear combination of both; thus the **hyperspherical associated Legendre functions** (9.1046c) are defined as a linear combination of (9.1045a–c) with coefficients $(C_{11}, C_{12}, C_{21}, C_{22})$ such that for $\lambda = 0$ the associated Legendre functions (9.1045a, b) are obtained:

$$P_{\nu,0}^{\mu}(x) = P_\nu^\mu(x): \qquad R_{\nu,0}^{\mu}(x) = R_\nu^\mu(x): \qquad \begin{bmatrix} P_{\nu,\lambda}^{\mu}(x) \\ R_{\nu,\lambda}^{\mu}(x) \end{bmatrix} = \begin{bmatrix} C_{11} & C_{12} \\ C_{21} & C_{22} \end{bmatrix} \begin{bmatrix} A_{\nu,\lambda}^{\mu}(x) \\ B_{\nu,\lambda}^{\mu}(x) \end{bmatrix}; \qquad (9.1046a–c)$$

the constants can be determined from (9.1046c) at two points, for example $x = 0$ and $x = 1$. Thus *the general integral of the hyperspherical associated Legendre differential equation (9.1037b) is (standard CDXXIV) a linear combination (9.1047c) with arbitrary constants $C_{1,2}$ of the* ***first (second) modified hyperspherical associated Legendre functions*** *(9.1045a) [(9.1045b)] of the first kind:*

$$\beta \neq -\frac{1}{2}, -\frac{3}{2}, -\frac{5}{2} \ldots: \qquad |x| < 1: \quad y(x) = C_1\, A^{\mu}_{\nu,\lambda}(x) + C_2\, B^{\mu}_{\nu,\lambda}(x); \tag{9.1047a–c}$$

the solution is absolutely convergent in the unit disk (9.963a, b) and also uniformly convergent in a closed sub-disk (9.963c–e). On the unit circle $|x| = 1$ the convergence at the special points $x^2 = 1$ or $x = \pm 1$ (at all other points) is specified by (9.964a–e [(9.965a–f)] with g given by (9.1042d). The roots (9.1043a) specify the coefficients (9.1044a, b) of the Gaussian hypergeometric functions in (9.1045a, b) for which γ is not an integer.

In the (standard CDCCV) particular case (9.1048a) of the associated Legendre differential equation (9.1027b) the parameters in (9.1043a; 9.1042d; 9.1044a, b) simplify to (9.1048a–d):

$$\lambda = 0: \qquad \vartheta_{\pm} = \pm\frac{\mu}{4}, \qquad g = 1 \mp \frac{\mu}{2}, \qquad \alpha, \beta = \frac{1 \pm \mu}{4} \pm \frac{1}{2}\sqrt{\nu^2 + \nu + \frac{1}{4}}, \tag{9.1048a–e}$$

in the further particular case of the Legendre differential equation (9.1018b) there are (9.1049a, b) the further simplifications (9.1049a–e):

$$\lambda = 0 = \mu: \qquad \vartheta_{\pm} = 0, \qquad g = 1, \qquad \alpha, \beta = \frac{1}{4} \pm \frac{1}{2}\sqrt{\nu^2 + \nu + \frac{1}{4}}. \tag{9.1049a–e}$$

The solutions (9.1048a–e) [(9.1049a–e)] in (9.1045a, b) of the Legendre (associated Legendre) differential equation (9.1008b) [(9.1027b)] are linear combinations (9.1012a) [(9.1033c)] of the Legendre (9.1012b, c) [associated Legendre (9.1031a, b; 9.1032b–d)] functions. The solutions (9.1045a, b) in the general integral (9.1047a, b) are Gaussian hypergeometric series (9.971a–e) around the origin that is a regular point, hence are analytic functions; the singularities of the hyperspherical associated Legendre differential equation (9.1037b) at $x = \pm 1$ are the special points on the boundary of convergence, and thus there is (9.1042d) absolute convergence (9.964e; 9.965f) for (9.1050a); the factors in (9.1045a) [(9.1045b)] are singular at $x = \pm 1$ for (9.1050b) [(9.1050c) and thus the singularity of the solution is specified by the leading term in (9.1045a) [(9.1045b)] if (9.1050b) [(9.1050c)] hold:

$$\operatorname{Re}(\vartheta) < -\frac{1}{4}\operatorname{Re}(\lambda); \qquad \operatorname{Re}(\vartheta) < 0, \qquad \operatorname{Re}(\vartheta) < -\frac{1}{2}. \tag{9.1050a–c}$$

If (9.1050a) and the reverse of (9.1050b, c) hold there are no singularities at $x = \pm 1, \theta = 0, \pi$. If (9.1050a) does not hold the Gaussian hypergeometric series in (9.1045a, b) do not converge, and the leading terms alone do not represent the singularities at $x = \pm 1$.

For example, *if (9.1051a–c) hold (standard CDXXVI) the general integral of the hyperspherical associated differential equation (9.1037b) [(9.1036b)] finite (9.1051f) in the interval (9.1051d) [sphere (9.1051e)] is (9.1051g) [(9.1051h)]:*

$$0 > \operatorname{Re}(\vartheta) > -\frac{1}{2}, \quad \operatorname{Re}(\vartheta) < -\frac{1}{4}\operatorname{Re}(\lambda), \ -1 \le x \le +1 \Leftrightarrow 0 \le \theta \le \pi, \ y(x) = w(\theta) < \infty, \tag{9.1051a–f}$$

$$y(x) = B^{\mu}_{\nu,\lambda}(x) = A\left(1 - x^2\right)^{\vartheta + 1/2} F\left(\alpha + \frac{1}{2}, \beta + \frac{1}{2}; \frac{3}{2}; x^2\right), \tag{9.1051g}$$

$$w(\theta) = B^{\mu}_{\nu,\lambda}(\cos\theta) = A \sin^{1+2\vartheta}\theta \, F\left(\alpha + \frac{1}{2}, \beta + \frac{1}{2}; \frac{3}{2}; \cos^2\theta\right). \tag{9.1051h}$$

If the interval (9.1051d) [sphere (9.1051e)] was open $-1 < x < +1$ *(excluded the axis* $0 < \theta < \pi$*) then the linear combination (9.1047c) of solutions (9.1045a, c) would apply.* The hyperspherical associated Legendre functions (notes 9.23–9.24) are (Diagram 9.3): (i) equivalent to the Gaussian hypergeometric functions because both have three parameters; (ii–iv) the associated (ultra/hypersherical) Legendre functions [note 9.22 (9.21/9.25)] and original Legendre functions (note 9.20) are respectively two and one parameter particular cases of the Gaussian hypergeometric functions. Similarly, the Jacobi functions (notes 9.26) have three parameters that are equivalent to the Gaussian hypergeometric functions whereas the Chebychev functions of the first (second) type [note 9.27 (9.28)] are particular one parameter cases.

Concerning the hierarchy of Legendre functions in Diagram 9.2 the hyperspherical associated Legendre differential equation (9.1035a, b) ≡ (9.1037a, b) has three parameters and includes as particular two parameter cases the associated (9.1026a, b) ≡ (9.1027a, b) [hyperspherical (9.1036a, b) ≡ (9.1052a, b)] Legendre differential equations; both have in turn as a particular one parameter case the Legendre differential equation (9.1006a–c; 9.1008a, b). The latter is also a particular one parameter case of the ultraspherical Legendre differential equation (9.1019a, b) ≡ (9.1018b, c) that has two parameters but is not included in the hyperspherical associated Legendre differential equation (9.1035a, b) ≡ (9.1036a, b) that has three parameters. Of these five related differential equations, only (9.1037b) with $\mu = 0$, that is the hyperspherical Legendre differential equation (9.1036a, b) ≡ (9.1052a, b) of degree ν and dimension λ:

$$y(x) = P_{\nu,\lambda}(x): \qquad \left(1 - x^2\right) y'' - (2 + \lambda)\, x y' + \nu(\nu + 1)\, y = 0, \tag{9.1052a, b}$$

remains to be considered in detail (note 9.25) using a method distinct from (close to) that in the notes 9.23–9.24 (9.20–9.22).

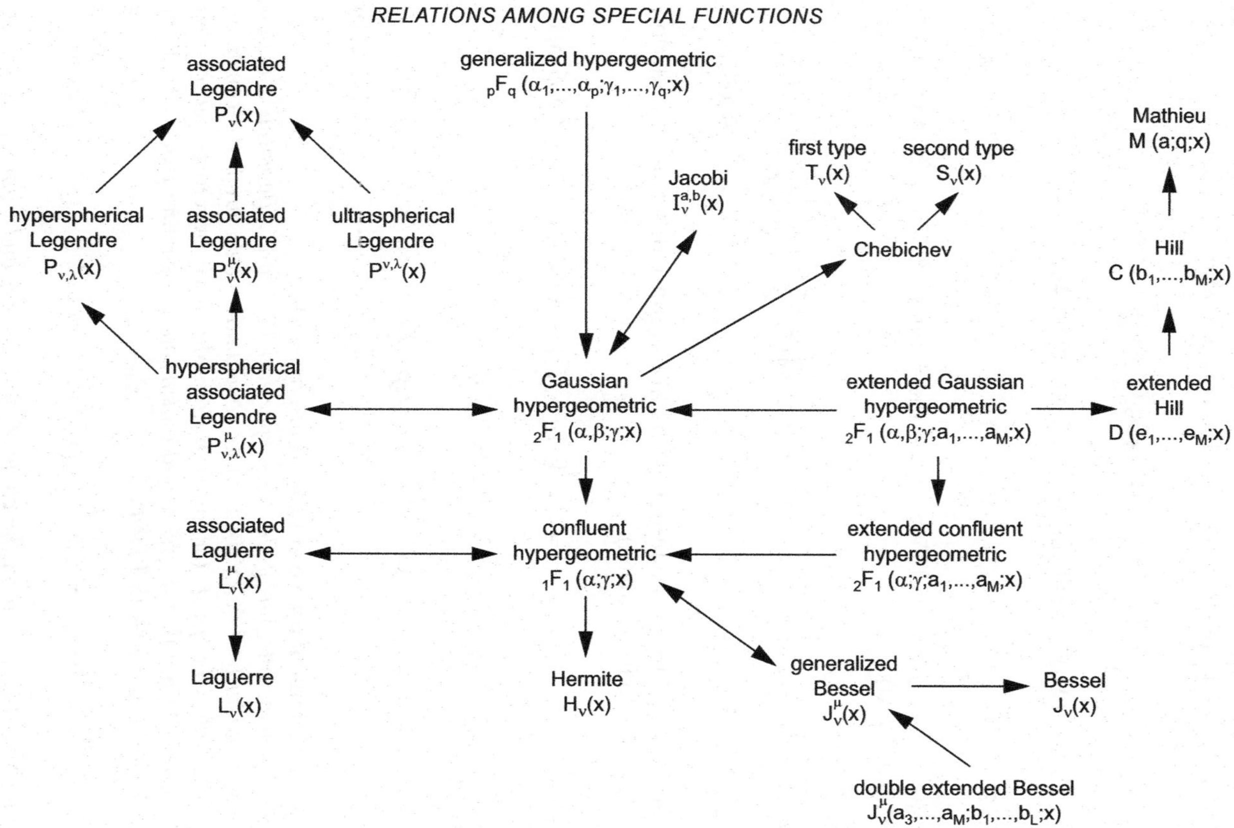

DIAGRAM 9.2
Relations among some special functions and the corresponding linear unforced second-order differential equations with variable coefficients.

NOTE 9.25: Hyperspherical Legendre Differential Equation (Campos & Cunha 2012)

The change of independent variable (9.1009c–e) transforms (9.1052b) to (9.977b) a Gaussian hypergeometric differential equation (9.1053):

$$\xi(1-\xi)z''+\left[(1+\lambda/2)-(2+\lambda)\xi\right]z'+\nu(\nu+1)z=0, \qquad (9.1053)$$

with parameters (9.1054a–c) leading (9.974b) to (9.1054d):

$$\gamma=1+\lambda/2,\quad \alpha+\beta=1+\lambda,\quad \alpha\beta=-\nu(\nu+1): \qquad g=1-\lambda/2. \qquad (9.1054\text{a–d})$$

The parameters α,β in (9.1054b, c) are the roots of (9.1055a, b) and hence given by (9.1053c, d):

$$0=(X-\alpha)(X-\beta)=X^2-(1+\lambda)X-\nu(\nu+1):\quad \alpha,\beta=\frac{1+\lambda}{2}\pm\sqrt{\left(\frac{1+\lambda}{2}\right)^2+\nu(\nu+1)}. \qquad (9.1055\text{a–d})$$

One solution (9.971b) of the hyperspherical Legendre differential equation (9.1052b) is (9.1056b) for (9.1056a):

$$\lambda\neq-2,-4\ldots: \qquad P_{\nu,\lambda}(x)=F\left(\alpha,\beta;1+\lambda/2;(1-x)/2\right), \qquad (9.1056\text{a, b})$$

and another (9.981d, e) is (9.1057b) for (9.1057a):

$$\lambda\neq0,2,4,\ldots:\quad R_{\nu,\lambda}(x)\equiv(1-x)^{-\lambda/2}F\left(\alpha-\lambda/2,\beta-\lambda/2;1-\lambda/2\,;(1-x)/2\right); \qquad (9.1057\text{a, b})$$

otherwise functions of the second kind are needed.

Thus *the general integral of the hyperspherical Legendre differential equation (9.1052b) is (standard CDXXVII) a linear combination with arbitrary constants (A,B) of (9.1058c) the* ***first (second) hyperspherical Legendre functions*** *(9.1056a, b) [(9.1057a, b)] of degree* ν *and dimension* λ *assuming that* $\lambda/2$ *not an integer (9.1056a; 9.1057a)* ≡ *(9.1058a):*

$$\lambda\neq0,\pm2,\pm4,\ldots: \qquad 1<|1-x|<2: \qquad y(x)=A\,P_{\nu,\lambda}(x)+B\,R_{\nu,\lambda}(x). \qquad (9.1058\text{a–c})$$

valid: (i) for (9.1013a–f) and on the circle of convergence; and (ii/iii) at the special point $x=-1$ *(other points) the convergence is specified by (9.964a–e) [(9.965a–f)] with (9.1054d). In particular (standard CDXXVIII) if (9.1059a) holds the solution of the hyperspherical associated Legendre differential equation (9.1052b) simplifies*

(9.1059d) to the first term of (9.1058c) and is absolutely (and uniformly) convergent for (9.1059b) [(9.1059c)]:

$$\mathrm{Re}(\lambda) > 0: \quad 0 \le |1-x| \le 2: \quad A.C.; \quad 1-\varepsilon \le |1-x| \le 2-\delta : T.C.; y(x) = A\,P_{\nu,\lambda}(x). \tag{9.1059a–d}$$

The alternatives to the Gaussian hypergeometric function (9.971a–c) with three parameters are the hyperspherical associated Legendre functions (notes 9.23–9.24) and the Jacobi functions (note 9.26) that also have three parameters.

NOTE 9.26: Jacobi (1859) Functions and Differential Equation

The ***Jacobi functions (1859)*** *with variable x, degree ν, and parameters (a, b) are related (standard CDXXIX) to the Gaussian hypergeometric functions by:*

$$a \ne -1,-2,\ldots: \qquad I_\nu^{a,b}(x) \equiv \binom{\nu+a}{\nu} F\left(-\nu, \nu+a+b+1; a+1; (1-x)/2\right); \tag{9.1060}$$

they satisfy (9.1061e) a Gaussian hypergeometric differential equation (9.977b) with parameters (9.1061a–d) and variables (9.1009c–e):

$$\alpha = -\nu,\ \beta = \nu+a+b+1,\ \gamma = 1+a,\ g = 1-b:$$
$$\xi(1-\xi)\,z'' + \left[1+a-(a+b+2)\xi\right] z' + \nu(\nu+a+b+1)\, z = 0. \tag{9.1061a–e}$$

The change of independent variable (9.1009c, e) leads to the **Jacobi differential equation** (9.1062a, b) with degree ν and parameters (a, b):

$$y(x) = I_\nu^{a,b}(x): \quad \left(1-x^2\right) y'' + \left[b-a-(a+b+2)x\right] y' + \nu(\nu+a+b+1)\, y = 0. \tag{9.1062a, b}$$

Another solution (9.981d, e) of (9.1062b) is:

$$a \ne 0,1,2,\ldots: \quad (1-x)^{-a} F\left(-\nu-a, \nu+1+b; 1-a; (1-x)/2\right)$$
$$= (1-x)^{-a} F\left(-\bar\nu, \bar\nu+\bar a+\bar b+1; 1+\bar a; (1-x)/2\right), \tag{9.1063a, b}$$

that is satisfied by (9.1064a–c):

$$\bar a = -a, \bar\nu = \nu+a, \bar b = b: (1-x)^{-a}\, I_{\bar\nu}^{\bar a,\bar b}(x) \binom{\bar\nu+\bar a}{\bar\nu}^{-1} = (1-x)^{-a}\, I_{a+\nu}^{-a,b}(x) \binom{\nu}{a+\nu}^{-1}, \tag{9.1064a–d}$$

leading to the second solution (9.1064d) where the last constant factor can be omitted. Thus *the general integral of the Jacobi differential equation (9.1062b) for a not an integer (9.1065a) is (standard CDXXX) a linear combination (9.1065b) with arbitrary constants (A,B) of the Jacobi functions (9.1060):*

$$a \neq 0, \pm 1, \pm 2, \ldots: \qquad y(x) = A\, I_\nu^{a,b}(x) + B\,(1-x)^{-a}\, I_{\nu+a}^{-a,b}(x), \tag{9.1065a, b}$$

valid for (9.1013a–f) with convergence on the boundary point $x = -1$ (other boundary points) given by (9.964a–e) [(9.965a–f)] with (9.1061d). Two particular one-parameter cases of the Gaussian hypergeometric function are the Chebychev polynomials of the first (second) type (subsection II.5.6.7), that are solutions of the corresponding differential equations [notes 9.27 (9.28)].

NOTE 9.27: Chebychev (1859) Differential Equation of the First Type

The **Chebychev function of first type** (1859) defined by:

$$x = \cos\theta: \qquad T_\nu(x) = T_\nu(\cos\theta) = \cos(\nu\theta) = \cos(\nu\, arc\cos x), \tag{9.1066a–d}$$

generalizing to complex ν the polynomials (II.5.129a) of positive integer degree n and suppressing a constant factor 2^{1-n}. Adding the identities (II.5.47a) ≡ (9.1067a, b):

$$\cos[(\nu \pm 1)\theta] = \cos(\nu\theta)\cos\theta \mp \sin(\nu\theta)\sin(\theta), \tag{9.1067a, b}$$

leads to (9.1068a) that is (9.1066a, c) the **recurrence formula** (9.1068b) for the Chebychev functions of the first type:

$$\cos[(\nu+1)\,\theta] + \cos[(\nu-1)\,\theta] = 2\cos\theta\cos(\nu\theta): T_{\nu+1}(x) = 2x\,T_\nu(x) - T_{\nu-1}(x). \tag{9.1068a, b}$$

Differentiating (9.1066c) leads to (9.1069a):

$$T_\nu'(x) = \frac{d[\cos(\nu\theta)]}{d[\cos(\theta)]} = \frac{d[\cos(\nu\theta)]/d\theta}{d[\cos(\theta)]/d\theta} = \nu\frac{\sin(\nu\theta)}{\sin\theta}, \tag{9.1069a}$$

$$\sin^2\theta\, T_\nu'(x) = \nu\sin(\nu\theta)\sin\theta = \nu\{\cos[(\nu-1)x] - \cos\theta\cos(\nu\theta)\}, \tag{9.1069b, c}$$

that is equivalent to (9.1069a) ≡ (9.1069b) and by (9.1067b) leads to (9.1069c). The latter is (9.1066a, c) the **differentiation formula** for the Chebychev functions of the first type (9.1070a):

$$(1-x^2)\,T_\nu' = -\nu x T_\nu + \nu T_{\nu-1} = \nu x T_\nu - \nu T_{\nu+1}, \tag{9.1070a, b}$$

with (9.1068b) used in (9.1070b).

The (standard CDXXXI) recurrence (9.1068b) and differentiation (9.1070a, b) formulas for the Chebychev functions of the first type (9.1066a–c) may be eliminated into a second-order linear differential equation for (9.1066c) alone as follows: (i) differentiation of (9.1070b) leads to (9.1071a); (ii) substitution of (9.1070a) with ν replaced by $\nu+1$ leads to (9.1071b); (iii) substituting (9.1070b) leads to (9.1071c) that simplifies to (9.1071d):

$$\left(1-x^2\right)T_\nu''-x(2+\nu)T_\nu'-\nu T_\nu=-\nu T_{\nu+1}'=-\frac{\nu(\nu+1)}{1-x^2}\left(T_\nu-xT_{\nu+1}\right)$$
$$=-\frac{\nu+1}{1-x^2}\left\{\nu T_\nu+x\left[\left(1-x^2\right)T_\nu'-\nu xT_\nu\right]\right\}=-(\nu+1)\left(\nu T_\nu+xT_\nu'\right); \tag{9.1071a–d}$$

and (iv) simplifying (9.1071d) leads to the **Chebychev differential equation of the first type** and degree ν:

$$y(x)\equiv T_\nu(x):\qquad \left(1-x^2\right)y''-xy'+\nu^2 y=0. \tag{9.1072a, b}$$

The change of independent variable (9.1009d, e) leads to (9.1073a):

$$\xi(1-\xi)\,z''+(1/2-\xi)\,z'+\nu^2 z=0, \tag{9.1073a}$$

that is a Gaussian hypergeometric differential equation (9.977b) with parameters (9.1073b–d) implying (9.1073e, f):

$$\gamma=1/2\,,\ \alpha+\beta=0,\ \alpha\beta=-\nu^2:\qquad \alpha=-\nu\,,\ \beta=\nu,\ g=3/2, \tag{9.1073b–g}$$

and (9.974b) also (9.1073g).

From (9.1073b, e, f; 9.1009c, e) it follows that the *first (second) Chebychev functions of the first type are related (standard CDXXXII) to the Gaussian hypergeometric functions by (9.1074a, b):*

$$T_\nu(x)=F\left(-\nu,\nu;3/2;(1-x)/2\right);$$
$$S_\nu(x)=(1-x)^{1/2}\,F\left(-\nu+1/2,\nu+1/2;3/2;(1-x)/2\right), \tag{9.1074a, b}$$

a second linearly independent solution of the Chebychev differential equation (9.1072b) is (9.981e) also of the first kind (9.1074b). In (9.1074a) there could be a constant factor; since the Gaussian hypergeometric series (9.871b) [Chebychev function of the first type (9.1066d)] both take the value unity (9.1075b) [≡(9.1075c–e)] at the point unity (9.1076a) the factor is also unity:

$$x=1:\qquad F(-\nu,\nu;3/2;0)=1=T_\nu(1)=\cos\left(\nu\arccos 1\right)=\cos 0. \tag{9.1075a–e}$$

Thus *the general integral (standard CDXXXIII) of the Chebychev differential equation (9.1072b) is a linear combination (9.1076c) with arbitrary constants (A, B) of the* **first (second) Chebychev functions of the first type** *and degree* ν *both of the first kind (9.1074a) [(9.1074b)]:*

$$|x-1|\le 2;\varepsilon\le|x-1|\le 2-\delta: \qquad y(x)=A\,T_\nu(x)+B\,S_\nu(x), \tag{9.1076a–c}$$

that converge absolutely (and uniformly) in (Figure 9.18b) the closed disk (9.1076a) [the closed sub-disk (9.1076b)] because (9.1073g) satisfies (9.964e; 9.965f). *The second function of the first kind (standard CDXXXIV) vanishes (9.1074b) at the north pole $x=1$ of a sphere $\theta=0$; the first function of the first kind (9.1074a) ν positive integer $\nu=n$ reduces to a polynomial (9.1005a–c) of degree n.* The analysis is similar for the Chebychev differential equation of the first (second) type [note 9.26 (9.27)].

NOTE 9.28: Chebychev (1947) Differential Equation of the Second Type

The ***Chebychev functions of the second type*** *(9.947) and degree* ν *are defined by (9.1077a–d):*

$$x=\cos\theta: \qquad U_\nu(x)=U_\nu(\cos\theta)=\frac{\sin[(\nu+1)\theta]}{\sin\theta}=\frac{\sin[(\nu+1)arc\cos x]}{\sqrt{1-x^2}}, \tag{9.1077a–d}$$

where was omitted the coefficient $2^{1-\nu}$ relative to the polynomials (II.5.129b). Adding the identities (II.5.47b) ≡ (9.1078a, b):

$$\sin\{[(\nu+1)\pm1]\theta\}=\sin[(\nu+1)\theta]\cos\theta\pm\cos[(\nu+1)\theta]\sin\theta, \tag{9.1078a, b}$$

leads to (9.1079a) that is the **recurrence formula** (9.1079b) for the Chebychev function of the second type:

$$\sin[(\nu+2)\theta]+\sin(\nu\theta)=2\cos\theta\sin[(\nu+1)\theta]: U_{\nu+1}(x)=2xU_\nu(x)-U_{\nu-1}(x), \tag{9.1079a, b}$$

that coincides with the recurrence formula for the first type (9.1068b) ≡ (9.1079b). The differentiation of (9.1077c) leads to (9.1080a):

$$U'_\nu(x)=\frac{d}{d(\cos\theta)}\left\{\frac{\sin[(\nu+1)\theta]}{\sin\theta}\right\}=-\frac{1}{\sin\theta}\frac{d}{d\theta}\left\{\frac{\sin[(\nu+1)\theta]}{\sin\theta}\right\}, \tag{9.1080a, b}$$

that is equivalent to (9.1080b) ≡ (9.1081a):

$$\begin{aligned}\sin^2\theta U_\nu' &= \frac{\cos\theta}{\sin\theta}\sin[(\nu+1)\theta] - (\nu+1)\cos[(\nu+1)\theta] \\ &= \cos\theta U_\nu + (\nu+1)\frac{\sin(\nu\theta) - \cos\theta\sin[(\nu+1)\theta]}{\sin\theta} \\ &= \cos\theta U_\nu + (\nu+1)[U_{\nu-1} - \cos\theta U_\nu],\end{aligned} \tag{9.1081a–c}$$

that is rewritten (9.1081b) using (9.1078b), thus leading to (9.1081c) ≡ (9.1082a):

$$\left(1-x^2\right)U_\nu' = -\nu x U_\nu + (\nu+1)U_{\nu-1} = (\nu+2)\,xU_\nu - (\nu+1)\,U_{\nu+1}; \tag{9.1082a, b}$$

substitution of (9.1079b) in (9.1082a) leads to (9.1082b). Thus (9.1082a, b) is the **differentiation formula** for the Chebychev functions of the second type.

The *recurrence (9.1079a, b) and differentiation (9.1082a, b) formulas (standard CDXXV) for the Chebychev functions of the second type (9.1077a–d)* may be eliminated into a second-order linear differential equation as follows: (i) differentiation (9.1082b) leads to (9.1083a); (ii) substitution of (9.1082a) with $\nu+1$ instead of ν yields (9.1083b); and (iii) using (9.1082b) leads to (9.1083c) that simplifies to (9.1083d):

$$\left(1-x^2\right)U_\nu'' - (\nu+4)\,x\,U_\nu' - (\nu+2)\,U_\nu = -(\nu+1)U_{\nu+1}'. \tag{9.1083a}$$

$$= -\frac{(\nu+1)(\nu+2)}{1-x^2}U_\nu + \frac{(\nu+1)^2}{1-x^2}xU_{\nu+1}, \tag{9.1083b}$$

$$= -\frac{(\nu+1)(\nu+2)}{1-x^2}U_\nu - \frac{(\nu+1)}{1-x^2}x\left[\left(1-x^2\right)U_\nu' - (\nu+2)xU_\nu\right], \tag{9.1083c}$$

$$= -(v+1)(v+2)U_v - (v+1)xU_v'. \tag{9.1083d}$$

From (9.1083d) ≡ (9.1084b) follows the **Chebychev differential equation of the second type** with degree ν:

$$y(x) \equiv U_\nu(x): \qquad \left(1-x^2\right)y'' - 3xy' + \nu(\nu+2)y = 0. \tag{9.1084a, b}$$

The change of variable (9.9109c, e) leads to (9.1085a):

$$\xi(1-\xi)\,z'' + (3/2 - 3\xi)\,z' + \nu(\nu+2)\,z = 0, \tag{9.1085a}$$

that is a Gaussian hypergeometric differential equation (9.977b) with parameters (9.1085b–d):

$$\gamma = 3/2, \quad \alpha+\beta = 2, \quad \alpha\beta = -\nu(\nu+2); \quad \alpha = -\nu, \beta = \nu+2, \quad g = 1/2, \tag{9.1085b–g}$$

from (9.1085c, d) follow (9.1085e, f) and (9.974b) also (9.1085g).

From (9.1085b, e, f; 9.1009c, e) it follows that *the first (9.1086a) [second (9.1086b)] Chebychev functions (standard CDXXXVI) of the second type are related to the Gaussian hypergeometric function by:*

$$U_\nu(x) = (\nu+1) F(-\nu, \nu+2; 3/2; (1-x)/2), \tag{9.1086a}$$

$$V_\nu(x) = (1-x)^{-1/2} F(-\nu-1/2, \nu+3/2; 1/2; (1-x)/2), \tag{9.1086b}$$

that follow from (9.971b) [(9.981e)]. The constant factor in (9.1086a) can be obtained comparing the values at the origin (9.1088a) of the Gaussian hypergeometric (Chebychev) function of the first kind (9.971b) [type (9.1077a–d)] that are (9.1087b) [(9.1087c–d)] in the ratio $1+\nu$:

$$x = 0: \quad F(-\nu, \nu+2; 3/2; 0) = 1, \quad U_\nu(1) = \lim_{\theta \to 0} \frac{\sin[(\nu+1)\theta]}{\sin\theta} = \nu+1. \tag{9.1087a–d}$$

Thus *the general integral of the Chebychev differential equation of the second type (9.1084b) is (standard CDXXXVII) a linear combination (9.1088b) with arbitrary constants (A,B) of the two functions of the first kind (9.1086a, b) where the second is singular at the point unity:*

$$|1-x| < 2: \qquad y(x) = A\, U_\nu(x) + B\, V_\nu(x). \tag{9.1088a, b}$$

The solution (9.1088b) is valid for (9.1013a–f) and on the boundary of convergence (9.1085g) shows that it diverges (9.964b) [converges conditionally (9.965e)] at the special point $x = -1, \xi = 1, \theta = \pi$ (all other points). Thus *a solution of the Chebychev differential equation of the second type (9.1084b) that is (standard CDXXXVIII) finite (9.1089c) in the closed interval (9.1089a) or sphere (9.1089b) must be specified by a terminating series, that must (9.1086a) ≡ (9.1089e) with ν positive integer:*

$$-1 \le x \le +1 \quad \Leftrightarrow \quad 0 \le \theta \le \pi: \quad y(x) < \infty, \nu = n \in |N: \quad y(x) = A U_n(x). \tag{9.1089a–e}$$

The Legendre polynomials (9.1016a–d) ≡ (9.1090b) [Chebychev polynomials of the first (9.1074a) ≡ (9.1090c) and second (9.1086a) ≡ (9.1090d) type] are all particular cases (standard CDXXIX) of terminating (9.1005a–c) Gaussian hypergeometric series (9.971a–c):

$$n \in| N: \quad F(-n, n+p; q; (1-x)/2) = \begin{cases} P_n(x) & \text{for} \quad p = 1 = q, \\ T_n(x) & \text{for} \quad p = 0, q = \dfrac{3}{2} \\ U_n(x) & \text{for} \quad p = 2, q = \dfrac{3}{2} \end{cases}. \tag{9.1090a–d}$$

The Gaussian (confluent) hypergeometric differential equation [notes 9.14–9.19 (9.29)] both include a number of important particular cases [notes 9.20–9.28 (9.30–9.33)].

NOTE 9.29: Confluent Hypergeometric Differential Equation (Kummer 1839)

The Gaussian (9.971b, c) [confluent (9.1091c, d)] series are the particular cases ${}_2F_1\left({}_1F_1\right)$ of the generalized hypergeometric series:

$$\gamma \neq 0, -1, -2, \ldots: \quad |x| < \infty:$$

$${}_1F_1(\alpha; \gamma; x) = 1 + \sum_{k=1}^{\infty} \frac{\alpha \ldots (\alpha + k - 1)}{j \ldots (j + k - 1)} \frac{x^k}{k!} = \frac{\Gamma(\gamma)}{\Gamma(\alpha)} \sum_{k=1}^{\infty} \frac{\Gamma(\alpha + k)}{\Gamma(\gamma + k)} \frac{x^k}{k!}; \tag{9.1091a–d}$$

the series (9.1091c, d) has infinite radius of convergence (9.1091b) and defines (Kummer 1836) the **confluent hypergeometric function** of variable x with upper (lower) parameter $\alpha(\gamma)$ that has simple poles for the integer values of γ excluded in (9.1091a). The confluent (Gaussian) hypergeometric functions are related by:

$$F(\alpha; \gamma; x) = \lim_{\beta \to \infty} F\left(\alpha, \beta; \gamma; \frac{x}{\beta}\right), \tag{9.1092}$$

that is proved by the two-stage process of (i) replacing x by x/β and then (ii) letting $\beta \to \infty$, to eliminate the factor:

$$\lim_{\beta \to \infty} \frac{\beta \ldots (\beta + k - 1)}{\beta^k} = \lim_{\beta \to \infty} \left(1 + \frac{1}{\beta}\right) \ldots \left(1 + \frac{k-1}{\beta}\right) = 1, \tag{9.1093a, b}$$

from the Gaussian hypergeometric series:

$$F\left(\alpha,\beta;\gamma;\frac{x}{\beta}\right)=1+\sum_{k=1}^{\infty}\frac{\alpha....(\alpha+k-1)}{j....(j+k-1)}\frac{x^k}{k!}\frac{\beta....(\beta+k-1)}{\beta^k}, \tag{9.1094}$$

leading to the confluent hypergeometric series (9.1091c). The same two-stage limit process applied to the Gaussian hypergeometric differential equation (9.971b) leads to:

$$\lim_{\beta\to\infty}\left[x\left(1-\frac{x}{\beta}\right)y''+\left(\gamma-\frac{\alpha+\beta+1}{\beta}x\right)y'-\alpha y\right]=xy''+(\gamma-x)\,y'-\alpha y, \tag{9.1095}$$

the confluent hypergeometric differential equation (9.1095) ≡ (9.869a, c) considered before (subsections 9.9.4–9.9.8).

The confluent hypergeometric function is specified by the power series (9.1091c) ≡ (9.1096a) with coefficients (9.1096b, c) ≡ (9.890a, b):

$$F(\alpha;\gamma;x)=\sum_{k=0}^{\infty}c_k\,x^k; \qquad c_0=1, \qquad c_k=\frac{\alpha....\,(\alpha+k-1)}{k!\gamma....(\gamma+k-1)}; \tag{9.1096a–c}$$

comparing (9.1096c) ≡ (9.1097a) with (9.873c) ≡ (9.1097b) leads to the polynomials (9.1097c, d):

$$\frac{\alpha+k-1}{k(\gamma+k-1)}=\frac{c_k}{c_{k-1}}=\frac{Q_1(k+a-1)}{P_2(k+a)}: \quad Q_1(a)=(a+\alpha), \quad P_2(a)=a(a+\gamma-1). \tag{9.1097a–d}$$

Thus the confluent hypergeometric function (9.1096a–c) must be a solution (9.935a–c) of the differential equation:

$$0=\left\{x\frac{d}{dx}\left(x\frac{d}{dx}+\gamma-1\right)-x\left(x\frac{d}{dx}+\alpha\right)\right\}y(x)=x\left[xy''+(\gamma-x)y'-\alpha y\right], \tag{9.1098}$$

leading to the confluent hypergeometric differential equation (9.1095) in square brackets in (9.1098) with parameters (α,β). The Gaussian (confluent) hypergeometric differential equations (9.977b) [(9.1095) ≡ (9.869c)] both have a regular singularity at the origin, with the same indices (9.973a, b) [≡ (9.887d, e)] and the corresponding linearly independent particular integrals of the first kind are (9.971a–c) [(9.891a–c)] and (9.981d, e) [(9.893a, b)]. The main difference is that the Gaussian ${}_2F_1$ (confluent ${}_1F_1$) hypergeometric functions correspond to ${}_pF_q$ with $p=q+1\,(p=q)$ and thus the nearest singularity to the origin is at the point unity $x=1$ (point at infinity $x=\infty$) implying a unit (9.982b) [infinite (9.894b)] radius of convergence. Thus *the general integral (standard CDXL) of the Gaussian (confluent) hypergeometric differential equation (9.977b) [(9.869b) ≡ (9.1095)] is a linear combination (9.982c) [(9.894c)] of Gaussian (confluent) hypergeometric functions of the first kind (9.971a–c; 9.981a–e) [(9.891a–c; 9.893a, b)] with unit (9.963a–e; 9.964a–e; 9.965a–f; 9.974b) [infinite (9.894b)] radius of convergence valid for γ not an integer (9.982a) [≡ (9.894a)].* The case of γ integer leads to Gaussian and confluent hypergeometric functions of the second kind (notes 9.16–9.18) that are similar suppressing the terms with the parameter β in the latter case; for example *for γ a positive integer (9.983a, b) [(9.1099a)] the (standard CDXLI) general integral (9.983c) [(9.1099b)]:*

$$\gamma=1,2,\ldots; \qquad y(x)=A\,F(\alpha;n;x)+B\,G(\alpha;n;x), \tag{9.1099a, b}$$

of the Gaussian (9.977b) [confluent (9.1095)] hypergeometric differential equation is a linear combination of functions of the first (9.971a–c) [(9.1091a–d)] and second (9.993; 9.992; 9.986b; 9.990) [(9.1100)] kinds:

$$\begin{aligned} G(\alpha;n;x) &= (-)^n \frac{(\alpha+1-n)\ldots(\alpha-1)}{n!(n-1)!}\log x\,F(\alpha;n;x) \\ &\quad + x^{1-n}\left[1+\sum_{k=1}^{n-2}\frac{(-x)^k}{k!n!}(\alpha+1-n)\ldots(\alpha+k-n)\right] \\ &\quad + \frac{(-)^n}{n!}\sum_{j=0}^{\infty} x^j \frac{(\alpha+1-n)\ldots(\alpha+j-1)}{j!(n+j-1)!} \\ &\quad [\psi(\alpha+j)+2\psi(1)-\psi(\alpha+1-n)-\psi(1+j)-\psi(n+j)]. \end{aligned} \tag{9.1100}$$

The confluent hypergeometric differential equation (note 9.28) has the Laguerre (associated Laguerre) differential equation [note 9.29 (9.30)] as a particular (equivalent) case with one (two) parameters.

NOTE 9.30: Laguerre (1879) Functions and Differential Equation

The **Laguerre function of the first kind** (1879) of degree ν is defined by (9.1101c):

$$\alpha=-\nu,\gamma=1: \qquad L_\nu(x)=\frac{e^{i\pi\nu}}{\Gamma(1+\nu)}F(-\nu;1;x), \tag{9.1101a–c}$$

that satisfies (9.1102a) a confluent hypergeometric differential equation (9.1022) with parameters (9.1101a, b):

$$xy''+(1-x)y'+\nu y=0; \qquad N_\nu(x)=\frac{e^{i\pi\nu}}{\Gamma(1+\nu)}G(-\nu;1;x), \tag{9.1102a, b}$$

a second linearly independent solution (9.983a–c) is (9.1102b) a **Laguerre function of the second kind** and degree ν. Thus *the Laguerre functions of degree ν of the first (second) kind are (standard CDXLII) related by (9.1101c) [(9.1102b)] to the confluent hypergeometric function of the first (9.1091a–d) [second (9.1100)] kind.* Thus *the general integral (standard CDXLIII) of the Laguerre differential equation (9.1102a) is a linear combination (9.1103b) with arbitrary constants (A,B) of the Laguerre functions of the first (9.1101c) [second (9.1102b)] kinds valid in the finite complex plane (9.1103a):*

$$|x|<\infty: \qquad y(x)=A\,L_\nu(x)+B\,N_\nu(x); \tag{9.1103a, b}$$

a solution finite (standard CDXLIV) at the origin (9.1104a) involves only the Laguerre function of the first kind (9.1104b):

$$y(0)<\infty; \quad y(x)=A L_\nu(x); \quad n\in|N: \quad y(x)=A\frac{(-)^n}{n!}F(-n;1;x), \tag{9.1104a–d}$$

that reduces (9.1005a–c) to a polynomial (9.1104d) for positive integer degree (9.1104c). The associated Laguerre function (note 9.31) is a generalization of the Laguerre function (note 9.30) from 1 to 2 parameters, and thus is equivalent to the confluent hypergeometric function (note 9.28).

NOTE 9.31: Associated Laguerre Differential Equation

The **associated Laguerre function** *of degree ν and order μ is related (standard CDXLV) to the confluent hypergeometric function by (9.1105c, d):*

$$\alpha=-\nu, \gamma=1+\mu; \mu\neq-1,-2,\ldots: \qquad L_\nu^\mu(x)=\frac{e^{i\pi\nu}}{\Gamma(1+\nu)}F(-\nu;1+\mu;x), \tag{9.1105a–c}$$

that satisfies (9.1106) a confluent hypergeometric differential equation (9.1095) with parameters (9.1105a, b):

$$xy''+(1+\mu-x)y'+\nu y=0. \tag{9.1106}$$

A second linearly independent solution (9.981d, e) is (9.1107a, b):

$$\mu\neq 0,1,2,\ldots: \qquad x^{-\mu}\frac{e^{-i\pi(\nu+\mu)}}{\Gamma(1-\mu-\nu)}F(-\nu-\mu;1-\mu;x)=x^{-\mu}L_{\nu-\mu}^{-\mu}(x). \tag{9.1107a, b}$$

Thus *the general integral of the* **associated Laguerre differential equation** *(9.1106) is (standard CDXLVI) a linear combination (9.1108c) with arbitrary constants (A,B) of the Laguerre functions of the first kind (9.1105c; 9.1107b) valid in the finite complex plane (9.1108b) for non-integer order (9.1108a):*

$$\mu \neq 0,\pm 1,\pm,2,\ldots: \qquad |x|<\infty: \qquad y(x)=A\,L_\nu^\mu(x)+B\,x^{-\mu}L_{\nu-\mu}^{-\mu}(x). \qquad (9.1108\text{a–c})$$

For (9.1109a) the solution finite at the origin (9.1109a) involves (standard CDXLVII) only the first associated Laguerre function (9.1109b) that is a polynomial of degree n for non-negative integer order $\nu=n$:

$$\operatorname{Re}(\mu)>0, \qquad y(0)<\infty: \qquad y(x)=A\,L_\nu^\mu(x). \qquad (9.1109\text{a–c})$$

The general integral in the case of positive integer order μ *involves functions of the second kind that have a logarithmic singularity at the origin.* The one parameter particular cases of the confluent hypergeometric differential equation (note 9.28) include the Laguerre (Hermite) differential equations [note 9.29(9.31)].

NOTE 9.32: Hermite (1864) Functions and Differential Equation

The **Hermite differential equation (1864)** of degree ν is (III.1.206) ≡ (9.1110b):

$$y(x)=H_\nu(x): \qquad y''-2xy'+2\nu y=0, \qquad (9.1110\text{a, b})$$

that is satisfied by the Hermite functions (9.1110a) with complex degree ν, that for positive integer degree reduce to the Hermite polynomials (subsection III.1.1.6 and note III.1.14). The transformation to a confluent hypergeometric differential equation requires changes of dependent and independent variables. The change of dependent variable (9.1111a) leads (9.516a–c) from (9.1110b) to the differential equation (9.1111b):

$$y(x)=x^a\,j(x): \quad x^2j''+2x\left(a-x^2\right)j'+\left[a(a-1)+2(\nu-a)\,x^2\right]j=0. \qquad (9.1111\text{a, b})$$

The choice (9.1036a) for the arbitrary constant leads (9.1112b) from (9.1111b) to the differential equation (9.1112c):

$$a=1: \qquad y(x)=x\,j(x): \qquad x\,j''+2\left(1-x^2\right)j'+2(\nu-1)\,x\,j=0. \qquad (9.1112\text{a–c})$$

The change of independent variable (9.1113a) ≡ (9.1038a–d) leads (9.1113b) from (9.1112c) to the differential equation (9.1113c):

$$\zeta\equiv x^2, \qquad j(x)=h(\zeta): \qquad \zeta h''+\left(\frac{3}{2}-\zeta\right)h'+\frac{\nu-1}{2}h=0; \qquad (9.1113\text{a–c})$$

the differential equations (9.1113c) is of the confluent hypergeometric type (9.1095) with parameters (9.1114a, b):

$$\alpha = \frac{1-\nu}{2}, \quad \gamma = \frac{3}{2}: \qquad h(\zeta) = F\left(1/2-\nu/2;3/2;x^2\right), \tag{9.1114a–c}$$

leading to the solution (9.1114c).

Substitution of (9.1110a; 9.1112b; 9.1113a, b; 9.1114c) relates (standard CDXLVIII) *the* ***first Hermite function*** *of variable x and degree* ν *to (9.1115) the confluent hypergeometric function with variable (9.1113a) and parameters (9.1114a, b):*

$$H_\nu(x) = 2^\nu x F\left(1/2-\nu/2;3/2;x^2\right). \tag{9.1115}$$

The constant coefficient 2^ν in (9.1115) is introduced for consistency with the Hermite polynomials (III.1.18) ≡ (9.1116b) for positive integer order (9.1116a):

$$\nu = 1,2,3,\ldots = n \in |N: \qquad H_n(x) = (-)^n e^{x^2} \frac{d^n}{dx^n}\left(e^{-x^2}\right); \qquad H_1(x) = 2x. \tag{9.1116a–c}$$

For example, setting $n = 1$ in (9.1116b) and (9.1115) leads to the same result (9.1116c), proving that 2^ν is the correct multiplying constant in (9.1115). A second linearly independent solution of the confluent hypergeometric differential equation (9.1113c) with parameters (9.1114a, b) is (9.893b) leading (9.1115) to (9.1117a):

$$2^\nu x\left(x^2\right)^{-1/2} F\left(-\nu/2;1/2;x^2\right) = 2^\nu F\left(-\nu/2;1/2;x^2\right) \equiv I_\nu(x), \tag{9.1117a, b}$$

that relates the **second Hermite function** (9.1117b) of degree ν *to (standard CDXLIX) hypergeometric function of the first kind.* Thus *the general integral of the Hermite differential equation (9.1110b) is (standard CDL) a linear combination (9.1118b) with arbitrary constants (A,B) of the first (9.1115) [second (9.1117b)] Hermite function, both of the first kind and valid in the finite complex x-plane (9.1117a):*

$$|x| < \infty: \qquad y(x) = A\, H_\nu(x) + B\, I_\nu(x). \tag{9.1118a, b}$$

Several examples have been (will be) given [notes 9.20–9.32 (9.35–9.38)] of sub (super) hypergeometric differential equations [note 9.33 (9.34)] that reduce (do not reduce) to the generalized, Gaussian, or confluent hypergeometric differential equations (notes 9.9–9.19).

NOTE 9.33: Subhypergeometric and Bessel Differential Equations

The **subhypergeometric differential equations** *are (standard CDLI) those that can be reduced to generalized, Gaussian, or confluent hypergeometric differential equations because they fall in one of two groups: (a) differential equations of any order N with up to three regular singularities that are reducible to generalized (Gaussian)* *hypergeometric type [notes 9.9–9.13 (9.14–9.19)] for order larger than (equal to) two; and (b) differential equations of second-order with one regular singularity and irregular singularity of degree one that are reducible to the confluent hypergeometric type (note 9.29; subsections 9.9.4–9.9.8).* The examples of the first (a) [second (b)] set include notes 9.20–9.28 (9.30–9.32)] the Legendre, Ultraspherical, hyperspherical and associated Legendre, hyperspherical associated Legendre, Jacobi, and two types of Chebychev (Laguerre, associated Laguerre, Hermite, Bessel, and generalized Bessel) functions.

The last statement is proved next: *the original (generalized) Bessel differential equation (9.430b) [(9.428a–f)] has solution in terms of the generalized (original) Bessel function (9.448) [(9.510a)] that can be obtained [standard CCCLXXXIX (CDLII)] from the Gaussian (confluent) hypergeometric function (9.971a–c) [(9.1091a–d)] via the relations (9.1118) [(9.896b)]:*

$$J_\nu(x) = \frac{(x/2)^\nu}{\Gamma(1+\nu)} \lim_{\alpha,\beta\to\infty} F\left(\alpha,\beta;1+\nu;-\frac{x^2}{4\alpha\beta}\right). \tag{9.1119a}$$

The proof of (9.1119a) is made noting that the Gaussian hypergeometric series (9.971b, c) is uniformly convergent with regard to α,β, and thus the limit can be taken term by term in (9.971a) ≡ (9.1119b):

$$\begin{aligned}
&\lim_{\alpha,\beta\to\infty} F\left(\alpha,\beta;1+\nu;-\frac{x^2}{4\alpha\beta}\right)\\
&= \Gamma(1+\nu)\sum_{k=0}^{\infty} \frac{(-x^2/4)^k}{k!\,\Gamma(1+\nu+k)} \lim_{\alpha,\beta\to\infty} \frac{\alpha\ldots(\alpha+k-1)\beta\ldots(\beta+k-1)}{\alpha^k\beta^k} \qquad \text{(9.1119b–d)}\\
&= \Gamma(1+\nu)\sum_{k=0}^{\infty} \frac{(-x^2/4)^k}{k\,!\,\Gamma(1+\nu+k)} = \Gamma(1+\nu)(x/2)^{-\nu} J_\nu(x),
\end{aligned}$$

where were used (9.1093a, b) in (9.1119c) and (9.510a) in (9.1119d). The opposite cases of superhypergeometric differential equations (note 9.34) include the Mathieu and Hill equations.

NOTE 9.34: Superhypergeometric and Generalized Hill Differential Equations

The **superhypergeometric differential equations** *are (standard CDLIII) those not reducible to generalized, Gaussian, or confluent hypergeometric differential equations because they have (a) either at least four regular singularities or (b) two regular and one irregular singularities or (c) two singularities, one of which is irregular of degree at least two or (d) an irregular singularity of degree at least three.* An example is the **generalized Hill differential equation** *(9.699a, b) ≡ (9.1120a, b):*

$$w(\theta) = D(b_0,\ldots,b_M;\cos\theta): \qquad \frac{d^2w}{d\theta^2} + \left[\sum_{\ell=0}^{M} b_\ell \cos(\ell\theta)\right] w = \theta, \tag{9.1120a, b}$$

that adds terms with cosines of odd multiplies of θ to the cosines with even multiples of θ in the original Hill differential equation (9.705a, b) and where M may be finite or infinite. Since the cosines of multiple angles can be expressed as powers of cosines by (II.5.110) ≡ (9.1121a):

$$\cos(\ell\theta) = \sum_{k=0}^{\leq \ell/2} \frac{(-)^k}{k!} \ell(\ell-k-1)...(\ell-2k+1) 2^{\ell-2k-1} \cos^{\ell-2k}\theta, \qquad (9.1121a)$$

the generalized Hill differential equation (9.1120b) can be rewritten (9.1122):

$$w'' + \left[\sum_{\ell=0}^{M} e_s \cos^s\theta\right] w = 0, \qquad (9.1122)$$

with the new coefficients e_s related to the former b_ℓ by:

$$\sum_{s=0}^{M} e_s \cos^s\theta = \sum_{\ell=0}^{M} b_\ell \sum_{k=0}^{\leq \ell/2} \frac{(-)^k}{k!} \ell(\ell-k-1)....(\ell-2k+1)\, 2^{\ell-2k-1} \cos^{\ell-2k}\theta, \quad (9.1123)$$

that is obtained equating (9.1122) ≡ (9.1120b) and using (9.1121a). Equating powers of $\cos\theta$ in (9.1123) leads to (9.1124a) and the restriction (9.1124b) that implies (9.1124c):

$$s = \ell - 2k: \qquad 0 \leq s + 2k = \ell \leq M \quad \Rightarrow \quad 0 \leq k \leq \frac{M-s}{2}. \qquad (9.1124a\text{–}c)$$

Using (9.1124b, c) in (9.1123) leads to (9.1125):

$$2^{1-s} e_s = \sum_{k=0}^{\leq (M-s)/2} b_{s+2k} \frac{(-)^k}{k!} (s+2k)(s+k-1) .... (s+1), \qquad (9.1125)$$

as the relation between the coefficients in the equivalent forms (9.1120b) ≡ (9.1122) of the generalized Hill differential equation.

The change of independent variable (9.1007a–d) in (9.1122) leads to the differential equation (9.1126a, b):

$$y(x) = D(e,....,e_M;x): \qquad \left(1-x^2\right) y'' - xy' + \sum_{s=0}^{M} e_s x^s y = 0. \qquad (9.1126a, b)$$

The further change of independent variable (9.1009c–e) leads to (9.1127a, b):

$$z(\xi) = y(x): \qquad \xi(1-\xi) z'' + (1/2-\xi) z' + \sum_{m=0}^{M} f_m \xi^m z = 0, \qquad (9.1127a, b)$$

where the coefficients in (9.1127b) are related to those in (9.1126b) by (9.1128a):

$$\sum_{m=0}^{M} f_m \, \xi^m = \sum_{s=0}^{M} e_s \left(1-2\xi\right)^s = \sum_{s=0}^{M} e_s \sum_{k=0}^{s} \left(-2\xi\right)^k \frac{s!}{k!(s-k)!}, \tag{9.1128a, b}$$

that implies (9.1128b) ≡ (9.1129a, b):

$$m = k: \qquad f_m = \sum_{s=m}^{M} e_s \frac{s!(-2)^m}{m!(s-m)!}. \tag{9.1129a, b}$$

The generalized Hill differential equation has (standard CDLIV) four equivalent forms (9.1120a, b) ≡ (9.1122; 9.1125) ≡ (9.1007a–d; 9.1126a, b) ≡ (9.1009c, e; 9.1127a, b; 9.1129b). The differential equation (9.1127b) has regular singularities at $\xi = 0,1$ like the Gaussian hypergeometric differential equation (9.977b), but unlike it the point at infinity is not a regular singularity but rather an irregular singularity of degree M. Thus the generalized Hill differential equation is not subhypergeometric since it is not included in the Gaussian hypergeometric differential equation (9.977b), but is a particular case of an extended form considered next (note 9.35).

NOTE 9.35: Extended Gaussian Hypergeometric Differential Equation (Campos 2000)

The **extended Gaussian hypergeometric differential equation** with variable x, upper (lower) parameters $\alpha, \beta(\gamma)$ and asymptotic coefficients $(A_1, \ldots., A_M)$ is defined by (9.1130a, b):

$$y(x) = \Gamma\left(\alpha, \beta; \gamma; A_1, \ldots., A_M; x\right):$$

$$x(1-x)y'' + \left[\gamma - (\alpha+\beta+1)x\right]y' - \left(\alpha\beta + \sum_{m=1}^{M} A_m \, x^m\right)y = 0. \tag{9.1130a, b}$$

where M is the degree of the irregular singularity at infinity and the singularities at $x = 0$ and $x = 1$ are regular. Thus the generalized Hill differential equation (9.127a, b) is the particular case (9.1131a–e) of the extended Gaussian differential equation (9.1130a, b):

$$\gamma = 1/2, \quad \alpha+\beta = 0, \quad \alpha\beta = -f_0, \quad m = 1, \ldots, M, \quad A_m = -f_m:$$

$$g = 3/2, \quad \alpha = \sqrt{-f_0} = -\beta, \tag{9.1131a–h}$$

implying (9.1311g, h) and also (9.1131f) by (9.974b). Hence *the generalized Hill function (9.1126a) is related (standard CDLV) by (9.1132):*

$$D(b_0,\ldots,b_M;x) = F\left(\sqrt{-f_0}, -\sqrt{-f_0}; 1/2; -f_1,\ldots,-f_M; (1-x)/2\right). \quad (9.1132)$$

to the extended Gaussian hypergeometric function (9.1130a, b) with parameters (9.1311a, d, e, g, h) and (9.1129b; 9.1125).

The Mathieu differential equation (4.89) ≡ (9.1133a, b):

$$w(\theta) = M(a,q;\cos\theta): \qquad w'' + \left(a + 2q - 2q\cos^2\theta\right)w = 0, \quad (9.1133a, b)$$

can be transformed (9.1007a–d) [(9.1009c, e)] to (9.1134a, b) [(9.1135a, b)]:

$$y(x) = M(a,q;\cos\theta): \qquad \left(1-x^2\right)y'' - xy' + \left(a + 2q - 2qx^2\right)y = 0, \quad (9.1134a, b)$$

$$y(x) = z(\xi): \qquad \xi(1-\xi)z'' + (1/2-\xi)z' + \left[a + 8q\xi(1-\xi)\right]z = 0. \quad (9.1135a, b)$$

The Mathieu differential equation has (standard CDLVI) four equivalent forms (4.89) ≡ (9.1133a, b) ≡ (9.1134a, b; 9.1007a–d) ≡ (9.1135a, b; 9.1009c–e). The latter *(9.1135b)* is an extended Gaussian hypergeometric differential equation (9.1130a, b) with parameters (9.1136a–e) leading to (9.1136f–h):

$$\gamma = 1/2, \alpha + \beta = 0, \alpha\beta = -a, A_1 = 8q = -A_2, \quad g = 3/2, \quad \alpha = \sqrt{-a} = -\beta. \quad (9.1136a–h)$$

Thus *the Mathieu differential equation (4.89) ≡ (9.1135a, b) is (standard CDLVII) the particular case (9.1136a–h) of the extended Gaussian hypergeometric differential equation (9.1130a, b) and the corresponding functions are related by (9.1137):*

$$M(a,q;x) = F\left(\sqrt{-a}, -\sqrt{-a}; 1/2; 8q, -8q; (1-x)/2\right). \quad (9.1137)$$

Thus the solutions (9.1137) [(9.1132)] of the Mathieu (4.89) ≡ (9.1133a, b) ≡ (9.1134a, b) ≡ (9.1135a, b) [generalized Hill (9.1120a, b) ≡ (9.1122; 9.1125) ≡ (9.1126; 9.1009c) ≡ (9.1127a, b; 9.1129b)] differential equations can be expressed in terms of extended Gaussian hypergeometric functions (note 9.36).

NOTE 9.36: Extended Gaussian Hypergeometric Functions (Campos 2001a)

The extended Gaussian hypergeometric differential equation (9.1130b) has a regular singularity at the origin and at the point unity, and hence a regular integral solution around the origin (9.937d) exists with radius of convergence unity (9.1138a) leading to (9.1138b):

$$|x|<1: \qquad 0=-\sum_{k=0}^{\infty} x^{k+a} c_k(a)\left[(a+k)(a+k+\alpha+\beta)+\alpha\beta\right]$$

$$+\sum_{j=0}^{\infty} x^{j+a-1} c_j(a)(a+j)(a+j+\gamma-1)-\sum_{\ell=0}^{\infty}\sum_{m=1}^{M} x^{\ell+a+m} c_\ell(a) A_m. \qquad \text{(9.1138a, b)}$$

The changes of index of summation (9.1139a, b) lead from (9.1138b) to (9.1139c):

$$j-1=k=\ell+m: \quad 0=\sum_{k=0}^{\infty} x^k$$

$$\left[(a+k+\alpha)(a+k+\beta)c_k(a)-(a+k+1)(a+k+\gamma)c_{k-1}(a)+\sum_{m=1}^{M} A_m\, c_{k-m}(a)\right]. \qquad \text{(9.1139a–c)}$$

Setting $k=0$ in (9.1139c) leads to the same indices (9.980a, b) as for the Gaussian hypergeometric differential equation, but the recurrence formula for the coefficients (9.980c) is no longer of two-term type in the extended case (9.1140a, b):

$$c_0(a)=1: \qquad (a+k+1)(a+k+\gamma)\, c_{k-1}(a)$$

$$=(a+k+\alpha)(a+k+\beta)c_k(a)+\sum_{m=1}^{M} A_m\, c_{k-m}(a). \qquad \text{(9.1140a, b)}$$

The convergence in the unit disk (9.896a–e) and on its boundary (9.964a–e; 9.965a–f) is the same for the extended and original Gaussian hypergeometric differential equations because the extra terms involving A_m in (9.1140b) are $O\left(k^{-2}\right)$, and do not affect (9.974a–c).

The index (9.980a) corresponds to the extended Gaussian hypergeometric series (9.1141b, c) with coefficients (9.1140a, b) for (9.1141a):

$$\gamma\neq 0,-1,-2,\ldots: \quad y_1(x)\equiv F(\alpha,\beta;\gamma;A_1,\ldots,A_M;x)=1+\sum_{k=1}^{\infty} x^k\, c_k(0); \qquad \text{(9.1141a–c)}$$

a second linearly independent solution (9.981a–e) is (9.1142b) for (9.1142a):

$$\gamma \neq 1,2, \dots: \qquad x^{1-\gamma} F(\alpha+1-\gamma, \beta+1-\gamma; 2-\gamma; A_1, \dots, A_M)$$
$$= x^{1-\gamma}\left[1+\sum_{k=1}^{\infty} x^k c_k(1-\gamma)\right] \equiv y_2(x). \qquad (9.1142a, b)$$

Thus *the general integral (standard CDLVIII) of the extended Gaussian hypergeometric differential equation (9.1130b) is a linear combination (9.1143b) with arbitrary constants (A,B) of the functions of the first kind (9.1141b, c; 9.1142b) for (9.1141a; 9.1142a) ≡ (9.1143a):*

$$\gamma \neq 0, \pm 1, \pm 2, \dots: \qquad y(x) = A\, y_1(x) + B\, y_2(x). \qquad (9.1143a, b)$$

If γ is an integer functions of the second kind are needed. The convergence conditions are specified by (9.963a–e; 9.964a–e; 9.965a–f; 9.974b). These results also apply to the Mathieu (4.89) ≡ (9.1133a, b) ≡ (9.1134a, b) ≡ (9.1135a, b) [generalized Hill (9.1120a, b) ≡ (9.1122; 9.1125) ≡ (9.1007c; 9.1126b) ≡ (9.1009c; 9.1127a, b; 9.1129b)] differential equations using (9.1136a–h; 9.1137) [(9.1131a–h)]. The extended forms apply [note(s) 9.36 (9.34–9.35)] both to the confluent (Gaussian) hypergeometric differential equations [(note(s) 9.28 (9.14–9.18)].

NOTE 9.37: Extended Confluent Hypergeometric Differential Equation (Campos 2001b)

The extended confluent hypergeometric differential equation with upper (lower) parameters $\alpha(\beta)$ and asymptotic parameters $A_1, \dots, A_M$ is defined by (9.1144a, b):

$$y(x) = F(\alpha; \gamma; A_1, \dots, A_m; x): \quad x y'' + (\gamma - x) y' - \left(\alpha + \sum_{m=1}^{M} A_m x^m\right) y = 0. \qquad (9.1144a, b)$$

The point at infinity is an irregular singularity of degree $M+1$, and the only other singularity at the origin leads to regular integral solutions in the finite complex plane (9.1145a):

$$|x| < \infty, \qquad \gamma \neq 0, \pm 1, \pm 1, \pm 2: \qquad y(x) = A\, y_1(x) + B\, y_2(x), \qquad (9.1145a–c)$$

consisting of functions of the first kind (9.1145c) for (9.1145b). One of the functions of the first kind is the **extended confluent hypergeometric series** (9.1146a–c):

$$\gamma \neq 1, 2, \dots: \qquad F(\alpha; \gamma; A_1, \dots A_M; x) = 1 + \sum_{k=1}^{\infty} x^k c_k(0) \equiv y_1(x), \qquad (9.1146a–c)$$

with recurrence formula for the coefficients (9.1147a, b):

$$c_0(a)=1,\ (a+k+1)(a+k+\gamma)c_{k+1}(a)=(a+k+\alpha)c_k(a)+\sum_{m=1}^{M}A_m\,c_{k-m}(a). \tag{9.1147a, b}$$

The second linearly independent integral is (9.1148a–c):

$$\gamma\neq 0,-1,-2,\ldots:\qquad x^{1-\gamma}F(\alpha+1-\gamma;2-\gamma;a_1,\ldots,a_M;x)$$

$$=x^{1-\gamma}\left[1+\sum_{k=1}^{\infty}x^k\,c_k(1-\gamma)\right]\equiv y_2(x). \tag{9.1148a–c}$$

Thus *the general integral (standard CDLIX) of the extended confluent hypergeometric differential equation (9.1144b) is a linear combination (9.1145c) with arbitrary constants (A, B) of the extended confluent hypergeometric functions of the first kinds (9.1146b, c; 9.1148b, c) with coefficients (9.1147a, b) valid in the finite complex x-plane (9.1145a) for (9.1146a; 9.1148a) ≡ (9.1145b). If γ is an integer functions of the second kind are needed.* The doubly (singly) extended differential equations are considered for the Bessel (Gaussian and confluent hypergeometric) differential equations [note(s) 9.37 (9.34–9.36)].

NOTE 9.38: Doubly Extended Bessel Differential Equation

The **singly (doubly) extended differential equations** *are obtained (standard CDLX) by multiplying the coefficient of the dependent variable (also of its derivative) by a polynomial of degree M(L), with the degree of the irregular singularity at infinity specified by M [the largest (9.1150e) of M and L–1].* For example, the **doubly extended Bessel differential equation** of order ν with asymtotic coefficients $A_3,\ldots,A_M$ and $B_2,\ldots,B_L$ is (9.1068a, b):

$$y(x)=J_\nu(A_3,\ldots,A_M;B_2,\ldots,B_L;x):$$

$$x^2y''+x\left(1+\sum_{\ell=2}^{L}B_\ell\,x^\ell\right)y'+\left(x^2-\nu^2+\sum_{m=3}^{M}A_m\,x^m\right)y=0. \tag{9.1149a, b}$$

The original Bessel differential equation (9.430b) omits all asymptotic coefficients (9.1150a, b) and the generalized Bessel differential equation (9.428a–f) has (9.1050d) only one non-zero asymptotic coefficient (9.1150c):

$$A_m=0=B_\ell;\quad B_2=-\frac{\mu}{2};\quad J_\nu^\mu(x)=J_\nu\left(0;-\frac{\mu}{2};x\right);\qquad S=\max(M,L-1). \tag{9.1150a–e}$$

the doubly extended Bessel differential equation (9.1149b) has an irregular singularity at infinity of degree (9.1150e).

The origin is the only other singularity, and it is regular, and thus a regular integral solution (9.937d) exists leading (9.1149b) to (9.1151):

$$\begin{aligned} 0 &= \sum_{k=0}^{\infty} c_k(a) x^{k+a}\left[(k+a)^2 - \nu^2\right] + \sum_{j=0}^{\infty} c_j(a)\, x^{j+a+2}\left[(j+a)B_2 + 1\right] \\ &+ \sum_{p=0}^{\infty} c_p(a) \sum_{\ell=3}^{L} B_\ell\, x^{a+p+\ell}(p+a) + \sum_{q=0}^{\infty} c_q(a) \sum_{m=3}^{\infty} A_m\, x^{a+q+m}. \end{aligned} \tag{9.1151}$$

The changes of index of summation (9.1152a–c) lead to (9.1152d):

$$k = j+2 = p+\ell = q+m: \qquad 0 = \sum_{k=0}^{\infty} x^k \left\{\left[(k+a)^2 - \nu^2\right] c_k(a) \right.$$

$$\left. + \left[1 + (k-2+a)B_2\right] c_{k-2}(a) + \sum_{\ell=3}^{L} (k-\ell+a)\, B_\ell\, c_{k-\ell}(a) + \sum_{m=3}^{M} A_m\, c_{k-m}(a) \right\}. \tag{9.1152a–d}$$

Setting $k = 0$ the indicial equation is the same (9.444a–e) as for the original and generalized Bessel differential equations.

The indices (9.444e) correspond to the solutions (9.1153b, c) for (9.1153a):

$$\pm\nu \neq 0,1,2,\ldots: \quad y_\pm(x) = \left(\frac{x}{2}\right)^{\pm\nu} \sum_{k=0}^{\infty} x^k\, c_k(\pm\nu) \equiv J_{\pm\nu}\left(A_3,\ldots,A_M; B_2,\ldots B_L; x\right), \tag{9.1153a–c}$$

with recurrence formula for the coefficients (9.1154a, b):

$$\begin{aligned} c_0(\pm\nu) = 1: \qquad k(k\pm 2\nu)\, c_k(\pm\nu) &= -\left[1 + (k-2\pm\nu)B_2\right] c_{k-2}(\pm\nu) \\ &- \sum_{\ell=3}^{L} (k-\ell\pm\nu)\, B_\ell\, c_{k-\ell}(\pm\nu) - \sum_{m=3}^{M} A_m\, c_{k-m}(\pm\nu). \end{aligned} \tag{9.1154a, b}$$

Thus *the doubly extended Bessel differential equation (9.1149b) has (standard CDLXI) general integral (9.1155c) that is a linear combination with arbitrary constants $C_\pm$ of the* ***doubly extended Bessel functions*** *of orders $\pm\nu$ of the first kind*

(9.1153b, c) with coefficients (9.1154a, b) valid in the finite complex x-plane (9.1155b) for (9.1153a) ≡ (9.1155a):

$$\nu \neq 0, \pm 1, \pm 2, , ...; \qquad |x| < \infty: \qquad y(x) = C_+ \, y_+(x) + c_- \, y_-(x). \tag{9.1155a–c}$$

If ν is an integer functions of the second kind are needed. The only case in which the recurrence formulas (9.1154b) for the coefficients reduce to two terms is (9.1150a–d) is the generalized Bessel differential equation (9.428a–f). A linear second-order differential equation (note 5.6) can be transformed [note 5.7 (5.8)] to self-adjoint (invariant) form (note 9.39); for example the invariant form of the confluent hypergeometric differential equation (note 9.39) leads to the Whittaker differential equation (note 9.40).

NOTE 9.39: Self-Adjoint and Invariant Differential Equations

A linear unforced second-order differential equation (5.235b) ≡ (9.1156a) has a ***transformation factor*** *(5.239b) ≡ (9.1156b):*

$$y'' + P(x)\, y' + Q(x)\, y = 0: \qquad R(x) = \exp\left\{ \int^x P(\xi)\, d\xi \right\}, \tag{9.1156a, b}$$

such (standard CDLXII) that: (i) multiplication of the differential equation (9.1156a) by the transformation factor (9.1156b) leads (9.1157a) to the ***self-adjoint form*** *(9.1157b) of the differential equation (9.1157c):*

$$0 = \exp\left(\int P dx\right)\left[y'' + Py' + Q\right] = \left[\exp\left(\int P dx\right) y'\right]' + \exp\left(\int P dx\right) Qy = (Ry')' + RQy; \tag{9.1157a–c}$$

(ii) performing a change of dependent variable (5.242a) ≡ (9.1158a) that consists of multiplication by the square root of the transformation factor (9.1156b) leads to the ***invariant form*** *(5.242b; 5.243a) ≡ (9.1158b) of the differential equation:*

$$v(x) = y(x)\sqrt{R(x)}: \qquad v'' + \left\{ Q(x) - \frac{P'(x)}{2} - \left[\frac{P(x)}{2}\right]^2 \right\} v = 0, \tag{9.1158a, b}$$

that omits the first-order derivative. For example the confluent hypergeometric differential equation (9.1095) ≡ (9.1156a) has coefficients (9.1159a, b) and (9.1156b) transformation factor (9.1159a–e):

$$P(x) = \frac{\gamma}{x} - 1, \quad Q(x) = -\frac{\alpha}{x}: \quad R(x) = \exp\left\{ \int \left(\frac{\gamma}{\xi} - 1\right) d\xi \right\} = \exp(\gamma \log x - x) = x^\gamma e^{-x}: \tag{9.1159a–e}$$

(i) multiplication by (9.1159e) leads to the self-adjoint form (9.1160a–c):

$$y(x)=F(\alpha;\gamma;x):\quad 0=x^{\gamma}e^{-x}\left[y''+\left(\frac{\gamma}{x}-1\right)y'-\frac{\alpha}{x}y\right]=\left[x^{\gamma}e^{-x}y'\right]'-\alpha e^{-x}x^{\gamma-1}y; \tag{9.1160a–c}$$

and (ii) the change of dependent variable (9.1161a) leads to the invariant form (9.1161b):

$$v(x)=e^{-x/2}x^{\gamma/2}F(\alpha;\gamma;x):\quad v''-\left(\frac{1}{4}+\frac{\alpha}{x}-\frac{\gamma}{2x}-\frac{\gamma}{2x^2}+\frac{\gamma^2}{4x^2}\right)v=0. \tag{9.1161a, b}$$

Thus *the confluent hypergeometric differential equation (9.1095) has (standard CDLXIII) the self-adjoint (9.1160a–c) [invariant (9.1161a, b)] forms.*

NOTE 9.40: Whittaker (1904) Functions and Differential Equation

The **Whittaker (1904) differential equation** (9.1162b), whose solutions are Whittaker functions (9.1162a) with parameters k, m:

$$v(x)=W_{k,m}(x):\qquad v''-\left(\frac{1}{4}-\frac{k}{x}+\frac{m^2}{x^2}-\frac{1}{4x^2}\right)v=0, \tag{9.1162a, b}$$

coincides with the invariant form of the confluent hypergeometric differential equation (9.1161b) with the identification of parameters (9.1163a, b), that leads to (9.1163c–e):

$$k=\frac{\gamma}{2}-\alpha,\qquad m^2-\frac{1}{4}=\frac{\gamma^2}{4}-\frac{\gamma}{2}:\qquad m=\frac{\gamma-1}{2},\qquad \gamma=2m+1,\quad \alpha=\frac{1}{2}+m-k. \tag{9.1163a–e}$$

Substitution of (9.1162a; 9.1163d, e) in (9.1161a) leads to (9.1164):

$$W_{k,m}(x)=e^{-x/2}x^{1/2+m}F(1/2+m-k;1+2m;x); \tag{9.1164}$$

$$F(\alpha;\gamma;x)=e^{x/2}x^{-\gamma/2}W_{\gamma/2-\alpha,\gamma/2-1/2}(x), \tag{9.1165}$$

and the inverse (9.1165) is obtained substituting (9.1162a; 9.1163a, c, d) in (9.1161a). Thus *the confluent hypergeometric (9.1091a–d) and Whittaker functions are (standard CDLXIV) related by (9.1164) ≡ (9.1165).* A second linearly independent solution of the confluent hypergeometric differential equation (9.1095) is (9.893b) ≡ (9.1166a) that: (i) leads to (9.1166b) using (9.1163d, e); (ii) coincides with (9.1164) exchanging m for $-m$ thus leading to (9.1066c):

$$e^{-x/2}\, x^{1/2+m}\, x^{1-\gamma} F(\alpha+1-\gamma;2-\gamma;x) = e^{-x/2}\, x^{1/2-m}\, F(1/2-m-k;1-2m;x) = W_{k,-m}(x). \tag{9.1166a–c}$$

Thus *the general integral of the Whittaker differential equation (9.1162b) is (standard CDLXV) a linear combination (9.1167c) with arbitrary constants (A,B) of Whittaker functions (9.1164) with parameters* $(k,\pm m)$:

$$2m \neq 0,\pm 1,\pm 2; \qquad |x| < \infty: \qquad v(x) = A\, W_{k,m}(x) + B\, W_{k,-m}(x), \tag{9.1167a–c}$$

valid in the finite complex plane (9.167b) for 2m not an integer (9.1167a). Since the confluent hypergeometric functions are related to both the Whittaker (note 9.40) and generalized Bessel (subsection 9.9.9) functions, the latter two are also related (note 9.41).

NOTE 9.41: Self-Adjoint and Invariant Generalized Bessel Differential Equations

The generalized Bessel function of degree ν and order μ is related to the confluent hypergeometric function by (9.896b) and hence (9.1165) to the Whittaker function by (9.1168b):

$$\mu \neq 0: \qquad J_\nu^\mu(x) = \frac{x^{-1/2+\nu/2}\, e^{x/2}}{2^{-\nu}\,\Gamma(1+\nu)}\, W_{1/2+1/\mu,\nu/2}\left(\frac{\mu x^2}{4}\right), \tag{9.1168a, b}$$

that excludes (9.1168a) the original Bessel function. The relations (9.1169a–e) among the pairs of parameters (μ,ν) and (k,m) and variables (x,ξ) in (9.1168b):

$$k = \frac{1}{2} + \frac{1}{\mu}, \quad \mu = \frac{2}{2k-1}, \quad \nu = 2m, \quad \xi = \frac{\mu x^2}{4}, \quad x = 2\sqrt{\frac{\xi}{\mu}}, \tag{9.1169a–e}$$

allow the inversion of (9.1168b) as (9.1170):

$$W_{k,m}(\xi) = \Gamma(1+2m)\, 2^{1/2-m} \left(\frac{\xi}{\mu}\right)^{1/4-m/2} e^{-\sqrt{\xi/\mu}}\, J_{2m}^{2/(2k-1)}\left(2\sqrt{\frac{\xi}{\mu}}\right). \tag{9.1170}$$

Thus *the generalized Bessel functions (9.448) and Whittaker functions are (standard CDLXVI) related by (9.1168b) ≡ (9.1170) that exclude (9.1168a) the original Bessel function.* The generalized Bessel differential equation (9.428f) in the form

(9.1156a) has coefficients (9.1171a, b) and leads (9.1156b) to the transformation factor (9.1171c–d):

$$P(x) = \frac{1}{x} - \frac{\mu x}{2}, \quad Q(x) = 1 - \frac{\nu^2}{x^2}: R(x) = \exp \int^x \left(\frac{1}{\xi} - \frac{\mu \xi}{2} \right) d\xi = x \exp\left(-\frac{\mu x^2}{4} \right): \tag{9.1171a–d}$$

(i) multiplying (9.428f) by the transformation factor (9.1171d) leads to the self-adjoint differential equation (9.1172a–c):

$$y(x) = J_\nu^\mu(x): \qquad x \exp\left(-\frac{\mu x^2}{4} \right) \left[y'' + \left(\frac{1}{x} - \frac{\mu x}{2} \right) y' + \left(1 - \frac{\nu^2}{x^2} \right) y \right]$$

$$= \left[x \exp\left(-\frac{\mu x^2}{4} \right) y' \right]' + \left(x - \frac{\nu^2}{x} \right) \exp\left(-\frac{\mu x^2}{4} \right) y; \tag{9.1172a–c}$$

and (ii) the change of dependent variable (9.1173a) leads (9.1158b) to the invariant differential equation (9.1173b):

$$v(x) = \sqrt{x} \exp\left(-\frac{\mu x^2}{8} \right) J_\nu^\mu(x): \quad v'' + \left[1 - \frac{\nu^2}{x^2} + \frac{1}{4x^2} + \frac{\mu}{2} \left(1 - \frac{\mu x^2}{8} \right) \right] v = 0. \tag{9.1173a, b}$$

Thus *the generalized Bessel differential equation (9.428a–f) has (standard CDLXVII) self-adjoint (9.1172a–c) [invariant (9.1173a, b)] forms, that for the original Bessel differential equation simplify to (9.1174) [(9.1175a, b)]:*

$$0 = x \left[y'' + \frac{1}{x} y' + \left(1 - \frac{\nu^2}{x^2} \right) y \right] = (x y')' + \left(x - \frac{\nu^2}{x} \right) y, \tag{9.1174}$$

$$v(x) = \sqrt{x}\, J_\nu(x): \qquad v'' + \left(1 + \frac{1 - 4\nu^2}{4x^2} \right) v = 0. \tag{9.1175a, b}$$

The self-adjoint and invariant forms of the linear second-order differential equations associated with the most important special functions are obtained in three sets: (i) confluent hypergeometric, Whittaker, and generalized Bessel (note 9.41); (ii) Gaussian hypergeometric, Jacobi, and various Legendre (note 9.42); and (iii) Chebychev, two Laguerre, and Hermite (note 9.43).

NOTE 9.42: Gaussian Hypergeometric, Jacobi, and Legendre Forms

The Gaussian hypergeometric differential equation (9.977b) can be written in the form (9.1156a) with coefficients (9.1176a–c) leading (9.1156b) to the transformation factor (9.1176d–e):

$$P(x) = \frac{\gamma}{x(1-x)} - \frac{\alpha+\beta+1}{1-x} = \frac{\gamma}{x} - \frac{\alpha+\beta+1-\gamma}{1-x}, \quad Q(x) = -\frac{\alpha\beta}{x(1-x)}: \tag{9.1176a–c}$$

$$R(x) = \exp\left\{\int^x \left(\frac{\gamma}{\xi} - \frac{\alpha+\beta+1-\gamma}{1-\xi}\right) d\xi\right\} = x^\gamma (1-x)^{\alpha+\beta+1-\gamma}; \tag{9.1176c, d}$$

the transformation factor (9.1176e) in (9.1157a, b) [(9.1158a, b)] leads (standard CDLXVIII) to the self-adjoint (invariant) forms of the Gaussian hypergeometric differential equation (9.977b) in the recollection 10.1. In the case of the hyperspherical associated Legendre differential equation (9.1037b) the coefficients (9.1177a, b) in (9.1156a) specify (9.1156b) the transformation factor (9.1177c–d):

$$P(x) = -\frac{(2+\lambda)\,x}{1-x^2}, \qquad Q(x) = \frac{\nu(\nu+1)}{1-x^2} - \frac{\mu^2}{\left(1-x^2\right)^2}: \tag{9.1177a, b}$$

$$R(x) = \exp\left\{-\left(\frac{1}{2}+\lambda\right)\int^x \frac{2\,\xi}{1-\xi^2}\, d\xi\right\} = \left(1-x^2\right)^{1/2+\lambda}; \tag{9.1177c, d}$$

the transformation factor (9.1177d) leads (standard CDLXIX) to the self-adjoint and invariant forms of the hyperspherical associated Legendre differential equation (9.1037b) in the recollection 10.1 that includes: (i) for $\lambda = 0$ the associated Legendre differential equation (9.1027b); (ii) for $\mu = 0$ the hyperspherical Legendre differential equation (9.1052b); and (iii) for $\lambda = 0 = \mu$ the original Legendre differential equation (9.1008b).

The ultraspherical Legendre differential equation (9.1018c) is not included in (9.1177a–d), and has (9.1156a) coefficients (9.1178a, b) of which the first is unchanged (9.1177a) ≡ (9.1178a) and the second is distinct (9.1177b) ≠ (9.1178b) so that the transformation factor (9.1177c) ≡ (9.1178c) does not change:

$$P(x) = -\frac{(2+\lambda)\,x}{1-x^2}, \qquad Q(x) = \frac{\nu(\nu+1+\lambda)}{1-x^2}: \qquad R(x) = \left(1-x^2\right)^{1/2+\lambda}; \tag{9.1178a–c}$$

from (9.1177c) ≡ (9.1178c) follow *[standard CDLXIX (CDLXX) the self-adjoint and invariant forms of the hyperspherical associated Legendre (9.1037b) [ultraspherical Legendre (9.1018c)] differential equation in the recollection 10.1.* The Jacobi differential equation (9.1062b) can be written in the form (9.1056a) with coefficients (9.1179a, b) specifying by (9.1156b) the transformation factor (9.1179c, d):

$$P(x) = \frac{b-a}{1-x^2} - x\frac{a+b+2}{1-x^2}, \qquad Q(x) = \nu\,\frac{\nu+a+b+1}{1-x^2}; \tag{9.1179a, b}$$

$$R(x) = \exp\left\{\int^x \left(\frac{b-a}{1-\xi^2} - \xi\frac{a+b+2}{1-\xi^2}\right)d\xi\right\} = \left(1-x^2\right)^{1+a/2+b/2}\exp\left[(b-a)\arg\tanh x\right]; \tag{9.1179c, d}$$

the transformation factor (9.1179d) leads *(standard CDLXXI) to the self-adjoint and invariant forms of the Jacobi differential equation (9.1062b) in the recollection 10.1.*

NOTE 9.43: Chebychev, Laguerre, and Hermite Forms

The first (9.1072b) [second (9.1084b)] Chebychev differential equations can be written in the form (9.1156a) with coefficients (9.1180a, b) specifying by (9.1156b) to the transformation factor (9.1180c, d):

$$P(x) = -\{1,3\}\frac{x}{1-x^2}, \quad Q(x) = \frac{\{\nu^2, \nu(\nu+2)\}}{1-x^2}: \tag{9.1180a–d}$$

$$R(x) = \exp\left[-\left\{\frac{1}{2},\frac{3}{2}\right\}\int^x \frac{2\xi}{1-\xi^2}d\xi\right] = \left(1-x^2\right)^{1/2,3/2}; \tag{9.1180c, d}$$

the transformation factor (9.1180d) leads [standard CDLXXII [(CDLXIII)] to the self-adjoint and invariant forms of the first (9.1072b) [second (9.1084b)] Chebychev differential equations in the recollection 10.1. The associated Laguerre differential equation (9.1106) can be written in the form (9.1156a) with coefficients (9.1181a, b) specifying by (9.1156b) the transformation factor (9.1181c, d):

$$P(x) = \frac{1+\mu}{x} - 1, \quad Q(x) = \frac{\nu}{x}: \quad R(x) = \exp\left\{\int^x \left(\frac{1+\mu}{\xi} - 1\right)\right\}d\xi = e^{-x}x^{1+\mu}; \tag{9.1181a–d}$$

the transformation factor (9.1181d) leads to (standard CDLXXIV) the self-adjoint and invariant forms of the associated Laguerre differential equation (9.1106) in the recollection 10.1.

The Hermite differential equation (9.1110b) can be written in the form (9.1156a) with coefficients (9.1182a, b) specifying by (9.1156b) the transformation factor (9.1182c, d):

$$P(x) = -2x, \quad Q(x) = 2\nu: \quad R(x) = \exp\left(-2\int^x \xi \, d\xi\right) = \exp\left(-x^2\right); \qquad \text{(9.1182a–d)}$$

the transformation factor (9.1182d) leads to (standard CDLXV) the self-adjoint and invariant forms of the Hermite differential equation (9.1110b) in the recollection 10.1. The Mathieu (4.89) ≡ (9.1133b) [generalized Hill (9.1120b) ≡ (9.1122; 9.1125)] differential equations are already in a form that is invariant, and hence self-adjoint. The invariant forms of the linear differential equations are most convenient to compare differential equations; that is, check if they can be transformed into each other (note 5.9). The self-adjoint (9.1157a, b) and invariant (9.1158a, b) forms are two of an infinite number of transformations of a linear second-order differential equation (9.1156a). The transformations of the first (second) class [note 9.44 (9.45)] applied to the generalized Bessel differential equation (9.428a–f) lead to a generic form with 11 (12) particular cases, adding to 25 transformations of the generalized Bessel differential equation.

NOTE 9.44: Transformations of the Generalized Bessel Differential Equation (Malmsten 1850, Lommel 1868)

Several transformations of the original Bessel differential equation (Malmsten 1850; Lommel 1868) are included *in the combined changes of independent and dependent variable (9.1183a) that (standard CDLXXVI) may be applied to the generalized Bessel differential equation (9.428f) leading to* ***the first class of transformed generalized Bessel differential equations*** (9.1183b):

$$y(x) = x^a J_\nu^\mu\left(c x^b\right): \quad x^2 y'' + \left(1 - 2a - \frac{1}{2}\mu b c^2 x^{2b}\right) x y' + \left[a^2 - b^2\nu^2 + b^2 c^2 x^{2b}\left(1 + \frac{\mu a}{2b}\right)\right] y = 0. \qquad \text{(9.1183a, b)}$$

The proof of (9.1183b) is made in two steps: (i) substitution of (9.1183a) in the generalized Bessel differential equation (9.428f) leads to (9.1184):

$$\left\{c^2 x^{2b} \frac{d^2}{d\left(c x^b\right)^2} + c x^b \left(1 - \frac{\mu c^2}{2} x^{2b}\right) \frac{d}{d\left(c x^b\right)} + c^2 x^{2b} - \nu^2\right\} x^{-a} y(x) = 0; \qquad \text{(9.1184)}$$

(ii) in (9.1184) appear the first (9.1185a–c) [second (9.1186a–c)] order derivatives:

$$\frac{d\left(x^{-a}y\right)}{d\left(cx^{b}\right)}=\frac{\left(x^{-a}y\right)'}{\left(cx^{b}\right)'}=\frac{x^{-a-1}}{bcx^{b-1}}\left(y'x-ay\right)=\frac{x^{-a-b}}{bc}\left(y'x-ay\right), \qquad (9.1185a–c)$$

$$\frac{d^2\left(x^{-a}y\right)}{d\left(cx^{b}\right)^2}=\frac{1}{bc}\frac{d}{d\left(cx^{b}\right)}\left[x^{-a-b}\left(y'x-ay\right)\right]=\frac{\left(x^{1-a-b}y'-ax^{-a-b}y\right)'}{bc\left(cx^{b}\right)'}$$

$$=\frac{x^{-a-2b}}{b^2c^2}\left[x^2y''+\left(1-2a-b\right)xy'+a\left(a+b\right)y\right]; \qquad (9.1186a–c)$$

and (iii) substitution of (9.1185c; 9.1186c) in (9.1184) proves (9.1183b).

The particular case (9.1187a) is excluded from (9.1183a), since in this case the differential equation (9.1183b) simplifies to (9.1187b):

$$c=0: \qquad 0=x^2y''+\left(1-2a\right)xy'+\left(a^2-b^2\nu^2\right)y=\left\{P_2\left(\delta\right)\right\}y\left(x\right), \qquad (9.1187a–c)$$

that has a polynomial (9.1187c) ≡ (9.1188b) of homogenous derivatives (9.1188a):

$$\delta\equiv x\frac{d}{dx}: \quad P_2\left(\delta\right)=\delta\left(\delta-1\right)+\left(1-2a\right)\delta+a^2-b^2\nu^2=\delta^2-2a\delta+a^2-b^2\nu^2. \qquad (9.1188a–c)$$

The polynomial (9.1188c) ≡ (9.1189a) has roots (9.1189b, c):

$$P_2\left(\delta\right)=\left(\delta-\alpha\right)\left(\delta-\beta\right): \qquad \alpha,\beta=a\pm b\nu, \qquad (9.1189a–c)$$

leading to two cases: (i) for equal (9.1190a) [unequal (9.1191a)] roots (9.1190b, c) [(9.1191b)] the general integral is (9.1190d) [(9.1191c)] where (A, B) are arbitrary constants:

$$b=0: \qquad \alpha=a=\beta: \qquad y\left(x\right)=x^a\left(Ax+B\right), \qquad (9.1190a–d)$$

$$b\neq0: \qquad \alpha\neq\beta: \qquad y\left(x\right)=x^a\left[A\cosh\left(b\nu x\right)+B\sinh\left(b\nu x\right)\right]. \qquad (9.1191a–c)$$

Thus *the differential equation (9.1183b) has (standard CDLXXVI) a general integral that is a linear combination of generalized Bessel functions (9.1183a) of degrees* $\pm\nu$ *for* ν *not an integer; for* ν *integer the generalized Neumann function* Y_ν^μ *replaces* $J_{-\nu}^\mu$. *In the exceptional case (9.1187a) there are distinct elementary solutions (9.1190a–d) and (9.1191a–c).* Eleven particular cases (standards CDLXXVII–CDLXXXVII) of (9.1183a, b) are listed in the recollection 10.1, followed by 12 particular cases of a second class of transformation of the generalized Bessel differential equation (note 9.45).

NOTE 9.45: Two Classes of Combined Changes of Variable (Lommel 1879, Pearson 1880)

Another class (Lommel 1879, Pearson 1980) distinct from (9.1183a, b) that can also be extended from the original (9.430b) to the generalized (9.428f) Bessel differential equation is the combined changes of independent and dependent variable (9.1192d) involving two differentiable functions (9.1192a, b) leading to (standard CDLXXXVIII) the second class of transformed generalized Bessel differential equations (9.1192c, e):

$$f, g \in D(|C); \qquad h(x) = 2\frac{f'}{f} + \frac{g''}{g'} - \frac{g'}{g} + \frac{\mu g' g}{2};$$

$$y(x) = f(x)\, J_\nu^\mu(g(x)): \quad y'' - hy' + \left(h\frac{f'}{f} - \frac{f''}{f} + g'^2 - \nu^2 \frac{g'^2}{g^2}\right) y = 0. \tag{9.1192a–e}$$

The proof of (9.1192c, e) is made as for (9.1193b) in three steps: (i) substitution of (9.1192d) in the generalized Bessel differential equation (9.428f) leads to (9.1193):

$$\left\{g^2 \frac{d^2}{dg^2} + g\left(1 - \frac{\mu g^2}{2}\right)\frac{d}{dg} + g^2 - \nu^2\right\}\frac{y(x)}{f(x)} = 0; \tag{9.1193}$$

(ii) in (9.1193) appear the first (9.1194a, b) [second (9.1195a–c)] order derivatives:

$$\frac{d}{dg}\left(\frac{y}{f}\right) = \frac{(y/f)'}{g'} = \frac{y'}{g'f} - \frac{f'y}{g'f^2}, \tag{9.1194a, b}$$

$$\frac{d^2}{dg^2}\left(\frac{y}{f}\right) = \frac{1}{g'}\left[\frac{d}{dg}\left(\frac{y}{f}\right)\right]' = \frac{1}{g'}\left(\frac{y'}{g'f} - \frac{f'y}{g'f^2}\right)'$$
$$= \frac{y''}{g'^2 f} - \left(2\frac{f'}{f} + \frac{g''}{g'}\right)\frac{y'}{g'^2 f} + \left(2\frac{f'}{f} + \frac{g''}{g'} - \frac{f''}{f'}\right)\frac{f'y}{g'^2 f^2}; \tag{9.1195a–c}$$

and (iii) substitution of (9.1194b; 9.1195c) in (9.1193) proves (9.1193c, e).

Twelve particular cases (standards CDLXXXLX–D) of (9.1192a–e) are listed in the recollection 10.1; together the 12 (13) cases of (9.1183a, b) [(9.1192a–e)], including one general case [standard CDLXXVI (CDLXXXVIII)] and 11 (12) particular cases [standard CDLXXVII–CDLXXXVII (CDLXXXIX–D] that add to 25 cases (standard CDLXXVII–D). One case (standard CDLXXXVI) is considered in more detail as an example. Choosing (9.1196a–d) in (9.1183a, b) leads to the differential equation (9.1196f) that is satisfied by (9.1196e) involving a generalized Bessel functions:

$$a=\frac{1}{2}, b=\frac{3}{2}, c=\frac{2}{3}, \nu=\frac{1}{3}: \ y(x)=\sqrt{x}\,J_{1/3}^{\mu}\left(\frac{2}{3}x^{3/2}\right), \ y''-\frac{1}{3}\mu x^2 y'+\left(1+\frac{\mu}{6}\right)xy=0. \tag{9.1196a–f}$$

The solution (9.1196e) involving the original Bessel function (9.1197a) is (9.1197b) and satisfies (standard CDLXXXVII) the differential equation (9.1197c):

$$\mu=0: \qquad y(x)=\sqrt{x}\,J_{1/3}\left(\frac{2}{3}x^{3/2}\right), \qquad y''+xy=0, \tag{9.1197a–c}$$

that coincides (9.310b) with the Airy differential equation of variable $-x$; thus the Bessel functions in (9.1196e) of orders $\pm 1/3$ equal $x^{-1/2}$ multiplied by a linear combination of Airy functions (9.310c) of variable $-x$:

$$J_{1/3}\left(\frac{2}{3}x^{3/2}\right)=x^{-1/2}\left[C_1\,Ai(-x)+C_2\,Bi(-x)\right]; \tag{9.1198}$$

the constants (C_1, C_2) are determined by evaluating both sides of (9.1198) for two values of x. The relations (Diagrams 9.2–9.3) among the special functions (L ist 9.1) are summarized next (note 9.46).

NOTE 9.46: Algebraic and Elementary/Higher Transcendental Functions

The classes of functions may be considered (Diagram 9.3) starting with the simplest, namely the (i) polynomials, whose ratios are (ii) the rational functions, that together form the algebraic functions (chapter I.31) that can be expressed exactly in finite terms. The transcendental functions (volume I) require infinite representations (volume II) such as power series (chapters I.23, I.25, I.27, and I.29) and series of fractions, infinite products, and continued fractions (chapters II.1, II.3, and II.9). The generalized functions (volume III) are actually functionals rather than functions. The simplest transcendental functions are the elementary cases of the exponential and logarithm (chapter II.3) and the circular and hyperbolic functions (chapters II.5 and II.7); the latter may be generalized (section 9.4). The other higher transcendental functions include the elliptic functions, including those of Jacobi and Weierstrass, and the hyperelliptic integrals (sections I.39.8–I.39.9) that are solutions of non-linear first-order differential equations. The auxiliary functions include the Euler gamma (note III.1.8 and subsection 9.5.13), digamma (subsections I.29.5.2 and 9.5.16), and beta (subsections 9.8.1–9.8.3) functions that appear in several contexts, including the special functions.

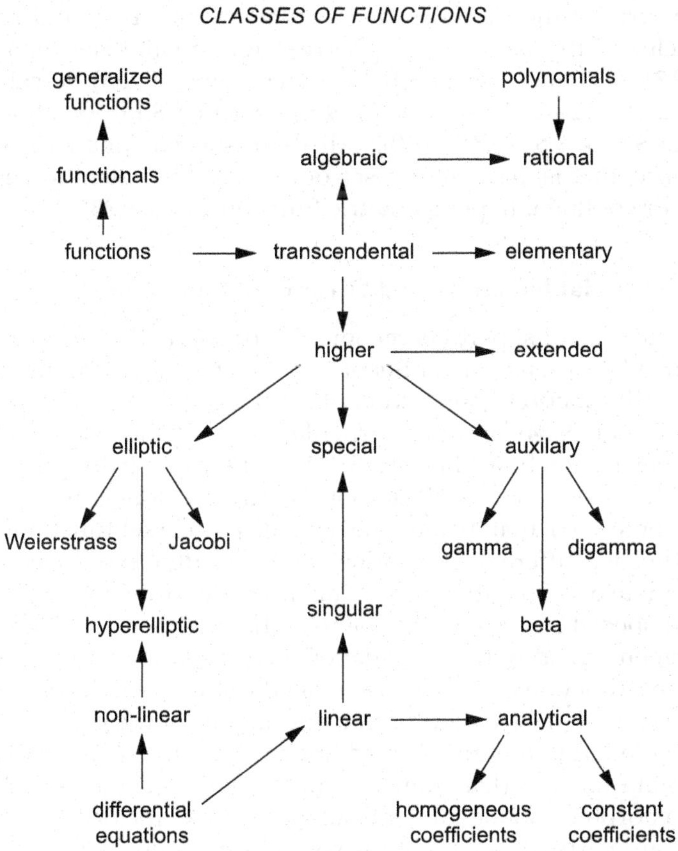

DIAGRAM 9.3
Classification of functions into classes, including algebraic, elementary, and higher transcendental functions, the latter including the special functions in Diagram 9.2.

The special functions (Diagram 9.2) are related to linear differential equations with variable coefficients; for example of order N for the generalized hypergeometric functions (example I.30.20, subsections II.1.9.1–II.1.9.4 and notes 9.9–9.13), including for the second-order the confluent (Gaussian) hypergeometric functions [subsections II.3.9.7–II.3.9.8, 9.9.4, 9.9.7–9.9.8, note 9.28 (section I.29.9, subsections II.3.9.2–II.3.9.5, notes 9.14–9.19)]. The Gaussian hypergeometric functions are equivalent to the hyperspherical associated Legendre functions (note 9.23) and include as particular cases the associated (hyperspherical) Legendre functions [note 9.22 (9.25)]. The Legendre functions (note 9.20) are a particular case of the preceding and a distinct generalization is the ultraspherical Legendre or Gegenbauer functions (note 9.21). The Gaussian hypergeometric functions are also equivalent to the Jacobi functions (note 9.26), and include the Chebychev functions of the first (second) type [note 9.27 (9.28)]. The confluent hypergeometric functions are a limiting form of the Gaussian hypergeometric function, and are equivalent to (includes) the associated Laguerre (Laguerre and Hermite) functions [notes(s) 9.31 (9.30 and 9.32) and the original (generalized) Bessel functions [subsections 9.5.22–9.5.26, 9.6.6–9.6.8, 9.6.15, 9.8.10–9.8.16, 9.9.9–9.9.12 (9.5.14–9.5.21, 9.6.9–9.6.14, 9.8.7–9.8.9, 9.9.9)]. All these special functions are subhypergeometric; that is, particular cases or at most equivalent to generalized, Gaussian, or confluent hypergeometric functions (note 9.33).

NOTE 9.47: Special Functions and Differential Equations

The opposite case of superhypergeometric functions that are not reducible to generalized, Gaussian, or confluent hypergeometric functions include the Mathieu (Hill) functions [subsections 4.3.2–4.3.11 (9.7.11–9.7.16)], that may be generalized (note 9.34), and are particular cases of the extended Gaussian hypergeometric function (notes 9.35–9.36). The extended confluent hypergeometric functions (note 9.37) do not include the doubly extended Bessel functions (note 9.38), that include the generalized Bessel functions. Any linear second-order differential equation can be written in self-adjoint (invariant) form [note 5.7 (5.8)], thus providing alternate forms (notes 9.39–9.43) in the case of special functions; for example, the invariant form of the confluent hypergeometric differential equation leads to the Whittaker differential equation and functions, that are also related to the generalized Bessel functions (notes 9.39–9.41). Two sets of transformations of the generalized Bessel differential equation are given as additional examples (notes 9.44–9.45). To the classes of functions (Diagram 9.3) can be added other (i) classes like analytic, meromorphic, monogenic, and sub-classes like the orthogonal polynomials that are particular cases of the special functions. To the Jacobian and Weierstrassian elliptic functions could be added the related theta functions. To the auxiliary functions could be added the zeta function, error functions, and exponential and Fresnel integrals.

List 9.1 of special functions is not complete, and omits important cases such as: (i–iii) the Weber/spheroidal/Lamé functions that arise from the separation of variables of the Laplacian operator respectively in parabolic cylinder/prolate and oblate spheroidal/ellipsoidal coordinates; (iv) the Heun functions that are the solutions of a linear second-order differential equations with four regular singularities. The aims of chapter 9 have been to present the methods of solution of linear differential equations, using as illustration mostly the original and generalized Bessel functions. The notes briefly mention related methods and a sample of some of the other more important special functions. The emphasis is on the solution of the differential equations; some properties of the special functions may be mentioned in passing as needed, whereas a more detailed study would require one or several separate volume(s): there are monographs on one special function (for example Bessel functions or spherical harmonics) and multi-volume works covering several higher transcendental functions in the bibliography at the end of this volume.

Conclusion 9

The (i) existence and (ii) unicity of solution of a differential equation, as well as other properties such as (iii) robustness with regard to perturbations of the initial conditions, and (iv) uniformity with regard to parameters, can be proved for fairly general classes of differential equations, even if explicit solutions are not available. The Lipschitz condition(s) leads to a contraction mapping (Figure 9.1) specifying a fixed point that is the unique solution; the region of convergence is a rectangle (Figure 9.2) in the plane of the dependent and independent variables. The robustness relative (bifurcation due) to initial conditions is demonstrated by the evolution as the independent variable increases [Figure 9.3 a(b)]. The qualitative methods (Diagram 9.1) applied to differential equations are also relevant (sections 4.8–4.9) to the stability of dynamical systems (Table 9.1 and Figure 9.4), both conservative (Table 9.2 and Figure 9.5) and non-conservative (Figures 9.6 and 9.7). Among the methods of solution of differential equations (Diagram 9.1) the focus is on infinite series, parametric integrals and continued fractions associated with higher transcendental (special) functions [Diagram 9.3 (9.2)].

The special functions are associated with the solution of linear differential equations with variable coefficients. In the general case of complex variables, two important points are: (i) whether the solutions or integrals are single- or multivalued functions (Figures 9.8–9.9); and (ii/iii) the type of the singularities of the differential equations (Figures 9.12–9.13) and of its solutions (Figures 9.10–9.11). The singularities of the coefficients of a linear differential equation (Tables 9.3–9.4) determine the type of power series solutions (Tables 9.7–9.9), for example for the original and generalized Bessel differential equation (Tables 9.5–9.6) and other special functions (Diagram 9.2). An alternative to the power series solutions is the use of integral transforms involving parametric integrals along paths in the complex plane (Figures 9.15–9.17). Other related topics include the solution of linear second-order differential equations using continued fractions, the auxiliary functions (Diagram 9.3) like the gamma and Beta functions (Figure 9.14), and regions and boundaries of convergence (Figure 9.18).

List 9.1 Notation for Some Special Functions

$Ai(x)$ – First Airy function: subsections 9.4.14, 9.4.18, note 9.45.

$A^{\mu}_{\nu,\lambda}(x)$ – First modified hyperspherical associated Legendre function of the first kind of degree ν, order μ, and dimension λ: notes 9.23–9.24.

$Bi(x)$ – Second Airy function: subsections 9.4.14, 9.4.18, note 9.45.

$B^{\mu}_{\nu,\lambda}(x)$ – Second modified hyperspherical associated Legendre function of the first kind of degree ν, order μ, and dimension λ: notes 9.23–9.24.

$C(b_1,\dots,b_M;x)$ = Hill function with parameters $b_1,\dots,b_M$: subsections 9.7.11–9.7.16.

$D(e_1,\dots,e_M;x)$ – Generalized Hill functions with parameters $e_1,\dots,e_M$: notes 9.34–9.35.

$E(\alpha,\beta;\gamma;x)$ – Preliminary Gaussian hypergeometric function with upper(lower) parameters $\alpha,\beta(\gamma)$: notes 9.16, 9.18.

$F(\alpha,\beta;x)$ – Confluent hypergeometric function of the first kind with upper(lower) parameter $\alpha(\beta)$: notes 9.28, 9.39, subsections 9.9.4, 9.9.7–9.9.8, and II.3.9.7 – II.3.9.8.

$F(\alpha,\beta;\gamma;x)$ – Gaussian hypergeometric function of the first kind with upper(lower) parameters $\alpha,\beta(\gamma)$; notes 9.14–9.19, 9.42, section I.29.9, subsections II.3.9.2 – II.3.9.5.

$F(\alpha_1,\dots,\alpha_p;\gamma_1,\dots,\gamma_q:x)$ – Generalized hypergeometric function with upper(lower) parameters $\alpha_1,\dots,\alpha_p(\gamma_1,\dots,\gamma_q)$: notes 9.9–9.13.

$F(\alpha;\gamma;A_1,\dots,A_M;x)$ – Extended confluent hypergeometric function with upper (lower) parameters $\alpha(\gamma)$, and asymptotic coefficients $A_1,\dots,A_M$: note 9.37.

$F(\alpha,\beta;\gamma;A_1,\dots,A_M;x)$ – Extended Gaussian hypergeometric function with upper (lower) parameters $\alpha,\beta(\gamma)$ and asymptotic coefficients $A_1,\dots,A_M$: notes 9.35–9.36.

$G(\alpha,\beta;\gamma;x)$ – Gaussian hypergeometric function of the second kind with upper(lower) parameters α,β: notes 9.16–9.18.

$H(\alpha,\beta;n;x)$ – Complementary Gaussian hypergeometric function with upper parameters $\alpha,\beta(\gamma)$: notes 9.17–9.18.

$H_\nu(x)$ – Hermite function of degree ν: notes 9.32, 9.43.

$h_\nu^{(1,2)}(x)$ – First and second spherical Hankel functions of degree ν: subsections 9.6.6–9.6.8.

$H_\nu^{(1,2)}(x)$ – First and second Hankel functions of degree ν: subsections 9.6.6–9.6.8, 9.8.13–9.8.15.

$H_{\mu,\nu}^{(1,2)}(x)$ – First and second generalized Hankel functions of degree ν and order μ: subsections 9.6.9–9.6.14.

$I_\nu^{a,b}(x)$ – Jacobi functions of degree ν and parameters α,β: notes 9.26, 9.42.

$j_\nu(x)$ – Spherical Bessel function of first kind and order ν subsections 9.5.23–9.5.26, 9.6.6–9.6.8.

$J_\nu(x)$ – Bessel function of order ν: subsections 9.5.22, 9.6.8, 9.8.10–9.8.11, 9.8.13–9.8.15, 9.9.10–9.9.12, notes 9.33, 9.41.

$J_\nu^\mu(x)$ – Generalized Bessel function of order ν and degree μ: subsections 9.5.12, 9.5.14–9.5.15, 9.8.7–9.8.9, 9.9.9, notes 9.41, 9.44–9.45.

$J_\nu(A_3,\dots,A_M,B_3,\dots,B_L;x)$ – Doubly extended Bessel function with asymptotic coefficients $(a_3,\dots,a_M,b_3,\dots,b_L;x)$: note 9.38.

$L_\nu(x)$ – Laguerre function of the first kind of degree ν: note 9.30.

$L_\nu^\mu(x)$ – Associated Laguerre function of degree ν and order μ: notes 9.31, 9.43.

$M(a;q;x)$ – Mathieu function of parameters a, q: note 9.35, subsections 4.3.2, 4.3.7–4.3.11.

$N_\nu(x)$ – Laguerre function of the second kind of degree ν: note 9.30.

$P_\nu(x)$ – Legendre function of the first kind of degree ν: note 9.20.

$P_\nu^\mu(x)$ – First associated Legendre function of degree ν and order μ: note 9.22.

$P_{\nu,\lambda}(x)$ – First hyperspherical Legendre function of degree ν and dimension λ: note 9.25.

$P^{\nu,\lambda}(x)$ – Ultraspherical Legendre function of degree ν and dimension λ: note 9.21.

$P_{\nu,\lambda}^\mu(x)$ – First hyperspherical associated Legendre function of the first kind, degree ν, order μ, and dimension λ: note 9.24, 9.42.

$Q_\nu(x)$ – Legendre function of the second kind of degree ν: note 9.20.

$R_\nu^\mu(x)$ – Second associated Legendre function of degree ν and order μ: note 9.22.

$R_{\nu,\lambda}(x)$ – Second hyperspherical Legendre function of degree ν and dimension λ: note 9.25.

$R_{\nu,\lambda}^\mu(x)$ – Second hyperspherical assuciated Legendre function of the first kind, degree ν, order μ, and dimension λ: note 9.24.

$S_\nu(x)$ – Second Chebychev function of the first type of order ν: note 9.27.

$T_\nu(x)$ – First Chebychev function of the first type of order ν: notes 9.27, 9.43.

$U_\nu(x)$ – First Chebychev function of the second type of order ν: notes 9.28, 9.43.

$V_\nu(x)$ – Second Chebychev function of the second type of order ν: note 9.28.

$X_n^\mu(x)$ – Preliminary generalized Neumann function of degree μ: subsection 9.5.17.

$y_\nu(x)$ – Spherical Neumann function of degree ν: subsections 9.5.23–9.5.26, 9.6.6–9.6.8.

$Y_\nu(x)$ – Neumann function of order ν: subsections 9.5.22, 9.9.10–9.9.12.

$Y_\nu^\mu(x)$ – Generalized Neumann function of order ν and degree μ: subsections 9.5.18–9.5.21.

$Z_n^\mu(x)$ – Complementary generalized Neumann function of degree μ: subsection 9.5.18.

Bibliography

The bibliography of *Singular Differential Equations and Special Functions*, that is the fifth book of the volume IV, *Ordinary Differential Equations with Applications to Trajectories and Oscillations*, and the eighth book of the series *Mathematics and Physics Applied to Science and Technology* adds the subject of "Special Functions." The books in the bibliography that have influenced the present volume the most are marked with one, two, or three asterisks.

Special Functions

Appell, P. *Les functions hypergeometriques*. Masson 1934, Paris.

Briot, C. H. and Bouquet, C. *Theorie des fonctions elliptiques*. Gauthier-Villars 1875, Paris.

Campbell, R. *L'equation de Mathieu*. Masson 1955, Paris.

Cayley, A. *Elliptic functions*. George Bell 1895, London, reprinted Dover 1961, New York.

Greenhill, A. G. *Elliptic functions*. 1882, reprinted Dover 1959, New York.

Hancock, H. *Elliptic functions*. 1909, reprinted Dover 1961, New York.

Hobson, E. W. *Spherical and ellipsoidal harmonics*. Cambridge University Press 1931, Cambridge, reprinted Dover 1965, New York.

Klein, F. *Vorlesungen ueber der hypergeometrische Funktion*. Teubner 1933, Leipzig.

Krazer, A. *Lehrbuch der thetafunktion*. Teubner 1903, Leipzig, reprinted Chelsea 1970, New York.

Laurent, H. *Theorie elementaire des fonctions elliptiques*. Gauthier-Villars 1880, Paris.

Luke, Y. L. *Integrals of Bessel functions*. McGraw-Hill 1962, New York, reprinted Dover 2014, New York.

MacRobert, T. M. *Spherical harmonics*. Pergamon Press 1927, 3rd edition 1967.

Mathews, G. B. and Gray, A. *Bessel functions*. MacMillan 1931, London.

McLachlan, N. W. *Bessel functions for engineers*. Oxford University Press 1934, Oxford.

Moon, P. & Spencer, D. E. *Field theory handbook*. Springer-Verlag 1971, Berlin.

Nielsen, N. *Handbuch der Gammafunktion*. 1906, reprinted Chelsea 1965, New York. 2 vols.

Ronveaux, A. (editor) *Heun's differential equations*. Oxford University Press 1995, Oxford.

Slater, L. J. *The confluent hypergeometric function*. McGraw-Hill 1970, New York.

Strutt, M. J. O. *Lamésche und Mathieusche Funktion*. Springer, Berlin 1937, reprinted Chelsea 1967, New York.

Tannery, J. and Molk, J. *Functions elliptiques*. Gauthier-villars 1893–1902, Paris, reprinted Chelsea 1972, New York. **4 vols.**

* Thomson, W. & Tait, P. G. *Treatise of natural philosophy*. Cambridge University Press 1931, Cambridge, **2 vols**.
Tricomi, F. G. *Funzioni ipergeometrici confluenti*. Cremenese 1965, Rome.
** Wang, Z. X. & Guo, Z. X. *Special functions* World Scientific 1998, Singapore.
* Watson, G. N. *Bessel functions*. Cambridge U. P. 1922, 2nd edition 1944, Cambridge.
** Whittaker, E. T. & Watson, G. N. *Course of modern analysis*. Cambridge University Press 1902, Cambridge, 4th edition 1927.

References

1766 Euler, L. De Motu Vibratorio Tympanorum. *Novi Commentari Academia Petropolitana* **10**, 243–260.
1772 Euler, L. *Novi commentary Academia Scientarum Imperialis Petropolitana* **16**.
1785 Legendre, A. M. Sur l'attraction des spheroides. *Mémoires de Mathématique et Physique presentés à l'Académie Royalle des Aciences par divers savants, 10.*
1812 Gauss, C. F. "Disquisitiones circam seriem infinitam ..." *Commentationes Societones Regiae Scientarum Göttensis Recentiores* (*Werke* **1**, 185).
1812 Hoene-Wronski, J. *Refutation de la théorie des fonctions analytiques de Lagrange.* Paris.
1812 Laplace, P. S. *Théorie des probabilités.* Gauthier-Villars, Paris.
1824 Bessel, F. W. Untersuchung der theils der planetarischen storungen welchear aus des Bewegung der Sonne entsteht. *Berliner Abhandlungen.*
1836 Kummer, E. E. Ueber die hypergeometrische reihe ... *Journal fur reine and angewandte Mathematik* **83**, 127–172.
1838 Airy, G. B. On the intensity of light near a caustic. *Transactions of the Cambridge Philosophical Society* **6**, 379–402.
1850 Malmsten, C. J. Théoremes sur l'équation differentielle ... *Cambridge and Dublin Mathematical Journal* **5**, 180–182.
1856 Weiertrass, K. T. W. Theorie des Abel'schen Functionen. *Journal fur Mathematik* **52**, 285–379.
1859 Chebychev, P. L. Sur les questions de minima, qui se ratachent à la representation approximative des fonctions. *Mémoires de l'Académie Scientique de St. Petersbourg* **7**, 199–291 (*Ouevres* **1**, 271–378).
1859 Jacobi, C. G. J. Untersuchungen über die Differentialglechung der hypergeometrischen Reihe. *Journal fur reine und angewande Mathematik* **56**, 149–165.
1864 Hermite, C. Sur un nouveau development en série de fonctions. *Comptes rendus de l'Académie des Sciences* **58**, 93–100+266+273 (*Ouevres* **2**, 293–308, Gauthiers Villars 1908).
1864 Lipshitz, R. De explicatione per series trignometricas instituenda functionum unices variablis arbitrarium, et praecipue earum, qua per variablis spatium finitum valorum maximum et minimum numerarum habent infinitum disquisitio. *Journal pur reine and angewandte Mathematik* **63**, 296–308.
1866 Fuchs, J. L. Zur Theorie der linearen differentialgleichungen mit verändlichen Koefflizienten. *Journal pur reine and angewande Mathematik* **66**, 121–160.

1866–8 Fuchs, J. L. Zur theorie des linearen Differentialgleichungen mit verändlichen Koeffizienten. Ergängzung, *Journal fur reine and angewanden Mathematik* **66**, 121–160; **68**, 354–385.
1867 Newmann, C. G. *Theorie der Bessel'schen Funktionen*, Teubner, Leipzig.
1868 Lommel, E. C. J. Zur Theorie der Bessel'schen Functionen. *Mathematische Annalen* **14**, 510–536.
1869 Hankel, H. Die Cylinderfunktionen erster and zweiter Art. *Mathematischen Annalen* **1**, 467–501.
1873 Frobenius, G. Ueber die Integration des linearen Differentialgleichungen durch Reihen. *Journal fur Reine and Angewanden Mathematik* **76**, 214–235.
1873 Mathieu, E. *Cours de Physique Mathematique*. Gautiers-Villars, Paris.
1879 Laguerre, E. Sur l'integrale $\int_x^\infty \xi^{-1} e^{-\xi} d\xi$. *Bulletin de la societé mathematique de France* **7**, 72–81 (*Ouevres* **1**, 428–437, reprinted Chelsea 1971).
1879 Lommel, E. C. J. *Studien über der Bessel'shen Functionen*. Teubner, Leipzig.
1880 Pearson, K. On the solution of some differential equations by Bessel functions. *Messenger* **9**, 127–131.
1883 Floquet, G. *Annales Scientifiques de l'École Normale Superieure* **12**, 47–88.
1883 Floquet, G. Sur les équations differentielles à coefficients periodiques. *Annales Scientifiques de l'École Normale Supérieure* **12**, 14–88.
1883 Thomé, L. W. *Journal fur Mathematik* **95**, 75.
1886 Hill, G.W. On the part of the motion of the lunar perigee which is a function of the mean motions of the sun and the moon. *Acta Mathematica* **8**, 1–36.
1886 Poincaré, H. Sur les integrales irreguliéres des equations differentielles. *Acta Mathematica* **8**, 295–344.
1886 Poincaré, H. Sur les determinants d'ordre infini. *Bulletin de la Societé Mathematique de France* **14**, 77–90.
1892 Lyapunov, A. "The general problem of stability of motion." *Communications of the Mathematical Society of Kharkov.*
1892 von Koch, H. Sur les determinants infinis et les equations differentielles ordinaires. *Acta Mathematica* **16**, 217–295.
1893 Picard, E. Sur l'application de la méthode des approximations sucessives à l'étude de certaines équations differentielles. *Journal de Mathématiques Pures et Appliqués* **9**, 217–272.
1896 Mellin, H. Ueber die fundamentale Wichtigkeit des Satzes ven Cauchy fur die theorie der Gamma -und hypergeometrischen Funktionen. *Acta Societarum Scientarum Fennica* **21**, 1–115.
1904 Whittaker, E. T. An expression of certain known functions as generalized hypergeometric functions. *Bulletin of the American Mathematical Society* **10**, 125–134.
1907 Foppl, F. *Vorlesungen uber technische Mechanik*. Teubner, Leipzig.
1907 Lyapunov, A. Probléme general de la stabilité du mouvement. *Annales de la Faculté de Sciences de Toulouse* **9**, 203–469.
1909 Bateman, H. The solution of linear differential equations by means of definite integrals. *Transactions of the Cambridge Philosophical Society* **21**, 171–196.
1938 Kontorovich, M. I. & Lebedev, N. N. A method for the solution of problems in diffraction theory and related topics. *Journal of Experimental and Theoretical Physics* **8**, 1192–1206 (in Russian).

1947 Chebychev, P. L. *Collected works* **2**, 25–51.
1953 Landau, L. D. & Lifshitz, E. F. 1953 *Fluid Mechanics*. Pergamon Press, Oxford.
1954 Lyapunov, A. *Collected works*. Moscow.
1966 Lyapunov, A. *Stability of motion*. Academic Press, New York.
2000 Campos, L. M. B. C. On the singularities and solutions of the extended hypergeometric equation. *Integral Transforms and Special Functions* **9**, 99–120.
2001 Campos, L. M. B. C. On the derivation of asymptotic expansions for special functions from the corresponding differential equations. *Integral Transforms and Special Functions* **12**, 227–236.
2001 Campos, L. M. B. C. On the extended hypergeometric equation and functions of arbitrary degree. *Integral Transforms and Special Functions* **11**, 233–256.
2001 Campos, L. M. B. C. On some solutions of the extended confluent hypergeometric differential equation. *Journal of Computational and Applied Mathematics* **137**, 177–200.
2012 Campos, L. M. B. C. & Cunha, F. S. R. P. On hyperspherical Legendre polynomials and higher dimensional multipole expansions. *Journal of Inequalities and Special Functions* **3**, 1–28.
2019 Campos, L. M. B. C., Moleino, F., Silva, M. & Paquim, J., "On regular integral solutions of a generalized Bessel differential equation", *Advances in Mathematical Physics* ID8919516, doi 10.1155/2018/8919516

Index

Absolute convergence, 184
Adjoint operator, 218–219
Airy differential equation, 88
Alternate natural integrals, 58
Analytical methods of solution, of differential equations, 244–245
Analytic asymptotic integrals, 78
Analytic coefficients, generalized circular/hyperbolic functions and
  Airy (1838) differential equation and functions, 88
  analytic, regular, and irregular integrals, 75–78, *77*
  calculation, 82–83
  complex non-integer values of parameter, 90–92
  differentiation of generalized cosine and sine functions, 92–93
  generalized circular cosine and sine, 88–90
  generalized circular differential equation, 90
  generalized hyperbolic cosine and sine, 86–88
  generalized hyperbolic differential equation, 85–86
  inequalities for generalized cosines and sines, 93–94
  linear autonomous system, 79–81
  linear differential equation, 81–82
  overview, 64–65
  point-at-infinity, singularities and integrals at, 78–79
  principal branch, branch-point, and branch-cut, 72–74
  recurrence relation, methods to obtain, 84–85
  regular points, poles, and essential singularities, 68–70
  regular points and regular/irregular singularities, **74,** 74–75
  Riemann surface sheets of multi-valued function, 70–72, *71*
  secant, cosecant, tangent, and cotangent, generalized, 94–95
  single-valued complex functions, singularities of, 65–68, *66, 67*
Analytic continuation, 76, 255–260
Analytic integrals, 74, 75–78, *77,* 179–181, **180**
Analytic point, 74
Arbitrary constants, 102
Associated Laguerre differential equation, 292–293
Associated Legendre differential equation, 274–276
Asymptotic coefficient, 78
Asymptotic expansions *vs.* convergent series, 148–150
Asymptotic integral(s)
  analytic, 78
  of cylindrical Bessel differential equation, 152–153
  irregular, 79
  normal, 142
  parametric discontinuity in, 165–166
  regular, 79
Asymptotic regular series solutions, 253–254
Asymptotic solution, 78
Asymptotic stability
  equilibria, 27
  Lyapunov theorem, proof of, 35
  natural integrals and, 56–57
Autonomous differential equation, 53
Autonomous differential system, fundamental solution, 48–49
Autonomous system; *see also* Generalized autonomous system; Linear autonomous system
  asymptotically, 31
  third Lyapunov theorem on, 52
  unsteady, 31

Autonomous systems and equilibria stability, 23–53
asymptotic stability (instability), 27
autonomous differential equation, stability of solutions of, 53
conservative forces, 29
damped oscillator
position-dependent parameters, 37–38
time-depending parameters, 38–39
eigenvalue, 43–44
exponential asymptotic growth/decay, 40–41, *42*
extended positive (negative) definite function, 28
fundamental solution, 48–49
linear autonomous system with constant coefficients, 45–46
linear differential equation with bounded coefficients, 44–45
linearized differential system near equilibrium point, 46–48
local/asymptotic stability/instability and indifference, *25*, 25–27, **27**
Lyapunov (1966) function and first theorem, 31–34, *33*
Lyapunov stability theorem
asymptotic stability, proof on, 35
instability, proof on, 36–37
proof of, 34–35
mathematical equilibrium and stability, 26
overview, 23–24
physical equilibrium and stability, *25*, 25–26
positive-definite quadratic forms, 50
positive/negative definite/semi-definite and indefinite function, **28**, 28–29, *30*
second Lyapunov theorem (1892), proof of, 41–43
stability function, and derivative of, 51
stable equilibrium, 26–27
steady differential system, 31
third Lyapunov theorem, 52
unconditionally unstable, 29
undamped oscillator with parametric resonance, 40
unsteady differential system, 29–31
Auxiliary functions, xxiv

Bateman kernel, partial differential equation for, 216–217
Bateman transform, 195–196
Bessel differential equation, 294–295
application, 212–213
cylindrical, 96–97, 134–135
asymptotic integrals of, 152–153
doubly extended, 301–303
generalized, 96–97, 118–121, 129–131
vs. original, 162–165, **163**
self-adjoint and invariant, 305–306
transformations of, 309–311
spherical, 97, 135–137
Wronskian of, 116–117
Bessel differential operator, 218–219
Bessel function, 168
asymptomatic expansion, 153–155
cylindrical, 96–97, 121
doubly extended, 302
generalized, 96–97, 121–123, 127, 130
integral representation, 210–212
integral representation, *214*, 214–216
numerical computation of, 168–169
second integral representation for, 223–224
spherical, 97, 121, 136–139, 140–141
Beta function, 196–198
gamma function and, 199–201
generalized permutation, 198–199
integrals evaluation via, 202–203
permutations and properties, 198–199
recurrence formula for, 197–198
Bifurcation, 166–167
Bilinear concomitant, 218–219
Boundary conditions, single-point, 82
Bounded coefficients, linear differential equation with, 44–45
Branch-cut, 72–74
Branch-point, 71, 72–74

Cauchy convergence principle, 185
Cauchy rule, 149
Change of index of summation, 106, 108, 141

Characteristic polynomials, 205, 248
Chebychev differential equation, 308–309
of first type, 284–286
of second type, 286–289
Chebychev functions, 247, *257*, 280, 313
Circles of convergence, 76
Circular/hyperbolic functions, generalized, *see* Generalized circular and hyperbolic functions
Coefficients of regular natural integrals, 98–99
Coincident indices, 109, 110
Complementary function, 127–128, 130
Complementary Gaussian hypergeometric function, 264–265
Complex continued fractions, convergence of, 238–240
Conditionally convergent, infinite determinant, 184
Confluent hypergeometric differential equation, 228–229, 289–291
generalized Bessel differential equation and, 231
Confluent hypergeometric function, continued fractions for, 230
Confluent hypergeometric series, 231–233
Conservative forces, autonomous systems, 29
Conservative system, stability of, **28**
Constant coefficients, 105
linear autonomous system with, 45–46
Continued fractions, as solutions of differential equations, 225–226
complex, convergence of, 238–240
confluent hypergeometric differential equation, 228–229
generalized Bessel differential equation and, 231
for confluent hypergeometric function, 230
confluent hypergeometric series, 231–233
for cylinder functions, 236–237
cylinder functions with integer order difference, 235–236
for generalized Bessel function, 233–234
logarithmic derivative of, 226–227
recurrence and differentiation relations for cylinder functions, 234–235
simple infinite, convergence of, 229–230
special, convergence of, 240–241
special limit periodic, 237–238
terminating, 227–228
Continuity, Lipschitz condition, 6–9
Contraction condition, *see* Lipschitz (contraction) condition
Contraction mapping, 2, 5–6; *see also* Lipschitz condition
Convergence; *see also specific types*
circles of, 76
of complex continued fractions, 238–240
of infinite determinants (types), 183–184
of series in the regular intervals, 113–115
of simple infinite continued fractions, 229–230
of special continued fractions, 240–241
of successive approximations, 4–5, *6*
uniform, to continuous solution, 9–10
Convergence theorem, for infinite determinants, 185
Convergent series *vs.* asymptotic expansions, 148–150
Cut-plane, 72
Cylinder functions
for continued fractions, 236–237
with integer order difference, 235–236
recurrence and differentiation relations for, 234–235
Cylindrical Bessel differential equation, asymptotic integrals of, 152–153
Cylindrical Hankel (1869) functions, 150–152

D'Alembert convergence test, 5
Damped harmonic oscillator, autonomous systems
  position-dependent parameters, 37–38
  time-depending parameters, 38–39
Dependent variable(s)
  combined changes of, 311–312
  continuity (contraction) condition on, 7–9, *8*
Diagonal matrices, linear differential equations, 57–58
Differentiability, 2
  Lipschitz condition, 6–7
Differential equation(s); *see also* Autonomous differential equation(s); Linear differential equation(s); *specific entries*
  approximate numerical and analytic, 244–245
  Airy (1838), 88
  of any order, 21–21
  associated Laguerre, 292–293
  Bessel differential equation, 152–153, 162–165
  Chebychev, 308–309
    of first type, 284–286
    of second type, 286–289
  combined theorem for, 22–23
  confluent hypergeometric, 289–291
  continued fractions as solutions of, *see* Continued fractions
  depression of degree of coefficients of, 207–208
  doubly extended Bessel, 301–303
  extended confluent hypergeometric, 300–301
  extended Gaussian hypergeometric, 297–300
  first-order, simultaneous system of, 16–17
  Gaussian hypergeometric, 260–261, 307–308
  generalized circular, 90
  generalized hyperbolic, 85–86
  generalized hypergeometric, 259
  Hermite, 293–294
  Hill differential equation, 186–189, 295–297
  hyperspherical associated Legendre, 276–278
  invariant second-order, 59, 62–63
  Jacobi functions and, 283–284, 307–308
  Laguerre functions and, 291–292
  methods of solution of, 244–245
  ordinary and partial, 245
  parametric uniformity and, 16
  qualitative theory of, 243
  second-order, *see* Second-order differential equation
  self-adjoint and invariant, 303–304
  singularity of, at point-at-infinity, 147–148
  solution of
    theorem of existence of, 10–11
    theorem of unicity of, 11–12
  special functions and, 314
  subhypergeometric, 294–295
  superhypergeometric, 295–297
  theorem of parametric uniformity, 16
  transformation into integral equation, 3–4
  Whittaker, 304–305
Differential system, stability function, 51
Differentiation formulas, 93
Digamma function, 123–125, 128, 264

Eigenintegrals; *see also* Integral(s)
  existence of, 170–172, *171*
Eigenvalue(s), 55
  autonomous system, 43–44
  coincident, 55–56
  distinct, 55–56
  existence of, 170–172, *171*
  of invariant second order equation, 62–63
Equilibrium point, linearized differential system near, 46–48
Equilibrium position, stability of, **27**
Equilibrium stability, autonomous systems and
  asymptotic stability (instability), 27
  autonomous differential equation, stability of solutions of, 53
  conservative forces, 29
  damped oscillator

position-dependent parameters, 37–38
time-depending parameters, 38–39
eigenvalue, 43–44
exponential asymptotic growth/ decay, 40–41, *42*
extended positive (negative) definite function, 28
fundamental solution, 48–49
linear autonomous system with constant coefficients, 45–46
linear differential equation with bounded coefficients, 44–45
linearized differential system near equilibrium point, 46–48
local/asymptotic stability/instability and indifference, *25*, 25–27, **27**
Lyapunov (1966) function and first theorem, 31–34, *33*
Lyapunov stability theorem
asymptotic stability, proof on, 35
instability, proof on, 36–37
proof of, 34–35
mathematical equilibrium and stability, 26
overview, 23–24
physical equilibrium and stability, *25*, 25–26
positive-definite quadratic forms, 50
positive/negative definite/semi-definite and indefinite function, **28**, 28–29, *30*
second Lyapunov theorem (1892), proof of, 41–43
stability function, and derivative of, 51
stable equilibrium, 26–27
steady differential system, 31
third Lyapunov theorem, 52
unconditionally unstable, 29
undamped oscillator with parametric resonance, 40
unsteady differential system, 29–31
Essential singularities, 68–70, 169–170
Eulerian integral
of first kind, *see* Gamma function
of second kind, *see* Beta function
Euler-Mascheroni constant, 118, 125
Existence; *see also* Theorem of existence
of eigenintegrals, 170–172, *171*
of eigenvalues, 170–172, *171*
Existence, unicity, and regularity theorems, 242–243
Existence, unicity, robustness, and uniformity, of solutions
combined theorem of, 19–20
continuity (contraction) condition on independent (dependent) variable, 7–9, *8*
contraction (Lipschitz) condition for several variables, 18–19
contraction mapping and fixed point, 5–6
differential equation, solution of
theorem of existence of, 10–11
theorem of unicity of, 11–12
theorem on uniformity and parameter in, 16
Lipschitz (contraction) condition, continuity, and differentiability, 6–7
Lipschitz condition and, 2–3
ordinary differential equation
of any order, 20–21
combined theorem for, 22–23
linear, 21–22
overview, 1–2
robustness relative to perturbed initial conditions, 12–14, 13f
simultaneous system of first-order differential equations, 16–17
successive approximations
convergence of, 4–5, *6*
rectangle as domain of, 11
vs. original and perturbed problems, 14–15
theorem of robustness, initial condition and, 15
transformation of differential into integral equation (Picard 1893), 3–4
uniform convergence to continuous solution, 9–10
Exponential asymptotic growth/decay, autonomous systems and stability of equilibria, 40–41, *42*
Exponential function, 5

Exponent(s), 55–56
Extended confluent hypergeometric differential equation, 300–301
Extended confluent hypergeometric series, 300
Extended Gaussian hypergeometric differential equation, 297–298
Extended Gaussian hypergeometric functions, 298–300
Extended matching coefficient, 133

First (second) cylindrical Hankel functions, 150
First Lyapunov stability theorem, 31–34, *33*, 38, 39
First-order differential equations, simultaneous system of, 16–17
First-order simultaneous equations, 2
First (second) spherical Hankel (1860) functions, 150
First (second) ultraspherical Legendre functions of the first kind, 273
Fixed point, 5–6
Floquet theory, 56–57, 243
Fourier (Laplace) transform, 203–204
Fourth Lyapunov theorem, proof of, 63–64
Fox transform, 204
Frobenius-Fuchs method, 110
Functions of the first kind, 98
Functions of the second kind, 98
Fundamental solution
  autonomous differential system, 48–49
  linear differential equations, 61–62

Gamma function, 117–118, 121, 123, 196
  and beta functions, 199–201
  integrals evaluation via, 202–203
Gaussian hypergeometric differential equation, 246–248, 307–308
  analytic and logarithmic cases, poles, and polynomials, 268–270
  general integral of, 266–268
Gaussian hypergeometric function, 247, 260–261N9.14
  complementary, 264–265
  of the first kind, 261–262
  preliminary, 263, 264–265
  of the second kind, 262–263
Gaussian hypergeometric series, 260–261
General integral, 96, 97, 99, 101–102, 107, 109, 120, 129–131
  in case of integer order, 129–131
  of Gaussian hypergeometric differential equation, 266–268
  of ultraspherical Legendre differential equation, 273
General integral transform (Bateman 1909), 204
Generalized autonomous system, 16, 31
Generalized Bessel differential equation, 116, 118–121, 129, 162–165, **163**
  application, 208–210, *210*
  confluent hypergeometric differential equation and, 231
  general integral in case of integer order, 129–131
  invariant, 305–306
  self-adjoint, 305–306
  transformations of, 309–311
  Wronskian of, 116
Generalized Bessel function, 121–123
  continued fractions for, 233–234
  integral representation, 210–212
  order and degree of, 121–123
  Wronskian of, 131–132
Generalized circular and hyperbolic functions
  analytic coefficients and
    Airy (1838) differential equation and functions, 88
    analytic, regular, and irregular integrals, 75–78, *77*
    calculation, 82–83
    complex non-integer values of parameter, 90–92
    cosine and sine, 86–88, 88–90
    cosines and sine, 93–94
    differentiation of generalized cosine and sine functions, 92–93
    generalized circular differential equation, 90

generalized hyperbolic differential equation, 85–86
linear autonomous system, 79–81
linear differential equation, 81–82
overview, 64–65
point-at-infinity, singularities and integrals at, 78–79
principal branch, branch-point, and branch-cut, 72–74
recurrence relation, methods to obtain, 84–85
regular points, poles, and essential singularities, 68–70
regular points and regular/irregular singularities, **74**, 74–75
Riemann surface sheets of multi-valued function, 70–72, *71*
secant, cosecant, tangent, and cotangent, 94–95
single-valued complex functions, singularities of, 65–68, *66*, *67*
cosine and sine, 85, 86–88, 88–90
differentiation of functions, 92–93
inequalities for, 93–94
secant, cosecant, tangent, and cotangent, 94–95
Generalized circular differential equation, 90
Generalized functions, xxiv; *see also specific entries*
Generalized Hankel function
of first kind, 155–158
of second kind, 158–160
Generalized Hill differential equation, 186, 295–297
Generalized hyperbolic cosine and sine, 86–88
Generalized hyperbolic differential equation, 85–86
Generalized hypergeometric asymptotic series, 255
Generalized hypergeometric differential equation, 259
Generalized hypergeometric functions of type ${}_2F_2$, 252–253
Generalized hypergeometric series, 251
Generalized Laplace transform, 195–196
in complex plane, 205–207
Generalized Neumann function, 125–126, 129, 130
with complex order, 133–134
Wronskian of, 131–132
Generalized permutation, beta function, 198–199
Growing/decaying and monotonic/oscillatory solutions, 60–61

Hankel functions
cylindrical, 150–152
generalized, 155–160
integral representations, 219–221, *220*
spherical, 150–152
Helmholtz equation, 135
Hermite differential equation, 293–294, 308–309
Hermite functions, 293–294
first Hermite function, 294
second Hermite function, 294
Heun differential equation, 247
Hill determinants
analytic evaluation of, 192–193
modified, 193
Hill differential equation
generalized, 186
with power coefficients, 188–189
with trigonometric coefficients, 187–188
Hill equation, 243
Hill infinite determinant, 192
Homogenous derivatives, method of two polynomials of, 249–251
Hyperspherical associated Legendre differential equation, 276–278
Hyperspherical Legendre differential equation, 282–283

Independent variable(s)
combined changes of, 311–312
continuity (contraction) condition on, 7–9, *8*
Indices, 172
differing by integer, 173–175
as roots of infinite determinant, 183
as roots of transcendental equation, 194–195
Indicial equation, 105–106

Infinite determinants, 169–170
  convergence of (types), 183–184
  convergence theorem for, 185
  Hill infinite determinant, 192
  indices as roots of, 183
Infinite linear system, for coefficients, 181–182, 189–192, *190*
Inhomogenous problem, 245–246
Initial condition(s)
  perturbation, robustness and, 12–14, *13*
  theorem of robustness and, 15
Instability, Lyapunov theorem, proof of, 36–37
Integer(s), case of indices differing by, 173–175
Integral equation, 2
  differential equation transformation into, 3–4
Integral representation
  Bessel function, *214*, 214–216, 223–224
  generalized Bessel function, 210–212
  Hankel functions, 219–221, *220*
  for Neumann function, 221–222
  parametric path, 203
Integral(s); *see also* Eigenintegrals; *specific entries*
  analytic, 74, 75–78, *77*, 179–181, **180**
  asymptotic, 78–79, 152–155, 165–166
  evaluation via beta and gamma functions, 202–203
  irregular, 75–78, *77*, 142–144, **143**, 172–173, 175–177, 179–181, **180**
  natural, 56–57, 58
  normal, existence near irregular singularities, 145–147
  at point-at-infinity, 78–79
  regular, 75–78, *77*, 142–144, **143**, 178–181, **180**
  Wronskians and alternative general, 160–162
Integral transforms, kernel and path of, 195–196, 203–204
  general, 204
  parametric path integral representation, 203
Interior and exterior of unit disk, analytic continuation between, 255–260
Invariant form, 303
Invariant second-order differential equation, 59
  eigenvalues of, 62–63
Irregular integral(s), 75–78, *77*, 179–181, **180**
  of first kind, 172–173
  of linear differential equation, 142–144, **143**
  of second kind, 175–177, **177**
Irregular singularities, **74**, 74–75
  of degree *M*, 145–146
  normal integral existence near, 145–147
  overview, 142
  regular integral near, 144–145
Iterated recurrence formula, 198

Jacobi differential equation, 283, 307–308
Jacobi functions, 283–284, 307–308
Jordan blocks, 57–58
Jordan matrix, 57–58

Kernel, 203
  adjoint operator and bilinear concomitant, 218–219
  Bateman kernel, partial differential equation for, 216–217
  integral transforms, 195–196, 203–204
  product kernels, 204

Laguerre functions, 291–292
  associated, 292–293
Laplace transform, generalized, 195–196, 205–207
Large variable, numerical computation for, 168–169
Laurent series, 66–68, *67*
  irregular integral of second kind, 176
  of two isolated singularities, 76–78, *77*
Legendre differential equation, 270–272, 307–308
  associated, 274–276
  hierarchy of, 278–281
  hyperspherical, 276–278, 282–283
  ultraspherical, 272–274, 307

Legendre functions, 278–281
of first kind, 271, 275
first modified hyperspherical associated, 279
hyperspherical associated, 278
modified hyperspherical associated, 278
Legendre polynomial, 272
ultraspherical, 274
Leibnitz chain rule, 82
Lemma of Wronskians, 132, 133
Linear autonomous system
with analytic coefficients, 79–81
with constant coefficients, 45–46
Linear differential equation(s), 21
with analytic coefficients, 81–82
with bounded coefficients, 44–45
with periodic coefficients
diagonal matrices and Jordan blocks, 57–58
distinct and coincident eigenvalues and exponents, 55–56
eigenvalues of invariant second order equation, 62–63
existence of periodic solutions, conditions for, 54–55
fourth Lyapunov (1907) theorem, proof of, 63–64
fundamental solution, 61–62
growing/decaying and monotonic/oscillatory solutions, 60–61
invariant second-order differential equation, 59
natural integrals and asymptotic stability, 56–57
overview, 54
with regular singularities (Fuchs 1868), 103–105
regular/irregular integrals of, 142–144, **143**
second-order, 84, 115, **143**
with variable coefficients, 245–246
Linear differential system, near equilibrium point, 46–48
Lipschitz (contraction) condition
continuity and differentiability, 6–7
described, 7
existence of solution and, 2–3
generalized of, 18
on independent (dependent) variable, 7–9, *8*
for several variables, 18–19
Lipschitz function, 2
Local stability/instability, 25–27
Logarithmic term, 127
Lyapunov function, 23–24, 31, 243; *see also* Autonomous systems and equilibria stability
calculation, 49
first theorem, 31–34, *33*
Lyapunov theorem(s), 24, 243
first theorem, *see* First Lyapunov stability theorem
fourth, *see* Fourth Lyapunov theorem
proof of, 34–35
asymptotic stability, 35
instability, 36–37
second, *see* Second Lyapunov theorem
third, *see* Third Lyapunov theorem
using, 24

Maclaurin series, 68, 81, 82, 107, 113
Markov chain, 2, 3, 17
Matching coefficient, 123
Mathematical equilibrium and stability, 26
Mathieu (Hill) differential equation, 247
Mathieu equation, 40, 185, 243
Mellin transform, 204
Mittag-Leffler theorem, 118
Modified Hill determinant, 193
Multiple pole of order M, 68
Multi-valued function, 70, 72
Riemann surface sheets of, 70–72, *71*

Natural integrals, 56–57
alternate, 58
asymptomatic stability and, 56–57
regular, 96–101, *see also* Regular integral
Neumann function, 129, 150
asymptomatic expansion, 153–155
generalized, 125–126, 129, 130, 131–132, 133–134

Neumann function (*continued*)
- integral representation, 221–222
- spherical, 138–139
- Wronskian of, 131–132

Non-Cartesian problem, 245–246
Non-integer (complex) values, of parameter, 85–86
Normal integral, 145
- existence near irregular singularities, 145–147

Numerical methods, 242

Ordinary differential equations, 245
- of any order, 20–21
- combined theorem for, 22–23
- linear, 21–22

Ordinary functions, xxiii
Ordinary point, 73

Parametric discontinuity, in asymptotic integrals, 165–166
Parametric resonance, by fundamental and harmonics, 186
Partial differential equation(s), 245; *see also* Differential equation(s)
- for Bateman kernel, 216–217

Period, 55
Periodic coefficients, linear differential equations with
- diagonal matrices and Jordan blocks, 57–58
- distinct and coincident eigenvalues and exponents, 55–56
- eigenvalues of invariant second order equation, 62–63
- existence of periodic solutions, conditions for, 54–55
- fourth Lyapunov (1907) theorem, proof of, 63–64
- fundamental solution, 61–62
- growing/decaying and monotonic/oscillatory solutions, 60–61
- invariant second-order differential equation, 59
- natural integrals and asymptotic stability, 56–57
- overview, 54

Perturbation expansions, 244
Physical equilibrium and stability, autonomous systems, *25*, 25–26
Picard method, 2, 4, 5, 17, 243
Pochhammer symbol, 106
Poincare theorems, 243
Point-at-infinity
- bifurcation for degree at, 166–167
- singularities and integrals at, 78–79
- singularity of differential equation at, 147–148

Poles, 68–70
Position-dependent parameters, damped oscillator with, 37–38
Positive-definite quadratic forms, autonomous systems, 50
Power coefficients, Hill differential equation with, 188–189
Preliminary function, 125, 126
Preliminary Gaussian hypergeometric function, 263, 264–265
Principal branch, 72–74
Product kernels, 204

Quadratic forms (positive-definite), autonomous systems, 50
Qualitative theory of differential equations, 243

Ray approximation, 244
Rayleigh formulas, 140
Rectangle, as domain of successive approximations, 11
Recurrence formula
- for beta function, 197–198
- for coefficients, 100, 106, 119
- iterated, 198

reductio ad absurdum method, 34
Regular asymptotic integral, 79
Regular integral(s), 75–78, *77*, 139, 179–181, **180**
- classification of, 139
- convergence of series in, 113–115
- of first and second kinds, 106–107
- indices and coefficients of, 98–99
- of linear differential equation, 142–144, **143**
- linear second-order differential equation and, 101–103
- near irregular singularities, 144–145

of second kind first type, 109–111, 178–179
of second kind second type, 111–113 178–179
Regular point(s), 68–70, **74,** 74–75
Regular singularity(ies), **74,** 74–75, 96–97
linear autonomous system with, 97–98
linear differential equation with, 103–105
second-order differential equation with, 107–109
Riemann's theorem, 34
Riemann surface sheets, of multi-valued function, 70–72, *71*
Robustness; *see also* Theorem of robustness
perturbed initial conditions and, 12–14, *13*
theorem of, 15

Schwartz group, 259
Second Lyapunov theorem, proof of, 41–43, 45
Second-order differential equation
invariant, 59
eigenvalues of, 62–63
linear, 84, **143**
Self-adjoint and invariant differential equations, 303–304
Self-adjoint form, 303
Simple infinite continued fractions, convergence of, 229–230
Simple pole, 68, 69
Simultaneous system, of first-order differential equations, 16–17
Single-point boundary conditions, 82
Single-valued complex functions, singularities of, 65–68, *66, 67*
Singularity(ies), 65–66
of differential equation at point-at-infinity, 147–148
essential, 68–70, 169–170
Laurent series, 66–68, *67,* 76–78, *77*
at point-at-infinity, 78–79
regular/irregular, **74,** 74–75, 144–147
of single-valued complex functions, 65–68, *66, 67*
Small variable, numerical computation for, 168–169
Solid displacement amplifier, 245
Special continued fractions, convergence of, 240–241
Special functions, 245–246, 246–248, 314
Special limit periodic continued fractions, 237–238
Spherical Bessel function, 137–139, 150
and elementary functions, 140–141
Spherical Hankel functions, 150–152
Spherical harmonics, 275
Spherical Neumann function, 138–139
Stability
autonomous differential equation, 53
equilibrium, *see* Equilibrium stability
Stability function; *see also* Lyapunov function
differential system, 51
Stable equilibrium, 26
Steady (autonomous) differential system, 31
Subhypergeometric differential equations, 294–295
Successive approximations, method of, 2–3
convergence of, 4–5, *6*
differential equation transformation into integral, 3–4
rectangle as domain of, 11
vs. original and perturbed problems, 14–15
Superhypergeometric differential equations, 295–297
Symmetry formula, 118

Terminating continued fractions, 227–228
Theorem of convergence of regular integrals, 113
Theorem of existence; *see also* Existence, unicity, robustness, and uniformity, of solutions
of solution of a differential equation, 10–11
Theorem of parametric uniformity, 16

Theorem of robustness; *see also* Existence, unicity, robustness, and uniformity, of solutions
  initial condition and, 15
Theorem of unicity, 2; *see also* Existence, unicity, robustness, and uniformity, of solutions
  of solution of differential equation, 11–12
Theorem on uniformity, parameter in differential equation, 16
Third Lyapunov theorem, 47–48
  on asymptomatic stability, 52
  on autonomous system, 52
Time-depending parameters, damped oscillator with, 38–39
Totally convergent, infinite determinant, 184
Transcendental equation, indices as roots of, 194–195
Transcendental functions, algebraic and elementary/higher, 312–314, *313*
Transformation factor, 303, 307
Trigonometric coefficients, Hill differential equation with, 187–188
Turning points, 244–245

Ultraspherical Legendre differential equation, 272–274
Ultraspherical Legendre functions of the first (second) kind, 273
Ultraspherical Legendre polynomial, 274
Unconditionally unstable, equilibrium, autonomous systems, 29
Undamped oscillator; *see also* Damped harmonic oscillator
  with parametric resonance, stability of, 40
Unicity, 10–12
Uniform convergence, 184
  to continuous solution, 9–10
Uniformity, 2
  parametric, 16
Unsteady autonomous system, 31
  differential system, 29–31
Unsteady problem, 245–246

Variable(s); *see also* Dependent variable(s); Independent variable(s)
  combined changes of, 311–312
  Lipschitz (contraction) condition, 18–19
  small and large, numerical computation for, 168–169

Wave envelope technique, 244
Wave problems, 245
Weierstrass infinite product, 118
Whittaker differential equation, 247, 304–305
Wronskian, 160–162
  of Bessel functions, 134
  of generalized Bessel functions, 121–122
  of generalized Bessel and Neumann functions, 131–132
  of generalized Hankel functions, 160–162
  of generalized Neumann functions, 162
  of linear second-order differential equation, 115–116